Topics in Anaesthesia and Critical Care

H.K.F. VAN SAENE, L. SILVESTRI, M.A. DE LA CAL (EDS.)
Infection Control in the Intensive Care Unit
1998, 380 pp, ISBN 3-540-75043-6

J. MILIC-EMILI (ED.)
Applied Physiology in Respiratory Mechanics
1998, 250 pp, ISBN 3-540-75041-X

Anestesia e Medicina Critica

G. SLAVICH
Elettrocardiografia Clinica
1997, 328 pp, ISBN 3-540-75050-9

G.L. ALATI, B. ALLARIA, G. BERLOT, A. GULLO, A. LUZZANI,
G. MARTINELLI, L. TORELLI
Anestesia e Malattie Concomitanti - Fisiopatologia e clinica del periodo perioperatorio
1997, 370 pp, ISBN 3-540-75048-7

B. ALLARIA, M.V. BALDASSARRE, A. GULLO, A. LUZZANI,
G. MANANI, G. MARTINELLI, A. PASETTO, L. TORELLI
Farmacologia Generale e Speciale in Anestesiologia Clinica
1997, 250 pp, ISBN 88-470-0001-7

Applied Physiology in Respiratory Mechanics

Springer-Verlag Italia Srl.

J. Milic-Emili (Ed.)

Applied Physiology in Respiratory Mechanics

Series edited by
Antonino Gullo

Springer

Prof. J. Milic-Emili
Respiratory Division
Meakins-Christie Laboratories
McGill University, Montreal - Canada

Series of ***Topics in Anaesthesia and Critical Care*** edited by
Prof. A. Gullo
Department of Anaesthesia, Intensive Care
and Pain Therapy
University of Trieste, Cattinara Hospital, Trieste - Italy

Die Deutsche Bibliothek - CIP-Einheitsaufnahme. **Milic-Emili, Joseph**: Applied Physiology in respiratory mechanics / J. Milic-Emili. Ser. ed. by Antonino Gullo.
(Topics in anaesthesia and critical care)

ISBN 978-88-470-2930-9 ISBN 978-88-470-2928-6 (eBook)
DOI 10.1007/978-88-470-2928-6

Originally published by Springer-Verlag Berlin Heidelberg New York in 1998

Cover design: Simona Colombo
Typesetting and lay-out: Graphostudio, Milano

SPIN 10572839

Preface

The close correlations between anatomo-functional data and clinical aspects are substantiated by the study and interpretation of the data of respiratory mechanics. This field has developed to such an extent that, today, it is hard to single out one researcher who is an expert of the whole sector, whereas super experts can be found among scholars who, thanks to their studies and continuous comparisons, have contributed to the widening of knowledge and the development of that part of research which correlates some basic disciplines with clinical medicine.

This notion is of paramount importance. Indeed, it has to be regarded as a starting point requiring a more precise definition. The analysis of data concerning ventilation parameters is based on the use of mathematical models that are necessary to simplify the complexity of the various clinical situations. For a correct application and interpretation of data, the most recent technological acquisitions in terms of ventilatory support require to be used as a function of simple mathematical models for the study, control and evolution of the lung diseases that concern the ICU.

Thus, the need has arisen to compare the experience acquired in the field of applied physiology and in the clinical sector.

In particular, in intensive care, the use of sophisticated respiratory function monitoring and support equipment stresses the need to analyse in depth various aspects of respiratory physiology: the machanisms of ventilation setting muscular fatigue, the static and dynamic properties of the respiratory system, respiratory work, gas exchange and pulmonary perfusion. Advanced research in the fields of the techniques supplying partial support to ventilation and applied pharmacology considerably benefits from a better understanding of the factors and mechanisms regulating the respiratory function.

It is therefore fundamental to stress the importance for ICU physicians to plan a clinical approach increasingly oriented towards a customized ventilatory support, adequately relying on applied research.

Antonino Gullo
Joseph Milic-Emili

Contents

Contributors

Andreose U.
Dept. of Anaesthesia and Intensive Care, Hospital of Padova, Italy.

Antonaglia V.
Dept. of Anaesthesia, Intensive Care and Pain Therapy, Cattinara Hospital, University of Trieste, Italy.

Arnulf I.
Dept. of Pneumology and Intensive Care, Pitié-Salpetriere Hospital, Paris, France.

Artigas A.
Dept. of Intensive Care, Parc Taulí Hospital, Sabadell, Spain.

Beltrame F.
Dept. of Anaesthesia, Intensive Care and Pain Therapy, Cattinara Hospital, University of Trieste, Italy.

Blanch L.
Dept. of Intensive Cae, Parc Taulí Hospital, Sabadell, Spain.

Brandolese R.
Dept. of Anaesthesia and Intensive Care, Hospital of Padova, Italy.

Brochard L.
Medical Intensive Care Unit, Henry Mondor Hospital, Creteil Cedex, France.

Cañete C.
Dept. of Pneumology, Bellvitge Universitary Hospital, Barcelona, Spain.

D'Angelo E.
Institute of Human Physiology I, University of Milan, Italy.

de Troyer A.
Laboratory of Cardiorespiratory Physiology, School of Medicine and Chest Service, Erasme University Hospital, Brussels, Belgium.

Derenne J. -Ph.
Dept. of Pneumology and Intensive Care, Pitié-Salpetriere Hospital, Paris, France.

Dreyfussl D.
Dept. of Intensive Care Medicale, Mourier Hospital, Colombes, Bichat, Paris, France.

Fernandez R.
Dept. of Intensive Care, Parc Taulí Hospital, Sabadell, Spain.

Fiore T.
Dept. of Anaesthesiology and Intensive Care, Policlinico Hospital, University of Bari, Italy.

Giuliani R.
Dept. of Anaesthesiology and Intensive Care, Policlinico Hospital, University of Bari, Italy.

Gommers D.
Dept. of Anaesthesiology, Erasmus University, Rotterdam, The Netherlands.

Grop A.
Dept. of Anaesthesia, Intensive Care and Pain Therapy, Cattinara Hospital, University of Trieste, Italy.

Gullo A.
Dept. of Anaesthesia, Intensive Care and Pain Therapy, Cattinara Hospital, University of Trieste, Italy.

Houmes R.J.
Dept. of Anaesthesiology, Erasmus University, Rotterdam, The Netherlands.

Jubran A.
Division of Pulmonary and Critical Care Medicine, Loyola University of Chicago, Stritch School of Medicine, Chicago, USA.

Lachmann B.
Dept. of Anaesthesiology, Erasmus University, Rotterdam, The Netherlands.

Laghi F.
Division of Pulmonary and Critical Care Medicine, Loyola University of Chicago, Stritch School of Medicine, Chicago, USA.

Lopez Aguilar J.
Dept. of Experimental Research, University Hospital of Bellvitge, Barcelona, Spain.

Lucangelo U.
Dept. of Anaesthesia, Intensive Care and Pain Therapy, Cattinara Hospital, University of Trieste, Italy.

Mascia L.
Dept. of Anaesthesiology and Intensive Care, Policlinico Hospital, University of Bari, Italy.

Milic-Emili J.
Respiratory Division, Meakins-Christie Laboratories, McGill University, Montreal, Canada.

Musch G.
Dept. of Anaesthesia and Intensive Care, University of Milan, S. Gerardo Hospital, Monza, Italy.

Nava S.
Division of Pneumology, Center of Montescano, I.R.C.C.S., Pavia, Italy.

Navajas D.
Laboratory of Biophysic and Bioengeneering, University of Barcelona, Spain.

Pesenti A.
Dept. of Anaesthesia and Intensive Care, University of Milan, S. Gerardo Hospital, Monza, Italy.

Ranieri V.M.
Dept. of Anaesthesiology and Intensive Care, Policlinico Hospital, University of Bari, Italy.

Robatto F.M.
Institute of Human Physiology, University of Milan, Italy.

Roca J.
Dept. of Pneumology, Clinic Hospital, University of Barcelona, Spain.

Romero F.J.
Dept. of Physics, Politecnic University of Valencia, Spain.

Romero P.V.
Dept. of Pneumology, Bellvitge Hospital, Barcelona, Spain.

Rubini F.
Division of Pneumology, Center of Montescano, I.R.C.C.S., Pavia, Italy.

Saumon G.
Dept. of Intensive Care Medicine, Louis Mourier Hospital, Colombes, Paris, France.

Saura P.
Dept of Intensive Care, Parc Taulí Hospital, Sabadell, Spain.

Similowski T.
Dept. of Pneumology and Intensive Care, Pitié-Salpetriere Hospital, Paris, France.

So K.L.
Dept. of Anaesthesiology, Erasmus University, Rotterdam, The Netherlands.

Sparacino M.E.
Dept. of Anaesthesia and Intensive Care, University of Milan, S. Gerardo Hospital, Monza, Italy.

Straus C.
Dept. of Pneumology and Intensive Care, Pitié-Salpetriere Hospital, Paris, France.

Tobin M.J.
Division of Pulmonary and Critical Care Medicine, Loyola University of Chicago, Stritch School of Medicine, Chicago, USA.

Versprille A.
Pathophysiological Laboratory, Department of Pulmonary Diseases, Erasmus University, Rotterdam, The Netherlands.

Chapter 1

Control of breathing: neural drive

C. Straus, I. Arnulf, T. Similowsky, J.-Ph. Derenne

Introduction

Breathing is a complex behaviour, governed by control systems hierarchically arranged to regulate ventilation. Their aim is to respond optimally to the prevailing metabolic needs and to various demands on the respiratory apparatus. Two aspects can grossly be identified. On the one hand, there is an automatic control system permanently aimed at maintaining the arterial pH, O_2 and CO_2 pressures (PaO_2, $PaCO_2$) within the normal range. This regulation is remarkably precise and can cope with major and rapid variations in metabolic needs or oxygen consumption. On the other hand, various systems can disrupt the automatic regulation in order to use the respiratory system in non respiratory tasks: speech is the main one in humans, but also include activities such as singing, swallowing, sucking, sniffing, sneezing, hiccough, vomiting, coughing, yawning, defaecating, straining and posture control.

Schematic description of the system

Three players contribute to the system which controls ventilation (Fig. 1):
- receptors (chemosensitive, barosensitive, stretch sensitive) collect various signals and transduce them as afferent parts of reflexes to the central controller;
- the central controller integrates these signals and generates neural drive; it is modulated by supra-pontine influences such as the degree of wakefulness, emotions and also voluntary commands of cortical origin;
- muscular effectors (*e.g.* upper airway dilatators, the diaphragm, intercostal and abdominal muscles etc.) receive this neural drive and produce forces. Applied to the passive respiratory system (lung, bronchial tree, chest wall) these forces are transformed into pressures finally dragging gas from the atmosphere to the alveoli where gas exchange between air and blood can occur.

Central controller

The central controller [1] is located in the brainstem and can be conceived to be of two main parts (Fig. 2), the first gating the activity of the second:
- a central pattern generator which can essentially be viewed as a timer that paces the rhythm, provided it receives some excitatory input from (chemo)

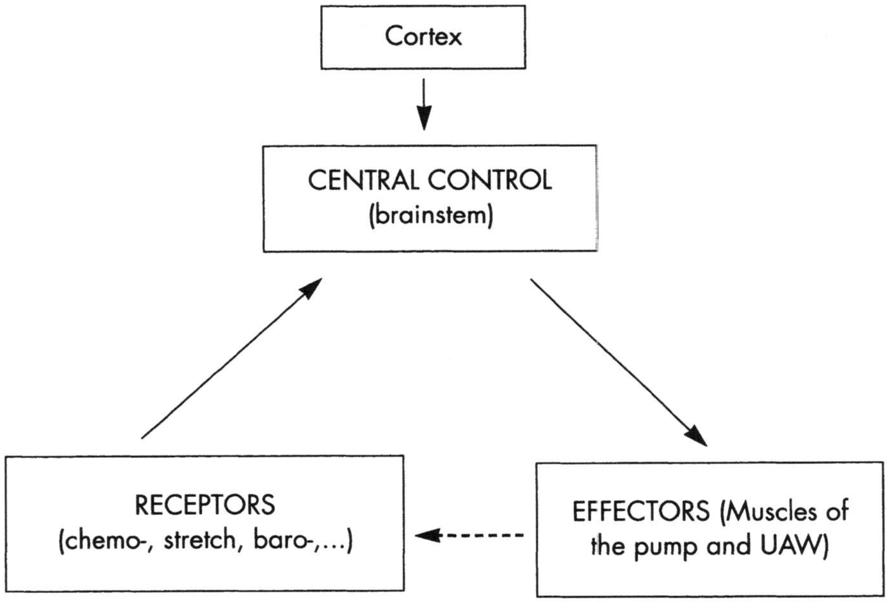

Fig. 1. The control systems of breathing

receptors and suprapontine influences. It is formed of parallel, self-sustaining oscillating networks organized as a set of coupled oscillators, widespread in the medulla, probably to secure continuous operation under all conditions;
- neuronal networks that shape the inspiratory bursts producing ramp-like activity for bulbo-spinal neurons and square wave pattern for upper airway motorneurons. Expiratory (E) and inspiratory (I) related neurons receive reciprocal inhibition and are located mainly in the dorso-medial and ventro-lateral parts of the medulla oblongata. The dorso-medial group contains the nucleus of Tractus Solitarius (NTS) and seems involved in the control of timing. The ventro-lateral group includes the nucleus Retroambigualis, the nucleus Paraambigualis and the nucleus Retrofacialis and appears to be more strongly involved in the control of inspiratory amplitude.

The neural drive generated by these networks consists of 3 phases : inspiratory phase, expiratory phase I and expiratory phase II.

The inspiratory motor activity has a sudden onset followed by a ramp-shaped increase in discharge rate, progressing until it is switched off. This activity is the result of three types of neuronal activity:
- early burst inspiratory neurons;
- inspiratory ramp neurons;
- late onset ("switch-off") neurons.

During expiratory phase I, which immediately follows switch off of inspiratory activity, a post-inspiratory inhibiting activity counteracts the initially strong elastic recoil of the chest and slows down the rate of exhalation in the first part

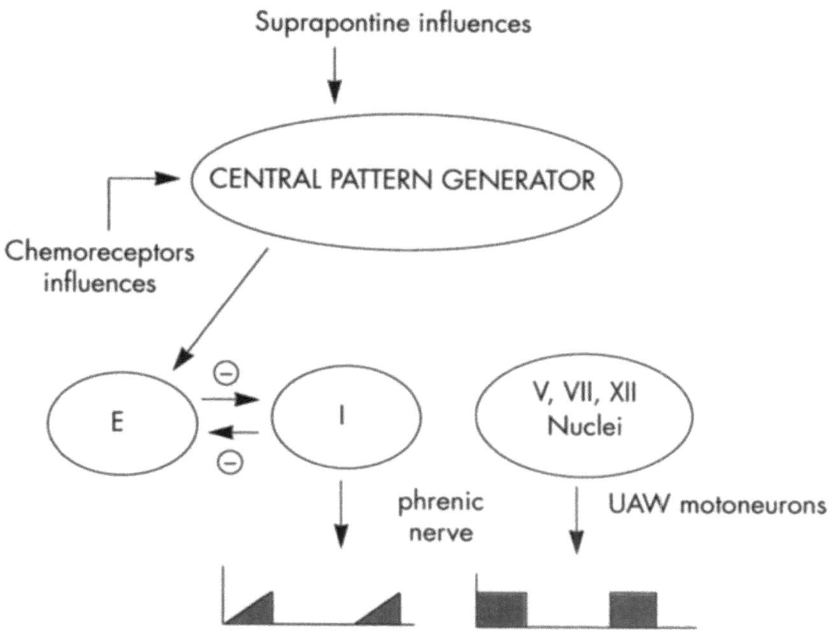

Fig. 2. Central control of breathing

of expiration. This activity is directly influenced by the degree of lung inflation.

During expiratory phase II the inspiratory muscles are inactive allowing passive expiration. Expiratory muscles, such as abdominal muscles and internal intercostals, are recruited only in cases of increased ventilatory drive by the activation of two types of neurons:
- early whole expiratory neurons;
- expiratory ramp neurons.

The upper airway dilator muscles are generally activated significantly earlier than the pump muscle in order to allow the airways to be dilated before any negative intrathoracic pressure is created. This illustrates the complexity of the system and the refined precision of its operating mode.

Receptors and reflexes

The receptor and reflexes of the control systems of breathing are described in Table 1.

1. The slow adaptative receptors are stretchreceptors located in airways in contact with smooth muscles. They are sensitive to pulmonary inflation: the bursts are transmitted through the myelinic large vagal fibers and are responsible for a reduction of respiratory frequency, via a reduction of expiration time. This phenomenon, now described as the Hering-Breuer reflex, plays a major role in some

Table 1. Receptors and reflex of the control sustems of breathing

Type of reflex	Receptors	Afferent	Effect	References
Hering Breuer	Stretch R (Slowly Adaptative R)	X (f IA)	inflation -> apnea	Hering & Breuer 1868
Pulmonary deflation	Irritant R (Rapidly Adaptative R)	X	Deflation / RF + bronchoconstriction + coughing	Guz 1970
J Reflex	J receptors	X (fc)	congestion / RF Ø arterial pressure	Paintal 1969
	Mechano R Chestwall	Intercostal nerves (f g)	/ intercostal burst	Euler 1974
Phrenico-Phrenic reflex	Mechano R Golgi		/ Phrenic EMG (position change)	Green 1974
Baro reflex	Baro R	IX	HTA -> Ø Vt	Grunstein 1975
Chemo reflex CO_2 /	Central chemo R (V4) and peripheral	IX	/ ventilation (linear)	
Chemo reflex H+ /	Central chemo R		/ ventilation	
Chemo reflex Ø O_2	Chemo R peripheral central (?)	IX	/ V non linear respiration depression	

animal species (rat, rabbit, etc.) but its importance in man is minor [2-4].

2. The rapidly adaptative receptors are irritant receptors located in airway epithelium. They are sensitive to various stimuli such as smoke, cold, dust, inflation and deflation; the bursts are transmitted through the vagal nerve and provoke cough, bronchoconstriction, tachycardia and polypnea (deflation reflex) [4, 5].

3. The J receptors, or C fiber receptors, are located in the bronchial and alveolar wall, probably close to small vessels; they are sensitive to capillary inflation and to interstitial oedema. Their bursts, through slow amyelinic vagal fibers, provoke cough, rapid and shallow respiration and at the most apnea [6].

4. The spindles are located in intercostal muscles and are responsible, through the gamma loop, for an enhancement in intercostal muscle activity when

stretched. Diaphragmatic receptors are essentially Golgi tendon organs [7-9].
5. The carotid baroreceptors when stimulated by an increased arterial pressure, induce reflex hypoventilation and apnea [10].
6. The aortic and central chemoreceptors are synergically stimulated by hypoxia and hypercapnia [11].

Heart-lungs transplantation in humans provide a model of complete vagal denervation. Studies in such patients indicate that the level and pattern of ventilation are well controlled in the absence of intrapulmonary afferent inputs, at least under resting and exercise conditions, therefore suggesting a minor role for intrapulmonary receptors [12-14].

How should the control of breathing be explored?

Clinicians confronted with respiratory abnormalities may wish to understand and quantify the part of central dysfunction. Abnormal blood gases with quasi-normal classical pulmonary function tests point to altered control of breathing. In such a situation voluntary hyperventilation is required to lower $PaCO_2$.

A combination of tests is available (Fig. 3) which can help identify the nature of the problem, and at times its level. None of these tests is perfect, each having its own sensitivity and specificity and each being more or less related to one or another aspect of the regulating system. A short description and critique of the main tests follows.

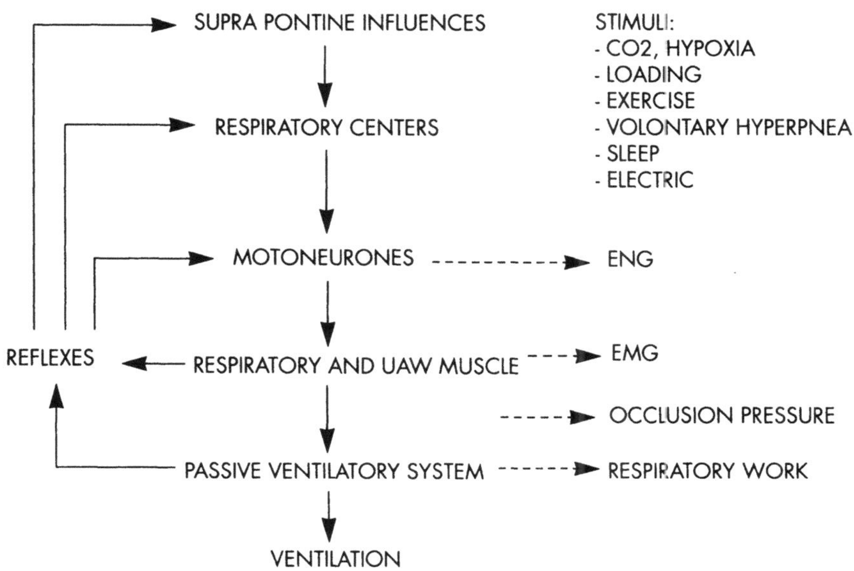

Fig. 3. Interaction levels between the control systems of breathing and the tests respiratory controller assessment

Respiratory drive and timing

Minute ventilation ($\dot{V}e$) is the product of the tidal volume (V_t) and the respiratory frequency (f):

$$\dot{V}e = V_t \cdot f \tag{1}$$

f is the inverse of total breath duration (T_{tot}):

$$f = \frac{1}{T_{tot}} \tag{2}$$

Therefore:

$$\dot{V}_E = \frac{V_t}{T_{tot}} \tag{3}$$

T_{tot} is the sum of inspiratory and expiratory duration (T_i and T_e):

$$T_{tot} = T_i + T_e \tag{4}$$

By multiplying the denominator and the numerator by T_i and T_e, Eq. 3 becomes:

$$\dot{V}_E = \frac{V_t}{T_i} \cdot \frac{T_i}{T_{tot}} = \frac{V_t}{T_e} \cdot \frac{T_e}{T_{tot}} \tag{5}$$

V_t/T_i is the mean inspiratory flow which is a mechanical transformation of central inspiratory drive. The fraction of inspiratory time to total respiratory cycle duration T_i/T_{tot} is a dimensionless index of "effective" respiratory timing [15]. T_i/T_{tot} is one of the major determinants of inspiratory muscle fatigue, particularly diaphragm fatigue [16, 17]. On the other hand, a reduction of minute ventilation due to a reduction of T_i/T_{tot} implies that the duration of expiration has increased in relation to that of inspiration. This may be due to central (bulbo-pontine) or peripheral influences (*e.g.* reflexes originating in the chest wall, lung and upper airway). A reduction in V_t/T_{tot} can be caused by decreased central inspiratory drive, neuromuscular inadequacy and increased impedance of the respiratory system [15]. Airway occlusion pressure can help differenciate if changes in respiratory system mechanics play a role or not in the reduction of V_t/T_i [15, 18]. Assessment of respiratory neural drive may also be provided by volume wave shape analysis [15, 19].

Work of breathing

The work of breathing is measured on the esophagal pressure-lung volume diagram. Minute ventilation, breathing frequency, lung compliance and airway resistance all influence the work of breathing and the energy demands of the respiratory muscles. A hyperstimulated central respiratory drive likewise imposes an increased inspiratory muscle work of breathing. Thus, work of breathing is an index of the output of the respiratory motor neurons. However, inspiratory work depends on lung volume and the force-velocity properties of the respiratory muscles [20]. Because the determination of the pressure-volume curve of the lungs requires the use of an esophagal catheter, the determination of the work of breathing is used in research rather than in clinical practice [21]. Being a composite index, it is difficult to interpret with respect to the control of breathing alone; however, this is possible if repeated measurements are made during a period of reasonable "mechanical steady state".

Airway occlusion pressure

Airway occlusion pressure is a simple non invasive means of respiratory controller assessment which was introduced in the 1970s [22, 23]. The airways are occluded at end expiration and mouth pressure is measured during the following inspiration. Since there is no flow or lung volume variation, if one neglects gas decompression (Boyle's law), mouth pressure is independent of the respiratory system compliance and resistance, and occlusion pressure is independent of the mechanical properties of the passive ventilatory system. In addition, there is no volume related vagal feedback and no Hering-Breuer reflex. Airway occlusion pressure is a global index of the inspiratory center activity which depends also on nervous transmission and respiratory muscle mechanics. It is correlated with electrical activity of the phrenic nerve in animals [24] and of the diaphragm in man and animals [25-27]. In anesthetized man airway occlusion pressure increases linearly with increasing alveolar PCO_2 (P_ACO_2). The shape of the pressure wave, defined as the ratio of pressure values measured at any fixed times after the onset of the occlusion pressure wave, remains identical at any P_ACO_2 [15]. Thus mouth pressure measured any time after occlusion is correlated with maximal pressure. This is a very relevant fact for clinical investigations because conscious man perceive occlusion after 150 to 200 ms. After this time, occlusion pressure will reflect the subject's reaction to the load. Before 150 ms, the pressure wave is reproducible and presumably independent of cortical influences [23]. The pressure developed 100 ms after the onset of the occlusion pressure wave is consequently used as a clinical index of the respiratory controller ($P_{0.1}$). Nevertheless, the interpretation of $P_{0.1}$ in clinical research is complex [28]. For instance:

- in chronic obstructive pulmonary disease (COPD) patients with high flow resistance and lung compliance, inequalities of time constants may alter the early part of the occlusion pressure wave by a small passive pressure transient associated with pendelluft or stress relaxation. Moreover, if the time constant is long, a phase shift between pressure and flow can occur which will markedly affect $P_{0.1}$, especially if, instead of a straight ramp, the driving pressure wave is convex or concave. Many situations can induce changes in the shape of the pressure wave. For example, in anesthetized humans, increasing lung volume with positive pressure makes the inspiratory pressure wave more concave [29];
- $P_{0.1}$ depends on respiratory muscle functions. An increase in lung volume will

shorten the diaphragm which will become less effective as a pressure generator. If the muscles are unequally damaged, as in quadriplegia for example, the loss of synergism can impair pressure generation and the ratio of occlusion pressure to neural drive can be altered.

$P_{0.1}$ remains a simple, reliable means for the clinical investigation of neural respiratory drive but the interpretation of variations of occlusion pressure is not always easy.

Response to CO_2

CO_2 inhalation is a means of testing the reflex loop between chemoreceptor stimulation, central control and ventilatory response. The CO_2 stimulus can be applied by two methods, *i.e.* steady-state and rebreathing. Response can be evaluated by looking at ventilation or occlusion pressure. The relationship between $PaCO_2$ and ventilation is usually linear [30].

Steady-state method

With this technique the subject inhales a mixture of CO_2 and expires freely. Ventilation is measured after reaching a so-called steady-sate 15-20 minutes later. At least two different $FiCO_2$ are used.

This technique is hindered by several problems: it is time consuming (15-20 min), requires invasive measurement of $PaCO_2$ and is not very precise (only 2 to 4 points to draw the relationship). Furthermore, "steady-state" is not stable, mainly because of central adaptation, i.e. $PaCO_2$ modifies ventilation but ventilation in turn modifies $PaCO_2$.

Rebreathing

The subject inspires from a bag containing a mixture of 50 % O_2, 7 % CO_2 and 43 % N_2 and expires, via a closed circuit, in to the same bag. Because all expired CO_2 is reinspired, the fractional inspiratory concentration of CO_2 ($FiCO_2$) keeps increasing. Equilibrium between pulmonary gas and container is reached after 30 seconds (Fig. 4). O_2 enrichment of the gas mixture suppresses the influence of the hypoxic drive.

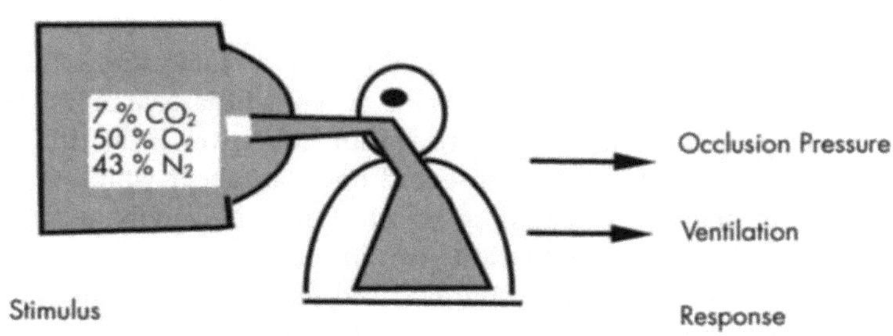

Fig. 4. Rebreathing technique

Compared to the so-called "steady-state" technique, the rebreathing method has several advantages: the test is short (4-5 min), does not require blood gas measurement (it relies on the assumption that $P_ACO_2 = PaCO_2$) and provides many points to describe the CO_2 response. Due to of the very principle of the test, ventilation cannot lower $PaCO_2$ and therefore the only parameter assessed is the influence of the latter on the former.

The CO_2 rebreathing method hence appears the method of choice to assess CO_2 response. It can be easily associated with the measurement of occlusion pressure. However, the interpretation of the results has limits. For example, the response to CO_2 may be genetically determined, as illustrated by the weak response in particular ethnic groups (New-Guinean) and certain families [31]. Particular physiological states are also associated with altered CO_2 response (athletes [32], premature infants [33]). CO_2 response is enhanced by metabolic acidosis and diminished by alcalosis [34]. It can be influenced by various drugs and hormones [30].

Response to O_2

Hypoxic stimulation of ventilation [35] can be realised in three ways:
- inhalation of pure N_2 for a few respiratory cycles [36];
- inhalation of a single low FiO_2 gas mixture;
- inhalation of successive gas mixtures with decreasing FiO_2 [37].

All these techniques require arterial puncture for PaO_2 measurement. CO_2 enrichment of the gas mixture is needed for the two last methods in order to avoid hyperventilation induced hypocapnia. The relationship between ventilation and PaO_2 is not linear, but rather curvilinear, which makes calculations more difficult.

Electromyography of the diaphragm

Neural drive output is transmitted to the respiratory muscles and their activation can be assessed by recording their electrical activity. Electromyography is a selective investigation tool which provides specific data about individual muscles. The electromyographic signal can be used rough or integrated. In man, the most important inspiratory muscle is the diaphragm. Diaphragmatic electromyogram in man can be obtained with a bipolar electrode introduced into the esophagus via the nose and positioned in contact with the diaphragm [38]. With this technique the electromyogram of the crural part of the diaphragm can be recorded, provided adequate signal treatment is used [39, 40]. Diaphragm EMG can also be recorded with surface electrodes positioned on the chest at the right 6-7th and left 7-8th intercostal spaces [41]. However, with this technique the electrical activity recorded arises from all muscle underlying the electrodes, that is the diaphragm but also intercostal and abdominal muscles. Lung volume, position of the electrodes, and other factors have been shown to affect the electromyogram signal [42]. For all these reasons, the usefulness of electromyograms to evaluate neural drive is limited. Between patients comparison is not possible and within patient comparison is conceivable only during a given recording session, all other factors being otherwise controlled for.

Phrenic nerve stimulation

The nature and integrity of neural drive pathways can be assessed by phrenic nerve stimulation. Phrenic nerve electrical percutaneous stimulation is relatively easy to perform in man. The stimulator is positioned at the posterior border of the sterno-mastoid muscle at the level of the upper margin of the thyroid cartilage. Mono- or bipolar electrodes deliver pulses of 0.1 to 0.2 ms and 5 to 60 mA [43]. After phrenic stimulation, diaphragm activation and contraction can be assessed by means of EMG recording [41], esophageal, transdiaphragmatic or mouth pressure measurements [44-46]. Phrenic nerve conduction time can be measured with surface EMG in both normal subjects and patients [47].

This technique has been used to extend to the diaphragm the twitch occlusion theory introduced by Merton [48]. Briefly, this theory states that muscle response to stimulation of its governing nerve linearly decreases with the intensity of a voluntary isometric contraction underlying the stimulation. If a voluntary effort is associated with complete suppression of response to stimulation, it is considered the result of maximal activation of all available muscle fibers. Bellemare and Bigland-Ritchie [44] demonstrated that a pattern similar to that described by Merton for a hand muscle could be demonstrated for the diaphragm. They concluded that maximal voluntary activation of the diaphragm was possible in normal subjects. This finding has been extended to patients with chronic obstructive pulmonary disease, demonstrating that voluntary activation was not a limiting factor of diaphragm performance in this setting [49]. Bellemare and Bigland-Ritchie [50] derived from diaphragm twitch occlusion a simple index to help differenciate the intrinsic function of the diaphragm from its activation by neural drive and assess the central component of diaphragmatic fatigue.

Transcutaneous bilateral electrical phrenic nerve stimulation is not always an easy technique, however. The exact localisation of the phrenic nerve at the neck may take up to 30 minutes [51] and sometimes be impossible [52]. Keeping the stimulus constant is difficult. Subject tolerance can be poor in the absence of strong motivation. Bilateral phrenic nerve stimulation can now be performed by use of cervical magnetic stimulation [53]; a painless, easy to perform and reliable method. As concerns assessment of phrenic conduction, both techniques seem equivalent.

Cortical involvement in respiratory neural drive

Breathing is essentially an automatic phenomenon. Among skeletal muscles, the diaphragm is peculiar in that it must cyclically contract 24-hour a day in order to sustain ventilation and maintain life. This activity is controlled by automatic brainstem mechanisms that also regulate respiratory homeostasis. Besides, everyone knows and experiences daily the fact that voluntary commands can disrupt the automatic control of breathing. Voluntary respiratory patterns can be generated, of which apnea diving and pulmonary function testing are examples. Above all, the diaphragm plays, together with other respiratory muscles, important roles in various non respiratory activities such as speech, singing, swallowing, posture etc. This supports a motor cortical representation of the diaphragm in man, associated with rapid conduction cortico-spinal pathways that have been evidenced in man by use of cortical electrical stimulation and diaphragmatic EMG [54].

Coupled with phrenic nerve stimulation, cortical stimulation provides a tool for respiratory cortico-spinal drive assessement. Cortical magnetic stimulation is easier to perform than electrical stimulation and is an efficient tool to assess cortico-diaphragmatic drive [55]. The localisation of the motor cortical diaphragmatic representation in man [56] and the unilaterality of the cortical motor area of each hemidiaphragm [57] have been reported with magnetic stimulation. However, these stimulation techniques do not investigate the respiratory controller activity, but help only in assessing neural pathways.

The involvement of the cerebral cortex in the generation of respiratory neural drive is suggested by several facts. Macefield and Gandevia [58] have shown that some respiratory movements may be associated with cortical "preparation", as demonstrated by the existence of premotor potentials. Colebatch et al. [59] have shown by use of positron emission tomography that the copying of a respiratory pattern from a pre-recorded oscilloscope signal was associated with activation of cortical areas both in the primary motor region but also in premotor areas. Murphy et al. [55] have, surprisingly enough, suggested a putative role for the cerebral cortex in CO_2 response by demonstrating CO_2 rebreathing-associated facilitation of diaphragm response to cortical magnetic stimulation.

Sleep and neural drive

Sleep is a natural condition during which neural drive to breathe varies and can be studied and separated in function of different sleep stages.

To simplify, during stable slow wave sleep cortical influences on ponto-bulbar centers are suppressed. Ventilation is very steady and is regulated solely by chemical stimuli. $PaCO_2$ is slightly increased and tidal volume is slightly decreased in line with an hypotonia related increase in upper airway resistance. Central respiratory CO_2 chemosensitivity does not decrease during sleep, although the ventilatory responses to hypercapnic and hypoxic stimuli are diminished [60]. Occlusion pressure response to hypercapnia is not reduced during NREM sleep [61].

During REM sleep, on the other hand, cortical influences on ponto-bulbar centers are maintained. As compared to wakefulness, the reactivity of these centers to chemo-, baro-, and mechano-stimuli is much delayed. This state could schematically correspond to some sort of "functional vagotomy". Neural drive then depends more on cortical influence than on afferent information.

Muscular atonia compromises rib cage inspiratory muscles. Ventilation is irregular with a succession of central apneas and periods of polypnea that are synchronized with rapid eye movement bursts. Mean tidal volume and respiratory frequency, hence minute ventilation, are similar to their NREM sleep values [62, 63]. From a physiological modelling point of view, NREM sleep provides a unique opportunity to study central chemosensitivity out of cortical control whereas REM sleep correponds to a model of ventilation devoid of reflex control arising from afferent impulses.

From a more practical point of view, ventilation is more fragile or, better, less well protected during sleep. As a result, any change in arterial blood gases or the work of breathing that would have been adequately compensated during wakefulness can be a problem during sleep. For example, during slow wave sleep the absence of descending output to upper airway muscles leads to increased upper airway resistance. Particularly in patients with impaired baseline load compensation capabilities, this can result in obstructive sleep apnea and hypoventilation (*e.g.* patients with kyphoscoliosis or thoracic neuromuscular disorders). REM sleep, on the other hand, is associated with respiratory deterioration in patients with compromised diaphragmatic function.

Neural drive during anesthesia

Almost all drugs used in anesthesia alter breathing efficiency as a side effect of their primary purpose. Assessment of these alterations rests on the measurement of various parameters such as minute ventilation, respiratory time components, occlusion pressure, end tidal PCO_2 ($PETCO_2$) and $PaCO_2$, this at baseline or after stimulation of the system by CO_2 increase or hypoxia.

In summary, inhalation anesthetics increase $PaC0_2$ and respiratory frequency, while minute ventilation and tidal volume are decreased. Response to CO_2 and to hypoxia are impaired. Enflurane, halothane and isoflurane depress V_t/T_i. Morphine-like agents and sedatives such as barbiturates or benzodiazepines increase $PaCO_2$, decrease respiratory frequency and alter response to CO_2 and hypoxia [64]. However, these observations do not necessarily imply that respiratory centers are impaired as a result of the pharmacological effects of the drugs. During halothane anesthesia, breathing is entirely due to the activity of the diaphragm, without the contribution of the accessory respiratory muscles [65] while isoflurane increases airway resistance [66]. These phenomena may help to explain the reduction in mean inspiratory flow (V_t/T_i) observed with these agents. Moreover, $P_{0.1}$ response to CO_2 is not depressed in patients under methoxyflurane anesthesia [15] or in coma due to voluntary intoxication with barbiturates and carbamates [67]. These considerations imply that mechanical factors are the major causes of the ventilatory depression caused by these drugs.

Respiratory drive in respiratory diseases

Chronic pulmonary diseases

a. *Chronic Obstructive Pulmonary Diseases (COPD)* are characterized by an increased airway resistance and by respiratory muscle impairment. Moreover, expiration of COPD patients is impaired by dynamic compression of the airways. T_e is increased and T_i is shortened causing a reduction in T_i/T_{tot}. However minute ventilation is normal and respiratory frequency is increased. T_i/T_{tot} is correlated with FEV_1, but there is no significant difference between hypercapnic and non-hypercapnic patients [68]. The ventilatory response to CO_2 is diminished in emphysematous patients in relation to the degree of airway obstruction [69]. This response tends to be more depressed in hypercapnic than in normocapnic patients [70]. Indeed, neuromuscular coupling seems to be altered in hypercapnic COPD patients [71]. $P_{0.1}$ and the integrated EMG of the diaphragm are increased in COPD patients suggesting that inspiratory neural drive is increased [68, 71]. In acute failure of COPD, V_t is low and respiratory frequency is high. Dead space (V_d) and V_d/V_t are increased leading to hypercapnia. Already above normal values at baseline in these patients, $P_{0.1}$ [72] and total inspiratory work of breathing [73] are further increased. It had long been postulated that oxygen administration in these patients resulted in decreased minute ventilation due to removal of the hypoxic drive, the hypercapnic one being already blunted. However, measurement of respiratory parameters in COPD patients experiencing acute respiratory failure has demonstrated that, after a transient decrease, minute ventilation promptly returns to its initial value. Oxygen induced hypercapnia cannot therefore be attributed to depressed neural drive, but rather is explained by impaired ventilation-perfusion characteristics of the lungs [74].

b. *Asthmatic patients* also exhibit an increased airway occlusion pressure although the shape of the ventilatory response to CO_2 is diminished [75]. Recent data in patients having survived near fatal asthma suggest that in some such cases response to hypoxia may be altered, whereas response to CO_2 can be normal or slightly decreased. These patients differed most of all from controls in their reduced capacity to detect added resistive loads [76]. This emphasizes the role of respiratory afferences in adequate adaptation to changing respiratory mechanical or chemical conditions.

c. *In patients with pulmonary fibrosis*, lung elastance is greatly increased. Both T_i and T_e are shorter than in normal subjects and minute ventilation is increased. V_t is almost normal and mean inspiratory flow (V_t/T_i) is increased while T_i/T_{tot} is normal [18]. The respiratory response to CO_2 is variable depending on the severity of the disease but airway occlusion pressure is always increased which seems to indicate that respiratory drive is increased [77].

Control of breathing in chest wall diseases

Many conditions such as kyphoscoliosis, obesity, thoracoplasty, ankylosing spondylitis (AS) or tetraplegia lead to chest wall deformation [78]. In all cases this deformation is associated with an increased elastic load of the respiratory system. In some cases other kinds of loads are present (*e.g.* mass loading in obesity), or there are concomitant alterations of the active respiratory system that hinder compensation (*e.g.* muscular paralysis in tetraplegia).

a. *Kyphoscoliosis* is characterized by a distortion of the rib cage and an increase of elastic loading. Increased stiffness of the chest wall requires more respiratory work to be done by the muscles, particularly the inspiratory ones, in order to adequately ventilate the lungs. This can be achieved through extrinsic (neural) compensation, *i. e.* increased neural drive, which is the most important mechanism. However, intrinsic compensation also exists that allows the system to take advantage of the mechanical changes (*e.g.* longer, therefore more efficient, diaphragm due to decreased in kyphoscoliosis). Kyphoscoliotic patients compensate for the load by using, as compared to normals, a larger percentage of their inspiratory muscle force for quiet breathing.

This condition leads to a higher risk of diaphragmatic fatigue and hypercapnia. During NREM sleep kyphoscoliosis is associated with hypoventilation.

b. *Ankylosing spondylitis (AS)* is particular in that increased elastic load of the rib cage is associated with increased, not decreased, functional residual capacity. The ventilatory and occlusion pressure responses to CO_2 rebreathing in patients with AS are similar to those observed in normal subjects, suggesting a normal or higher neuromuscular output [79].

Control of breathing in neuromuscular disease

Neuromuscular diseases are an heterogeneous group of diseases. The level of neural impairment is variable: it can be central (cortical, brainstem, spinal affections), peripheral (acute polyneuritis), neuromuscular (myasthenic syndrome) at muscular (dystrophia such as Duchenne's, myotonia such as Steinert's, and all congenital, metabolic and inflammatory muscles diseases).

Disorders of the lower motorneurons, such as amyotrophic lateral sclerosis, spinal muscular atrophies or poliomyelitis, are associated with a blunted hypercapnic ventilatory response. Volontary hyperventilation is normal [80]. This indicates that the behavioural pathway of the ventilatory drive is intact, at least during wakefulness, and that sleep is a condition exposing to hypercapnia.

Post-polio syndrome with chronic hypercapnia probably involves breathing control alterations since it results in kyphoscoliosis and diaphragmatic palsy. The role of long term metabolic dysfunction of surviving motorneurons has been postulated [81].

During acute polyneuritis related ventilatory failure T_i/T_{tot} remains low as if the respiratory controller was set in order to avoid respiratory muscle fatigue, even at the expense of alveolar ventilation. Neural drive appears reduced and muscle activation is decreased [82].

In myasthenia gravis ventilatory response after CO_2 rebreathing is lower than normal. $P_{0.1}$ is slightly above normal under baseline (room air) conditions, and slightly decreased during CO_2 rebreathing. Since all these abnormalities are corrected by administration of anticholinesterasic drugs whose action is peripheral in nature, alteration of respiratory drive is not likely to play a significant role in such diseases [83, 84].

In Duchenne's and Steinert's diseases the $P_{0.1}$ response to hypercapnia seems normal, although the minute ventilation, tidal volume and V_t/T_i responses to hypercapnia and hypoxia are reduced. Patients with Duchenne's dystrophia have obstructive sleep apnea associated with deep oxygen desaturations during REM sleep, conversely to patients with Steinert's myotonia who have a mild central sleep apnea syndrome. This central depressant effect on the respiratory center during Steinert's myotonia is associated with a high incidence of complications during anesthesia [85, 86].

Obesity

Obesity is not always associated with hypoventilation: most obese patients do not have arterial hypercapnia. Only in patients described below as Pickwickians is there evidence of impaired control of breathing.

The obesity-hypoventilation syndrome or Pickwick syndrome, is characterized by an increase in respiratory load from obesity, increased upper airway resistance and decreased lung compliance. Clinically it is associated with daytime sleepiness, cyanosis, polycythemia, right heart insufficiency, hypoxia and hypercapnia. It seems that central chemosensitivity is markedly decreased, and this is probably one of the rare conditions where neural drive of breathing is indeed profoundly impaired and the actual source of disease [87, 88].

Distinct from central sleep apnea syndrome is the obstructive sleep-apnea syndrome. It is a very common clinical entity, characterized by a normal awake ventilation, but recurrent cyclic apneas during light NREM and REM sleep. Upper airway instability, in other words pharyngeal collapse, is the main source of apnea. This condition leads to sleep fragmentation, excessive daytime sleepiness, systemic and pulmonary hypertension and cardiac arrhythmias. In these patients the diaphragm contracts more and more during the apneas, a reaction which increases the negative pharyngeal pressure and makes apnea longer. If anything, the respiratory centers during this phase can be viewed as struggling, and obviously not depressed. Neural inspiratory drive appears normal in the obstructive sleep apnea syndrome [89].

References

1. Euler von C (1991) Neural organization and rhythm generation. In: Crystal RG, West JB (eds) The lung. Raven Press Ltd, New York, 1307-1318
2. Guz A, Noble MIM, Eisele JH, Trenchard D (1970) The role of vagal inflation reflexes in man and other animals. In: Porter R (ed) Breathing: Hering-Breuer centenary syposium. Churchill, London 315-336
3. Hering E, Breuer J (1868) Die Selbsteuerung der Atmung durch den Nervus Vagus. S Ber Akad Wiss Wien 57920:672-677

4. Sant'Ambrogio G, Sant'Ambrogio FB (1991) Reflexes from the airway, lung, chest wall and limbs. In: Crystal RG, West JB (eds) The lung. Raven Press Ltd, New York 1383-1395
5. Green JF, Kaufman MP (1990) Pulmonary afferent control of breathing as end-expiratory lung volume decreases. J Appl Physiol 68:2186-2194
6. Paintal AS (1969) Mechanism of stimulation of type J pulmonary receptors. J Physiol 203:511-532
7. Euler von C (1974) On the role of proprioceptors in perception and execution of motor acts with special reference to breathing. In: Pengelly JD, Rebuck AS, Campbell EJM (eds) Loaded breathing. Don Mill, Longman, pp 139-164
8. Frazier DT, Revelette WR (1991) Role of phrenic afferents in the control of breathing. J Appl Physiol 70:491-496
9. Green M, Mead J, Sears TA (1974) Effect of loading on respiratory muscle control in man. In: Pengelly JD, Rebuck AS, Campbell EJM (eds) Loaded breathing. Don Mills, Longman:73-80
10. Grunstein MM, Derenne JP, Milic-Emili J (1975) Control of depth and frequency of breathing during baroreceptors stimulation in cats. J Appl Physiol 39:395-404
11. Cherniack NS (1991) Central chemoreceptors. In: Crystal RG, West JB (eds) The lung. Raven Press Ltd, New York, pp 1349-1357
12. Banner NR, Lloyd MH, Hamilton RD, Innes JA, Guz A, Yacoub MH (1989) Cardiopulmonary response to dynamic exercise after heart and combined heart-lung transplantation. Br Heart J 61:215-223
13. Sanders MH, Costantino JP, Owwens GR, et al (1989) Breathing during wakefulness and sleep after human heart-lung transplantation. Am Rev Respir Dis 140:45-51
14. Shea SA, Horner RL, Banner NR, et al (1988) The effect of human heart-lung transplantation at rest and during sleep. Respir Physiol 72:131-150
15. Derenne JP, Couture J, Iscoe S, Whitelaw W, Milic-Emili J (1976) Occlusion pressure in man rebreathing CO_2 under methoxyflurane anesthesia. J Appl Physiol 40:805-814
16. Bellemare F, Grassino A (1982) Effect of pressure and timing of contraction on human diaphragm fatigue. J Appl Physiol Respir Environ Exercice Physiol 53:1190-1195
17. Rochester DF (1985) The diaphragm: contractile properties and fatigue. J Clin Invest 75:1397-1402
18. Milic-Emili J (1982) Recent advances in clinical assessment of control of breathing. Lung 160:1-17
19. Derenne JP (1977) Méthodes d'investigation clinique des mécanismes régulateurs de la ventilation. Bull Europ Physiopath Resp 13:681-727
20. Roussos C, Campbell EJM (1986) Respiratory muscles energetics. In: Fishman AP, Macklem PT, Mead J, Geiger SR (eds) Handbook of physiology, section 3: The respiratory system, volume III, Mechanics of breathing part 2. American Physiological Society, Bethesda, pp 481-511
21. Kelsen SG, Fishman AP (1980) Clinical assessment of the regulation of ventilation. In: Fishman AP (ed) Assessment of pulmonary function. McGraw-Hill Inc, New York, pp, 247-255
22. Milic-Emili J, Whitelaw WA, Derenne JPh (1975) Occlusion pressure-simple measure of the respiratory center's output. N Engl J Med 293:1029-1030
23. Whitelaw WA, Derenne JPh, Milic-Emili J (1975) Occlusion pressure as a measure of respiratory centers output in conscious man. Respir Physiol 23:181-199
24. Evanich MJ, Bruce E, Eldridge FL, et al (1977) Workshop on assessment of respiratory control in humans. IV. Measurement of the electrical activity in respiratory muscles. Am Rev Respir Dis 115:541-544

25. Eldridge FL (1975) Relationship between respiratory nerve and muscle activity and muscle force output. Am Rev Respir Dis 111:907-908
26. Eldridge FL (1976) Quantification of electrical activity in the phrenic nerve in the study of ventilatory control. Chest 70:154-157
27. Lopata M, Evanich MJ, Lourenco R (1976) The electromyogram of the diaphragm in the investigation of human regulation of ventilation. Chest 70:162-165
28. Whitelaw WA, Derenne JP (1993) Airway occlusion pressure. J Appl Physiol 74:1475-1483
29. Derenne JP, Whitelaw W, Couture J, Milic-Emili J (1986) Load compensation during positive pressure breathing in anaesthetized man. Respir Physiol 65:303-314
30. Lambertsen CJ (1964) Effects of drugs and hormones on the respiratory response to carbon dioxide. In: Fishman AP, Macklem PT, Mead J, Geiger SR (eds) Handbook of Physiology. The Respiratory System. Section III, vol 1. American Physiological Society, Washington DC, 545-555
31. Beral V, Read DJC (1971) Insensitivity of respiratory center to carbon dioxide in the Enga people of New Guinea. Lancet 2:1290-1394
32. Lahiri S, Oelaney RG, Brody JS, et al (1976) Relative role of environnemental and genetic factors in respiratory adaptation to high altitude. Nature 261:133-135
33. Rigatto H, Verduzco R, Cates DB (1975) Effects of O_2 on the ventilatory responses to CO_2 in preterm infants. J Appl Physiol 39:896-899
34. Lambertsen CJ (1960) Carbon dioxide and respiration in acid base homeostasis. Anesthesiology 21:642-651
35. Milic-Emili J (1975) Clinical methods for assessing the ventilatory response to carbon dioxide and hypoxia. N Engl J Med 293:864
36. Dejours P, Labrousse Y, Raynaud J, Teillac A (1957) Stimulus oxygène chémo-reflexe de la ventilation à basse altitude (50 m) chez l'homme. J Physiol (Paris) 49:115-120
37. Rebuck AS, Campbell EJM (1973) A clinical method for assessing the ventilatory response to hypoxia. Am Rev Respir Dis 109:345-350
38. Delhez L (1965) Modalités chez l'homme normal de la réponse électrique des piliers du diaphragme à la stimulation électrique des nerfs phréniques par des chocs uniques. Arch Int Physiol 72:832-839
39. Beck J, Sinderby C, Grassino AE (1994) The influence of innervation zones on esophageal recordings of diaphragmatic EMG. Am J Resp Crit Care Med 149 [Suppl]: A131 (abstract)
40. Beck J, Sinderby C, Weinberg J, Grassino AE (1994) Effect of chest wall configuration on esophageal recordings of diaphragm EMG. Am J Resp Crit Care Med 149 [Suppl]: A131 (abstract)
41. Newsom Davis J (1967) Phrenic nerve conduction in man. J Neurol Neurosurg Psychiat 30:420-426
42. Grassino AE, Whitelaw WA, Milic-Emili J (1976) Influence of lung volume and electrode position on electromyography of the diaphragm. J Appl Physiol 40:971-975
43. Whittenberger JL, Sarnoff SJ, Hardenbergh E (1949) Electrophrenic respiration. II. Its use in man. J Clin Invest 28:124-128
44. Bellemare F, Bigland-Ritchie B (1984) Assessment of human diaphragmatic strength and activation using phrenic nerve stimulation. Respir Physiol 58:263-277
45. Similowski T, Yan S, Gauthier AP, Bellemare F, Macklem PT (1993) Assessment of diaphragm function using mouth pressure twitches in COPD patients. Am Rev Respir Dis 147:850-856
46. Yan S, Gauthier AP, Similowski T, Macklem PT, Bellemare F (1992) Evaluation of human diaphragm contractility using mouth pressure twtches. Am Rev Respir Dis 147:850-856
47. Zegers de Beyl D, De Troyer A (1982) Phrenic nerve conduction time measurement in pulmonary disorders. Acta Neurol Bel 82:91-98

48. Merton PA (1954) Voluntary strength and fatigue. J Physiol 67:553-564
49. Similowski T, Yan S, Gauthier AP, Macklem PT, Bellemare F (1991) Contractile properties of the human diaphragm during chronic hyperinflation. N Engl J Med 325:917-923
50. Bellemare F, Bigland-Ritchie B (1987) Central components of diaphragmatic fatigue assessed by phrenic nerve stimulation. J Appl Physiol 62:1307-1316
51. Mier A, Brophy C, Moxham J, Green M (1987) Phrenic nerve stimulation in normal subjects and in patients with diphragmatic weakness. Thorax 42:885-888
52. Newsom Davis J, Goldman M, Loh L (1976) Diaphragm function and alveolar hypoventilation. Q J Med 45:87-100
53. Similowski T, Fleury B, Launois S, Cathala HP, Bouche P, Derenne JPh (1989) Cervical magnetic stimulation: a new painless method for bilateral phrenic nerve stimulation in conscious humans. J Appl Physiol 67:1311-1318
54. Gandevia SC, Rothwell JC (1987) Activation of the human diaphragm from the motor cortex. J Physiol 384:109-118
55. Murphy K, Mier A, Adams L, Guz A (1990) Putative cerebral cortical involvement in the ventilatory response to inhaled CO_2 in conscious man. J Physiol 420:1-18
56. Maskill D, Murphy K, Mier A, Owen M, Guz A (1991) Motor cortical representation of the diaphragm in man. J Physiol 443:105-121
57. Similowski T, Catala M, Orcel B, Willer JC, Derenne JPh (1991) Unilaterality of the motor cortical representation of the human diaphragm. J Physiol 438:37P (abstract)
58. Macefield G, Gandevia SC (1991) The cortical drive to human respiratory muscles in the awake state assessed by premotor cerebral potentials. J Physiol 439:545-558
59 Colebatch JG, Adams L, Murphy K, et al (1991) Regional cerebral blood flow during volitional breathing in man. J Physiol 443:91-103
60. Parisi R, Edelman NH, Santiago TV (1992) Central respiratory CO_2 chemosensitivity does not decrease during sleep. Am Rev Respir Dis 145:832-836
61. White DP (1986) Occlusion pressure and ventilation during sleep in normal humans. J Appl Physiol 61:1279-1287
62. Douglas NJ (1985) Control of ventilation during sleep. Clin Chest Med 6:563-575
63. Remmers JE (1990) Sleeping and breathing. Chest 97 [Suppl] 3:77S-80S
64. Pavlin EJ, Hornbein TF (1986) Anesthesia and the control of ventilation. In: Fishman AP, Cherniack NS, Widdicombe JG, Geiger SR (eds) Handbook of physiology, section 3, The respiratory system, volume II, Control of breathing (part 2.) American Physiological Society, Bethesda, pp 793-815
65. Tusiewicz K, Bryan AC, Froese AB (1977) Contribution of changing rib cage-diaphragm interactions to the ventilatory depression of halothane anesthesia. Anesthesiology 47:327-337
66. Higgs BD, Carli F (1983) An analysis of the ventilatory response to carbon dioxide with halothane and isoflurane anesthesia. Anesthesiology 59:A487(abstract)
67. Launois S, Fleury B, Similowski T, et al (1990) The respiratory response to CO_2 and O_2 in patients with coma due to volontary intoxication with barbiturates and carbamates. Eur Respir J 3:566-572
68. Sorli J, Grassino A, Lorange G, Milic-Emili J (1978) Control of breathing in patients with chronic obstructive lung disease. Clin Sci Mol Med 54:295-304
69. Cherniack RM, Snidal DP (1956) The effect of obstruction to breathing on the ventilatory response to CO_2. J Clin Invest 35:1286-1290
70. Brodovsky D, Macdonnel JA, Cherniack RM (1960) The respiratory response to carbon dioxide in health and emphysema. J Clin Invest 39:724-729
71. Gorini M, Spinelli A, Gianni R, Duranti R, Gigliotti F, Scano G (1990) Neural respira-

tory drive and neuromuscular coupling in patients with chronic obstructive pulmonary disease. Chest 98:1179-1186
72. Derenne JP, Aubier M, Murciano D, Fournier M, Pariente R (1977) Contrôle de la respiration au cours des poussées d'insuffisance respiratoire aigüe des insuffisances respiratoires chroniques obstructives. Rev Fran Mal Resp 5:714-716
73. Fleury B, Murciano D, Talamo C, Aubier M, Pariente R, Milic-Emili J (1985) Work of breathing in patients with chronic obstructive pulmonary disease in acute respiratory failure. Am Rev Respir Dis 131:816-821
74. Derenne JP, Fleury B, Pariente R (1988) Acute respiratory failure of chronic obstructve pulmonary disease. Am Rev Respir Dis 138:1006-1033
75. Anthonisen NR (1976) Some steady-state effects of respiratory loads. Chest 70:168
76. Kikuchi Y, Okabe S, Tamura G, et al (1994) Chemosensitivity and perception of dyspnea in patients with a history of near-fatal asthma. N Engl J Med 330:1329-1334
77. Launois S, Clergue F, Medrano G, et al (1991) Contrôle de la respiration dans les fibroses pulmonaires. Rev Mal Resp 8:67-73
78. Tardif C, Sohier B, Derenne JPh (1993) Control of breathing in chest wall diseases. Monaldi Arch Chest Dis 48:83-86
79. Tsanaclis A, Grassino AE (1979) Diaphragm and intercostal muscle behaviour in ankylosing spondilitis during CO_2 rebreathing. Am Rev Respir Dis 119:366 (abstract)
80. Serisier DE, Mastaglia SL, Gibson J (1982) Respiratory muscle function and ventilatory control: I. In patients with motoneurone disease. II. In: patients with myotonic dystrophy. Q J Med 202:205-226
81. Lane DJ, Hazelman B, Nichols PJR (1974) Late onset respiratory failure in patients with previous poliomyelitis. Q J Med 172:551-568
82. Borel C, Tilford C, Nichols D, Hanley D, Traystman RJ (1991) Diaphragmatic performance during recovery from acute ventilatory failure in Guillain-Barre syndrome and myasthenia gravis. Chest 99:444-451
83. Scano G, Gigliotti F, Duranti R, Gorini M, Fanelli A, Marconi G (1993) Control of breathing in patients with neuromuscular diseases. Monaldi Arch Chest Dis 48:87-91
84. Spinelli A, Marconi G, Gorini M, Pizzi A, Scano G (1992) Control of breathing in patients with myasthenia gravis. Am Rev Respir Dis 145:1359-1365
85. Kaufman L (1960) Anaesthesia in dystrophia myotonica. Proc R Soc Med 53:183-188.
86. Begin R, Bureau MA, Lupien L, Lemieux B (1980) Control and modulation of respiration in Steinert's myotonic dystrophy. Am Rev Respir Dis 121:281-289
87. Burwell CS, Robin ED, Whaley RD (1956) Extreme obesity associated with alveolar hypoventilation - a Pickwickian sydrome. Am J Med 21:811-818
88. Sampson MG, Grassino A (1983) Neuromechanical properties in obese patients during carbon dioxide breathing. Am J Med 75:81-90
89. Lopata M, Onal E (1982) Mass loading, sleep apnea, and the pathogenesis of obesity hypoventilation. Am Rev Respir Dis 126:640-645

Chapter 2

Respiratory muscle function

A. DE TROYER

Introduction

The mechanical action of any skeletal muscle is essentially determined by the anatomy of the muscle and by the structures it has to displace when it contracts. The respiratory muscles are morphologically and functionally skeletal muscles, and their task is to rhythmically displace the chest wall and pump gas in and out of the lungs. Understanding the actions of the respiratory muscles, therefore, requires a clear understanding of their anatomy and of the mechanics of the chest wall.

This review will thus start with a discussion of the basic mechanical structure of the chest wall in humans. It will then analyze the actions of the muscles that displace the chest wall. For the sake of clarity, the functions of the diaphragm, the muscles of the rib cage and the muscles of the abdominal wall will be analyzed separately. It must be appreciated, however, that all these muscles normally work together in a coordinated manner; some of the most critical aspects of their mechanical interdependence will be emphasized here.

The chest wall

The chest wall can be thought of as consisting of two compartments, the rib cage and the abdomen, separated from each other by a thin musculotendinous structure, the diaphragm (Fig. 1). Expansion of the lungs can be accommodated by expansion of either the rib cage or the abdomen or both compartments simultaneously.

From a mechanical standpoint, the abdomen can be considered as a liquid-filled container. That is, if one neglects the 100-300 ml of abdominal gas volume, the abdominal contents are virtually incompressible. Consequently, any local inward displacement of its boundaries results in an equal outward displacement elsewhere. Many of these boundaries, however, such as the spine dorsally, the pelvis caudally, and the iliac crests laterally, are virtually immobile. The parts of the abdominal container that can be displaced are thus largely limited to the ventral abdominal wall and the diaphragm. When the diaphragm contracts during inspiration (see below), therefore, its descent usually results in an outward displacement of the ventral abdominal wall; conversely, when the abdominal muscles contract, they cause an outward displacement of the belly wall which results in a cranial motion of the diaphragm into the thoracic cavity.

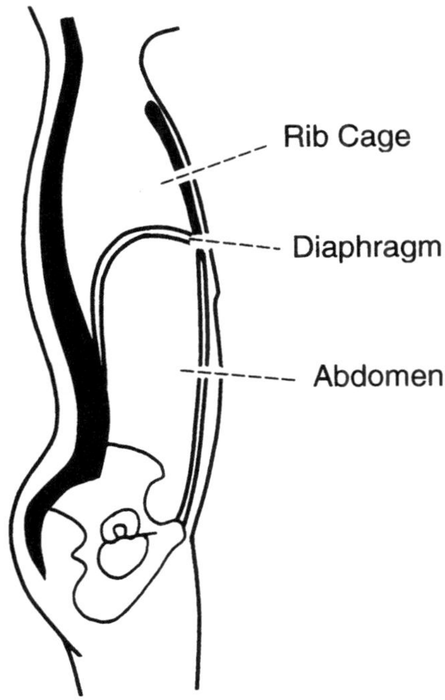

Fig. 1. Functional anatomy of the human chest wall at relaxed end-expiration (sagittal section)

Although the rib cage is a complicated structure, the ribs essentially move through a rotation around the axis defined by their articulations with the vertebral bodies and the transverse processes (Fig. 2). This movement is thus largely monoaxial. The axes of the necks of the ribs, however, are oriented laterally and dorsally. In addition, the plane of each rib (i.e., the plane defined by three points widely distributed on the arc of the rib) slopes downward from the back towards the front and also downward from the midline towards the side.

As a result, the displacements produced have three components: sagittal (dorsoventral), frontal (laterolateral) and axial (craniocaudal). Hence, when the ribs move axially in the cranial direction, there is usually an increase in the dorsoventral and lateral dimensions of the rib cage; the muscles which elevate the ribs are thus inspiratory in their action on the rib cage. Conversely, an axial motion of the ribs in the caudal direction is usually associated with a decrease in rib cage dimensions. The muscles that lower the ribs as their primary action therefore have an expiratory effect on the rib cage. It must be appreciated, however, that although the motion of the ribs in humans is essentially monoaxial, the costovertebral and costosternal articulations are lax enough to enable the rib cage to depart from a unitary behavior. Thus, significant deformations of the rib cage can occur under the influence of muscle contraction and pressure.

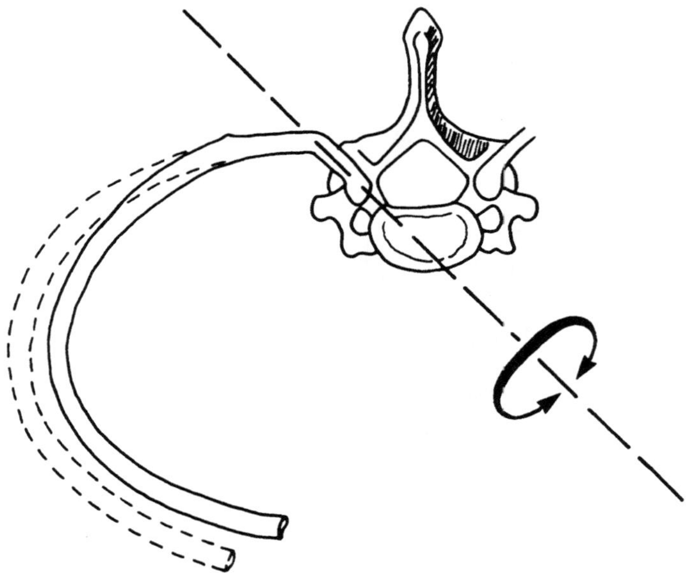

Fig. 2. Motion of the ribs in humans. The ribs move essentially through a rotation around the axis of the neck (broken axis and arrow), but their configuration is such that a rotation in an inspiratory direction causes increases in the anteroposterior and transverse diameters of the rib cage (dotted line)

The diaphragm

Functional anatomy

The diaphragm is anatomically unique among skeletal muscles in that its muscle fibres radiate from a central tendinous structure (the central tendon) to insert peripherally into skeletal structures. The crural (or vertebral) portion of the diaphragmatic muscle inserts in the ventrolateral aspect of the first three lumbar vertebrae and on the aponeurotic arcuate ligaments, and the costal portion inserts in the xiphoid process of the sternum and the upper margins of the lower six ribs. From their insertions the costal fibers run cranially so that they are directly apposed to the inner aspect of the lower rib cage; this is the so-called "zone of apposition" of the diaphragm to the rib cage [1] (Fig. 3). Although the older literature suggested the possibility of an intercostal motor innervation of some portions of the diaphragm, it has now been clearly established that its only motor supply is through the phrenic nerves which, in man, originate in the third, fourth, and fifth cervical segments.

Action of the diaphragm

As the muscle fibres of the diaphragm are activated during inspiration, they develop tension and shorten. As a result the axial length of the apposed diaphragm

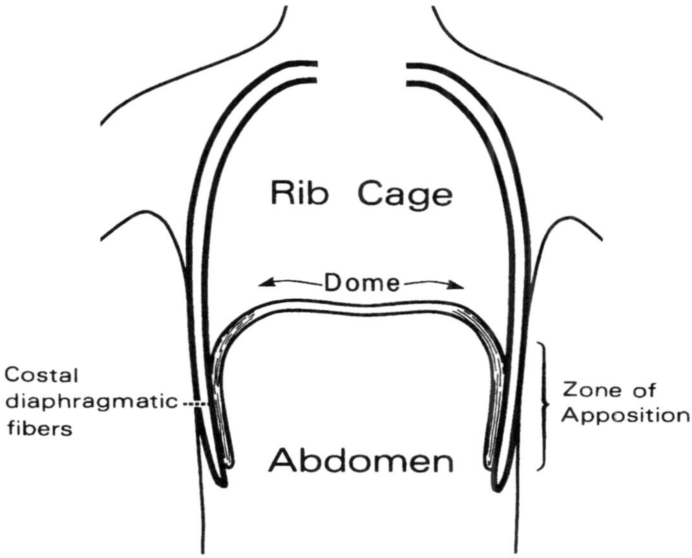

Fig. 3. Frontal section of the chest wall at end-expiration illustrating the functional anatomy of the diaphragm. Note the orientation of the costal diaphragmatic fibers; these fibers run cranially and are directly apposed to the inner aspect of the lower rib cage (zone of apposition)

diminishes and the dome of the diaphragm, which corresponds primarily to the central tendon, descends relative to the costal insertions of the muscle. The dome of the diaphragm remains relatively constant in size and shape during breathing, but its descent has two effects. Firstly, it expands the thoracic cavity along its craniocaudal axis. Hence, pleural pressure falls and, depending on whether the airways are open or closed, lung volume increases or alveolar pressure falls. Secondly, it produces a caudal displacement of the abdominal viscera and an increase in abdominal pressure which, in turn, pushes the ventral abdominal wall outwards.

In addition, because the muscle fibres of the costal diaphragm insert into the upper margins of the lower six ribs, they also apply a force on these ribs when they contract, and the cranial orientation of these fibres is such that this force is directed cranially. It has, therefore, the effect of lifting the ribs and rotating them outward. The fall in pleural pressure and the increase in abdominal pressure that results from diaphragmatic contraction, however, act on the rib cage simultaneously, which probably explains why the action of the diaphragm on the rib cage has been controversial for so long.

Action of the diaphragm on the rib cage

When the diaphragm in anesthetized dogs is activated selectively by electrical stimulation of the phrenic nerves, the upper ribs move caudally and the cross-sectional area of the upper portion of the rib cage decreases [2]. In contrast, the cross-sectional area of the lower portion of the rib cage increases. When a bilateral pneumothorax is subsequently introduced so that the fall in pleural pressure is eliminated, isolated contraction of the diaphragm causes a greater expansion of the lower rib cage, but the dimensions of the upper rib cage now remain unchanged [2]. It appears, therefore, that the diaphragm has two opposing effects on the rib cage when it contracts. On the one hand, it has an expiratory action on the upper rib cage, and the fact that this action is abolished by a pneumothorax indicates that it is due to the fall in pleural pressure. On the other hand, the diaphragm also has an inspiratory action on the lower rib cage. Measurements of chest wall motion in patients with traumatic transection of the lower cervical cord (in whom the diaphragm is often the only muscle active during quiet breathing [3, 4]) have shown that the action of the diaphragm on the human rib cage is essentially similar; in these patients, the lower rib cage thus expands during inspiration whereas the anteroposterior diameter of the upper rib cage decreases (Fig. 4).

Theoretical and experimental work has confirmed that the inspiratory action of the diaphragm on the lower rib cage results in part from the force the muscle applies on the ribs by way of its insertions; this force is conventionally referred to as the "insertional" force [5, 6]. This inspiratory action of the diaphragm, however, is also related to its apposition to the rib cage. The zone of apposition makes the lower rib cage, in effect, part of the abdominal container and measurements in dogs and rabbits have established that during breathing the changes in pressure in the pleural recess between the apposed diaphragm and the rib cage are almost equal to the changes in abdominal pressure. Pressure in the pleural recess rises, rather than falls, during inspiration, thus indicating that the rise in abdominal pressure is truly transmitted through the apposed diaphragm to expand the lower rib cage. This mechanism of diaphragmatic action has been called the "appositional" force.

Although the insertional and appositional forces make the normal diaphragm expand the lower rib cage, it should be appreciated that this action of the diaphragm is largely determined by the resistance provided by the abdominal contents to diaphragmatic descent. If this resistance is high (i.e., if abdominal compliance is low) the dome of the diaphragm descends less, so that the zone of apposition remains significant throughout inspiration and the rise in abdominal pressure is greater. Therefore, for a given diaphragmatic activation, the appositional force tending to expand the lower rib cage is increased. Conversely, if the resistance provided by the abdominal contents is small (if the abdomen is very compliant), the dome of the diaphragm descends more easily, the zone of apposition decreases more, and the rise in abdominal pressure is smaller. Consequently, the inspiratory action of the diaphragm on the rib cage is decreased. If the resistance provided by the abdominal contents were eliminated, not only would the zone of apposition disappear in the course of inspiration, but also the contracting diaphragmatic muscle fibres would become oriented transversely inward at their insertions onto the ribs. The insertional force would then have an expiratory, rather than inspiratory, action on the lower rib cage. Indeed, when a dog is eviscerated the diaphragm causes a decrease, rather than an increase, in lower rib cage dimensions [2, 5].

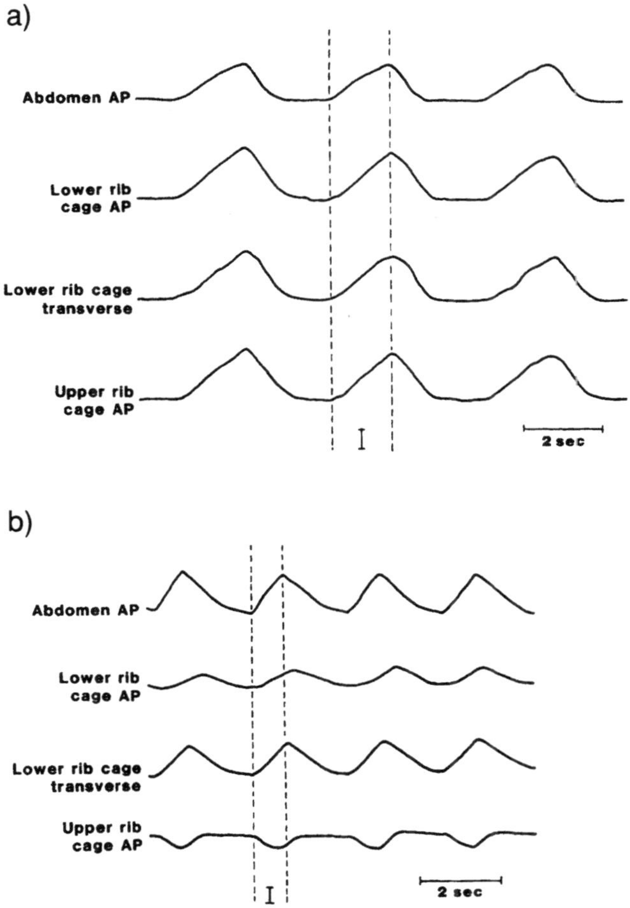

Fig. 4. Pattern of chest wall motion in a healthy subject (a) and a C5 tetraplegic patient (b) breathing at rest in the seated posture. The respiratory changes in anteroposterior (AP) diameter of the abdomen, lower rib cage (5th costalcartilage) and upper rib cage (manubrium sterni) are shown, as well as the changes in transverse diameter of the lower rib cage. In all traces an upward deflection corresponds to in increase in diameter, and a downward deflection corresponds to a decrease in diameter. I indicates the duration of inspiration

The muscles of the rib cage

The intercostal muscles

The intercostal muscles are two thin layers of muscle occupying each of the intercostal spaces. The external intercostals extend from the tubercles of the ribs dorsally to the costochondral junctions ventrally and their fibres are oriented obliquely caudal and ventrally from the rib above to the rib below. In contrast, the internal intercostals extend from the angles of the ribs dorsally to the sternocostal junctions ventrally and their fibres run obliquely caudal and dorsally from the rib above to the rib below. Thus, although the intercostal spaces contain two layers of intercostal muscle in their lateral portion, they contain a single layer in their ventral and dorsal portions. Dorsally from the angles of the ribs to the vertebrae the only fibres come from the external intercostal muscles, whereas ventrally, between the sternum and the chondrocostal junctions, the only fibres are those of the internal intercostal muscles. These latter, however, are particularly thick in this region of the rib cage, where they are conventionally called the "parasternal intercostals". All the intercostal muscles are innervated by the intercostal nerves.

The action of the intercostal muscles on the ribs is conventionally viewed according to the theory proposed by Hamberger in the mid 1700's [7]. As illustrated in Fig. 5, when an intercostal muscle contracts in one interspace, it pulls the upper rib down and the lower rib up. However, as the fibres of the external intercostal slope obliquely caudal and ventrally from the rib above to the one below, their lower insertion is more distant from the centre of rotation of the ribs (the vertebral articulations) than the upper one. When this muscle contracts, the torque acting on the lower rib is thus greater than that acting on the upper rib, and

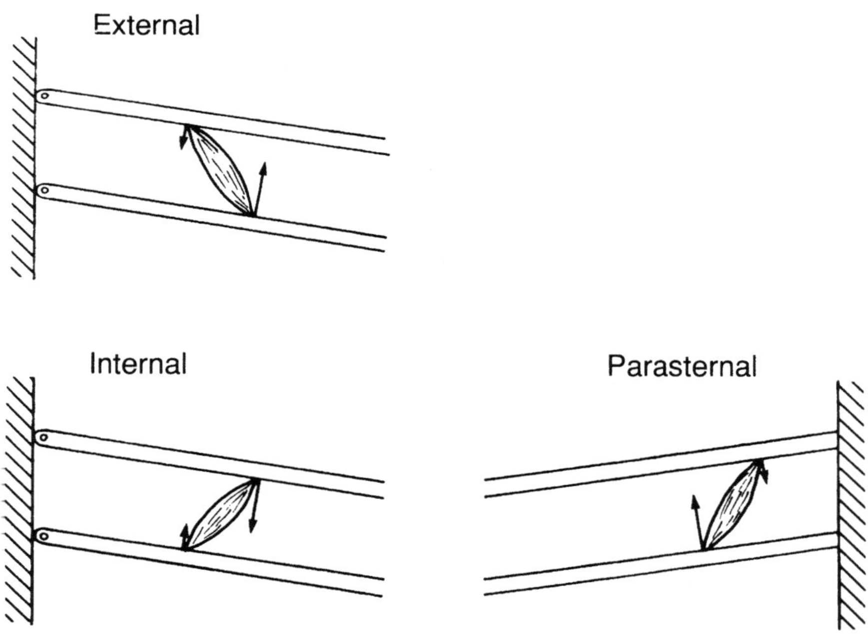

Fig. 5. Diagram illustrating the actions of the intercostal mucles as proposed by Hamberger [7]. The hatched area in the left panels represents the spine (dorsal view) and the hatched area in the lower right panel represents the sternum (ventral view). The two bars oriented obliquely represent two adjacent ribs. The external and internal intercostal muscles are depicted as single bundles and the torques acting on the ribs during contraction are represented by arrows

hence its net effect should be to raise the ribs. In contrast, the fibres of the internal intercostal run obliquely caudal and dorsally from the rib above to the one below. Therefore, their lower insertion is less distant from the centre of rotation of the ribs than the upper one and, as a result, when this muscle contracts, the torque acting on the lower rib is less than that acting on the upper rib, so that its net effect should be to lower the ribs. The parasternal intercostals are part of the internal intercostal layer, but their action should be referred to the sternum rather than to the vertebral column, their contraction should, therefore, raise the ribs.

This theory is an oversimplification and does not explain important features of intercostal muscle mechanics [8, 9]. A number of electromyographic recordings from intercostal nerves and muscles in animals have demonstrated that the parasternal intercostals and external intercostals are electrically active during the inspiratory phase of the breathing cycle; interestingly, the inspiratory activation of the external intercostals takes place mostly in the dorsal region of the rostral interspaces, where these muscles are thickest and have the greatest inspiratory mechanical advantage [9]. Normal humans at rest have similar phasic inspiratory activity in the parasternal intercostals and in the external intercostals of the most rostral interspaces [10, 11]. Furthermore, in the dog, when either the parasternal intercostal or the external intercostal in a given interspace is selectively activated by electrical stimulation it causes cranial displacement of the ribs into which it inserts [8]. In addition, when the diaphragm and all the external intercostals in dogs are denervated so that the parasternal intercostals are the only muscles active during inspiration, the ribs move cranially. Similarly, inspiratory cranial displacement of the ribs is seen when the canine diaphragm and parasternal intercostals have been paralyzed so that the external intercostals are the only muscles active during inspiration. Thus, both the parasternal intercostals and the external intercostals contract during inspiration, including resting breathing, to pull the ribs cranially and to expand the rib cage compartment of the chest wall. Studies in dogs have shown, however, that the contribution of the parasternal intercostals to resting breathing is much larger than that of the external intercostals [12].

The internal interosseous intercostals, on the other hand, have an expiratory action on the rib cage. In spontaneously breathing animals, these muscles contract during the expiratory phase of the breathing cycle, and in contrast to the external intercostals their contraction is confined to the caudal interspaces. In this way, they help the triangularis sterni (see below) to pull the ribs caudally and deflate the rib cage. As with the external intercostals, however, the contribution of the internal intercostals to resting breathing appears to be small [10].

The insertions and fiber orientations of the external and internal intercostal muscles would suggest that these muscles are also ideally suited to twist the rib cage [8]. Thus, contraction of the external intercostals on one side of the sternum would rotate the ribs in a transverse plane so that the upper ribs would move forward while the lower ribs would move backward. In contrast, contraction of the internal intercostals on one side of the sternum would move the upper ribs backward and the lower ribs forward. Recent studies in normal humans have shown that the external and internal interosseous intercostals are indeed actively involved in rotations of the thorax [13]. Specifically, the external intercostals on the right side of the chest are activated when the trunk is rotated to the left, whereas they are silent when the trunk is rotated to the right. Conversely, the internal intercostals on the right side of the chest are activated when the trunk is rotated to the right. Active use of these muscles during such postural movements is consistent with their abundant supply of muscle spindles.

The scalene muscles

The scalene muscles in man comprise three bundles that run from the transverse processes of the lower five cervical vertebrae to the upper surface of the first two ribs. When these muscles are selectively activated by electrical stimulation in dogs, they produce a marked cranial displacement of the ribs and sternum and cause an increase in rib cage anteroposterior diameter. Although the scalenes have traditionally been considered as "accessory" muscles of inspiration, studies with needle electrodes have established that in normal humans they invariably contract in concert with the diaphragm and the parasternal intercostals during inspiration [11, 14] (Fig. 6).

There is no clinical setting that causes paralysis of all the inspiratory muscles without also affecting the scalenes and, therefore, the isolated action of these muscles on the human rib cage cannot be precisely defined. Two observations, however, indicate that contraction of the scalenes is an important determinant of expansion of the upper rib cage during breathing. First, when normal subjects attempt to inspire with the diaphragm alone there is a marked, selective decrease in scalene activity associated with either less inspiratory increase or a paradoxical decrease in anteroposterior diameter of the upper rib cage [11]. Second, the

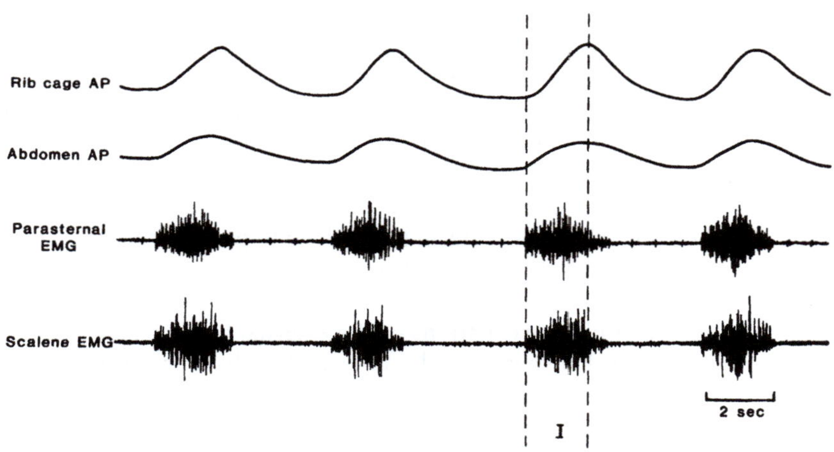

Fig. 6. Pattern of electrical activation of the scalene and paresternal intercostal muscles in normal humans. The subject shown here is breathing quietly in the seated position. The inspiration phase of the breathing cycle (I) is indicated by an increase in rib cage and abdomen anteroposterior (AP) diameter

inward inspiratory displacement of the upper rib cage characteristic of tetraplegia is usually not observed when scalene function is preserved after the lower cervical cord transection [4]. Since the scalenes are innervated from the lower five cervical segments, persistent inspiratory contraction is frequently seen in subjects with a transection at the C_7 level or below. In such subjects, the anteroposterior diameter of the upper rib cage tends to remain constant or to increase slightly during inspiration.

The sternocleidomastoids and other accessory muscles of inspiration

Many additional muscles, such as the pectoralis minor, the trapezius, the erector spinae, the serrati and the sternocleidomastoids, can elevate the ribs when they contract. These muscles, however, run between the shoulder girdle and the rib cage, the spine and the shoulder girdle or the head and the rib cage, and have primarily postural functions. In healthy individuals, they are active only during increased inspiratory efforts and in contrast to the scalenes, they are thus real "accessory" muscles of inspiration.

Of all these muscles only the sternocleidomastoids have been thoroughly studied. These descend from the mastoid process to the ventral surface of the manubrium sterni and the medial third of the clavicle and their action in man has been inferred from measurements of chest wall motion in patients with transection of the upper cervical cord. Indeed, in such patients the diaphragm, intercostals, scalenes and abdominal muscles are paralyzed, but the sternocleidomastoids (the motor innervation of which largely depends on the eleventh cranial nerve) are spared and contract forcefully during unassisted inspiration. When breathing spontaneously these patients show a marked inspiratory cranial displacement of the sternum and a large inspiratory expansion of the upper rib cage, particularly in its anteroposterior diameter. There is, however, a decrease in the transverse diameter of the lower rib cage [3, 15].

The triangularis sterni

The triangularis sterni, also called transversus thoracis, is a flat muscle that lies deep to the sternum and the parasternal intercostals. Its fibres originate from the dorsal aspect of the caudal half of the sternum and insert into the inner surface of the costal cartilages of ribs 3 to 7. The motor supply of the muscle comes from the intercostal nerves.

Although this muscle has long been neglected, it has an important respiratory function in quadrupeds [16]. In the dog and in the cat the triangularis sterni invariably contracts during the expiratory phase of the breathing cycle and this contraction acts to pull the ribs caudally and to deflate the rib cage below its neutral (resting) position. Consequently, when the muscle relaxes at the end of expiration there is passive rib cage expansion and an increase in lung volume that precedes the onset of inspiratory muscle contraction. In these animals the triangularis sterni thus shares the work of breathing with the inspiratory muscles and helps the parasternal intercostals produce the rhythmic inspiratory expansion of the rib cage [16].

In contrast to quadrupeds, the triangularis sterni in normal humans is usually inactive during resting breathing. However, it invariably contracts during voluntary or involuntary expiratory efforts such as coughing, laughing and speech. Normal humans, in fact, cannot produce expiratory efforts without contracting the triangularis sterni. Presumably, the muscle then acts in concert with the internal interosseous intercostals to deflate the rib cage and increase pleural pressure.

The abdominal muscles

Functional anatomy

The four abdominal muscles with significant respiratory function in man constitute the ventrolateral wall of the abdomen with the rectus abdominis being most ventral of these muscles. It originates from the ventral aspect of the sternum and the fifth, sixth and seventh costal cartilages, and runs caudally along the whole length of the abdominal wall to insert into the pubis. This muscle is enclosed in a sheath formed by the aponeuroses of the other three muscles. The most superficial of these is the external oblique which originates from fleshy digitations of the external surface of the lower eight ribs well above the costal margin, and directly covers the lower ribs and intercostal muscles. Its fibres radiate caudally to the iliac crest and inguinal ligament and medially to the linea alba. The internal oblique lies deep to the external obliques, its fibres arise from the iliac crest and inguinal ligament and diverge to insert on the costal margin and an aponeurosis contributing to the rectus sheath down to the pubis. The transversus abdominis is the deepest of the muscles of the lateral abdominal wall. It arises from the inner surface of the lower six ribs where it interdigitates with the costal insertions of the diaphragm. From this origin and from the lumbar fascia, the iliac crest and the inguinal ligament its fibres run circumferentially around the abdominal visceral mass and terminate ventrally in the rectus sheath.

Actions of the abdominal muscles

These four muscles have important functions as rotators and flexors of the trunk, but as respiratory muscles they have two principal actions. Firstly, as they contract they pull the abdominal wall inward and produce an increase in abdominal pressure. This causes the diaphragm to move cranially into the thoracic cavity, which in turn results in an increase in pleural pressure and a decrease in lung volume. Secondly, they displace the rib cage due to their insertions on the ribs. These insertions would suggest that the action of the abdominal muscles was to pull the lower ribs caudally and to deflate the cage, another expiratory action. Measurements of rib cage motion during separate stimulation of the four abdominal muscles in supine dogs have shown, however, that these muscles also have an inspiratory action on the rib cage [17]. Indeed, as previously discussed (Fig. 3), there is a large zone where the diaphragm is directly apposed to the rib cage which allows abdominal pressure to be transmitted to the lower rib cage. The rise in abdominal pressure that takes place when the abdominal muscles contract thus acts to expand the lower rib cage. Furthermore, the diaphragm, when forced cranially, is stretched, and this passive diaphragmatic tension tends to raise the lower ribs in the same way as does an active diaphragmatic contraction ("insertional" force).

The action of the abdominal muscles on the rib cage is thus determined by the balance between the insertional, expiratory force of the muscles and the inspiratory force related to the rise in abdominal pressure. Isolated contraction of the external oblique muscle in man produces a small caudal displacement of the sternum and a large decrease in the rib cage transverse diameter, but the rectus abdominis, while causing a marked caudal displacement of the sternum and a large decrease in the anteroposterior diameter of the rib cage, also produces a small increase in the rib cage transverse diameter [18]. The isolated actions of the internal oblique and transversus abdominis muscles on the human rib cage are not known. The anatomical arrangement of the transversus, however, would suggest that among the abdominal muscles this muscle has the smallest insertional, expiratory action on the ribs and is the most effective in increasing abdominal pressure. Therefore, isolated contraction of the transversus should produce little or no expiratory rib cage displacement.

Respiratory function of the abdominal muscles

Irrespective of their actions on the rib cage, the abdominal muscles are primarily expiratory muscles through their action on the diaphragm and the lung, and they play important roles in activities such as coughing and speaking. Their action, however, also enables them to assist inspiration. Thus, by contracting in phase with expiration and forcing the diaphragm cranially, the abdominal muscles can reduce lung volume below the neutral position of the respiratory system and hence, when they relax at end-expiration, can promote passive descent of the diaphragm so that lung volume increases before the onset of inspiratory muscle contraction. This effect, which is similar to that produced by the triangularis sterni in dogs, may prevent the inspiratory muscles from working disproportionately hard. Indeed, phasic expiratory contraction of the abdominal muscles occurs in healthy subjects whenever the demand placed on 'the inspiratory muscles is increased, such as during exercise, breathing CO_2-enriched gas mixtures, or breathing against increased inspiratory mechanical loads. It is noteworthy that in these conditions the transversus muscle is recruited during expiration well before activity can be recorded from either the rectus or the external oblique [19]. In view of the actions of these muscles, this differential recruitment also supports the notion that the effect of the abdominal muscles on abdominal pressure is more important for breathing than their action on the rib cage.

There is a second mechanism by which the abdominal muscles can assist inspiration. Most normal human subjects when adopting the standing posture develop tonic abdominal muscle activity unrelated to the phases of the breathing cycle, and studies in patients with transection of the upper cervical cord, in whom bilateral pacing of the phrenic nerves allows the degree of diaphragmatic activation to be maintained constant, have clearly illustrated the effect of this tonic abdominal contraction on inspiration [3]. When the patients were supine the unassisted paced diaphragm was able to generate an adequate tidal volume. However, when the patients were tilted head up or moved to the seated posture the weight of the abdominal viscera and the absence of abdominal muscle activity caused the belly wall to protrude. The tidal volume produced by pacing in this posture was markedly reduced relative to the supine posture but the reduction was significantly diminished when a pneumatic cuff was inflated around the abdomen to mimic tonic abdominal muscle contraction. Thus, by contracting throughout the breathing cycle in the standing posture, the abdominal muscles make the diaphragm longer at the onset of inspiration and prevent it from shortening excessively during inspiration; in accordance with the length-tension characteristics of the muscle, its ability to generate pressure is thus increased.

Conclusion

Although the diaphragm is the main respiratory muscle in man, it is not the only important contracting muscle. The diaphragm expands the abdomen and the lower rib cage, but the expansion of the cranial half of the rib cage is accomplished by other inspiratory muscles, in particular the scalenes and the parasternal intercostals. In normal subjects at rest the synchronous expansion of the abdominal and rib cage compartments of the chest wall thus results from the simultaneous contraction of these three inspiratory muscle groups and not from the isolated action of the diaphragm as previously thought. Additional muscles, such as the transversus abdominis and triangularis sterni, are also frequently involved in the act of breathing. These muscles are usually considered to be expiratory because they displace the respiratory system below its resting volume. By relaxing at end-expiration, however, they also cause an increase in lung volume, thereby reducing the load on the inspiratory muscles.

Moving the chest wall during breathing is thus a complex, integrated process that involves many muscles and the control mechanisms that promote coordinated use of these different muscles are critically important in maintaining alveolar ventilation within acceptable limits. These mechanisms play an important role in healthy subjects, particularly when the ventilatory requirements are increased, but they become absolutely essential to life in conditions where the diaphragm is less effective or paralyzed.

References

1. Mead J (1979) Functional significance of the area of apposition of diaphragm to rib cage. Am Rev Respir Dis 119:31-32
2. D'Angelo E, Sant'Ambrogio G (1974) Direct action of contracting diaphragm on the rib cage in rabbits and dogs. J Appl Physiol 36:715-719
3. Danon J, Druz WS, Goldberg NB, Sharp JT (1979) Function of the isolated paced diaphragm and the cervical accessory muscles in C1 quadriplegics. Am Rev Respir Dis 119:909-919
4. Estenne M, De Troyer A (1985) Relationship between respiratory muscle electromyogram and rib cage motion in tetraplegia. Am Rev Respir Dis 132:53-59
5. De Troyer A, Sampson M, Sigrist S, Macklem PT (1982) Action of costal and crural parts of the diaphragm on the rib cage in dog. J Appl Physiol 53:30-39
6. Loring SH, Mead J (1982) Action of the diaphragm on the rib cage inferred from a force-balance analysis. J Appl Physiol 53:756-760
7. Hamberger GE (1749) De Respirationis Mechanismo et usu genuino. Jena
8. De Troyer A, Kelly S, Macklem PT, Zin WA (1985) Mechanics of intercostal space and actions of external and internal intercostal muscles. J Clin Invest 75:850-857
9. Wilson TA, De Troyer A (1994) Respiratory effect of the intercostal muscles in the dog. J Appl Physiol 75:2636-2645
10. Taylor A (1960) The contribution of the intercostal muscles to the effort of respiration in man. J Physiol 151:390-402
11. De Troyer A, Estenne M (1984) Coordination between rib cage muscles and diaphragm during quiet breathing in humans. J Appl Physiol 57:899-906
12. De Troyer A (1991) The inspiratory elevation of the ribs in the dog: primary role of the parasternals. J Appl Physiol 70:1447-1455
13. Whitelaw WA, Ford GT, Rimmer KP, De Troyer A (1992) Intercostal muscles are used during rotation of the thorax in humans. J Appl Physiol 72:1940-1944
14. Raper AJ, Thompson WT Jr, Shapiro W, Patterson JLJr (1966) Scalene and sternomastoid muscle function. J Appl Physiol 21:497-502
15. De Troyer A, Estenne M, Vincken W (1986) Rib cage motion and muscle use in high tetraplegics. Am Rev Respir Dis 133:1115-1119
16. De Troyer A, Ninane V (1986) Triangularis sterni: a primary muscle of breathing in the dog. J Appl Physiol 60:14-21
17. De Troyer A, Sampson M, Sigrist S, Kelly S (1983) How the abdominal muscles act on the rib cage. J Appl Physiol 54:465-469
18. Mier A, Brophy C, Estenne M, Moxham J, Green M, De Troyer A (1985) Action of abdominal muscles on rib cage in humans. J Appl Physiol 58:1438-1443
19. De Troyer A, Estenne M, Ninane V, Van Gansbeke D, Gorini M (1990) Transversus abdominis muscle function in humans. J Appl Physiol 68:1010-1016

Chapter 3

Respiratory muscle dysfunction

S. NAVA, F. RUBINI

Introduction

The respiratory system consists of two main parts, the lung and the ventilatory pump. The latter is formed by the bony structure of the thorax, the central respiratory controllers, the inspiratory and expiratory muscles and the nerve innervating these muscles. Whereas failure of the lung leads to hypoxemia, failure of the ventilatory pump, in particular a dysfunction of the respiratory muscles, leads to hypercapnic respiratory failure. Respiratory muscle fatigue occurs when respiratory muscle endurance is exceeded; that is, when the load against which the muscles must contract requires too great an effort for too long [1]. Healthy people never approach this threshold, below which diaphragm fatigue does not occur. In contrast, patients with severe chronic obstructive pulmonary disease (COPD) neuromuscular diseases may be close to the threshold at rest and exceed it even with minor exertion [2, 3]. In September 1988 a workshop was held at Kansas State University to reassess the state of knowledge on respiratory muscle fatigue [4]. Muscle fatigue was defined as a condition in which there is a loss in the capacity for developing force and/or velocity of a muscle resulting from muscle activity and which is reversible by rest. Muscle weakness is a condition in which the capacity of a rested muscle to generate force is impaired.

According to Monod and Scherrer [5] the endurance time of a muscle (t_{lim}) during a constant isometric contraction is inversely proportional to the force developed, according to the following equation:

$$t_{lim} = \frac{K'}{F/F_{max}}$$

where K is a constant and F is the portion of maximal force that the muscle can develop. During an intermittent effort, like the respiratory muscles during spontaneous breathing, the time the contraction is maintained must be taken into account since this time is inversely proportional to t_{lim}. The tension-time index of the human diaphragm (TT_{di}) was used by Bellemare and Grassino [1] as a measure of diaphragmatic exertion against inspiratory loads. TT_{di} was defined as the product of the mean transdiaphragmatic pressure (P_{di}) developed during contraction (expressed as a fraction of maximal P_{di}) and the time of contraction relative to the total duration of the respiratory cycle (T_i/T_{tot}). The diaphragm develops fatigue in the course of repeated intermittents when TT_{di} exceeds values ranging from 0.15 to 0.18. Above this threshold the endurance time of the diaphragm is inversely related to TT_{di}. In the course of their experiments pleural (P_{pl}) and abdominal (P_{ab}) pressure changes were made to contribute equally to P_{di} during inspiration. However, in most situations [6] in which breathing is held against inspiratory loads the P_{pl} swing is larger than the abdominal one, suggesting increased recruitment of inspiratory muscles attached to the rib cage in addition to the diaphragm. Zocchi et al [7] have recently shown that when adopting this pattern of breathing the critical threshold of fatigue is higher than previously described by TT_{di} for diaphragm emphasis.

Three general types of fatigue have been described: central fatigue, transmission fatigue and contractile fatigue [8].

Central fatigue is a reversible decrease in central neural respiratory drive caused by overuse of the muscles. There are two kinds of central fatigue: 1) motivotional fatigue in which the level of respiratory effort drops off but can be restored by a voluntary super-effort. 2) non-motivational fatigue, where the muscle retains a normal response to electrical stimulation but no amount of exhortation can increase the level of respiratory effort. Transmission fatigue is a reversible, exertion-induced impairment in the transmission of neural impulses through nerves or across neuromuscular junctions. Possible locations are the axonal branch points, the neuromuscular junction itself and the muscle membrane. Contractile fatigue is a reversible impairment in the contractile response of the muscles to neural impulses which is not caused by drugs. This kind of fatigue can be divided into two types: a transient type known as high-frequency (reduced response to stimulation frequencies of 50 to 100 Hz), and a long-lasting form known as low frequency fatigue (reduced response to stimulation frequencies of 10 to 20 Hz). The transient high-frequency fatigue might be caused by accumulations of toxic metabolic by products of contraction, by altered calcium or by decreased ATP concentrations. The long lasting low-frequency fatigue is probably caused by minor muscle injury that must be repaired before normal function is restored.

To the clinician the identification of the etiology of ventilatory failure is fundamental to the appropriate therapeutic plan and in particular in assessing the supply of energy and the demands of the ventilatory muscles pump. Weakness and fatigue of the respiratory muscles are associated with several diseases and pathological conditions as follows.

a. Low Cardiac Ouput States. Aubier et al. [9] showed that cardiogenic shock in dogs resulted in failure of the ventilatory muscles, while Nava and Bellemare [10] demonstrated that the main cause of respiratory muscle fatigue in this condition depends on central factors. Whatever the main cause, the death of the animals resulted from ventilatory failure. Field et al. [11] extended these findings to critically ill patients requiring mechanical ventilation. They noted that these patients not only had an increased oxygen consumption by respiratory muscle, but also exhibited a diminished efficiency of the ventilatory pump. They postulated that mechanical ventilation in such a group would increase oxygen delivery to more vital organ systems.

b. Nutrition. It is clear that many patients with COPD are malnourished. An important consequence of malnutrition and weight loss is a significant decrease in respiratory muscle mass, with related weakness [12]. In addition, acute depletion of certain trace elements dramatically interferes with muscle performance. Hypophosphatemia [13] usually a consequence of increased excretion in patients with diminished stores, may result in ventilatory failure. Hypokaliemia and hypomagnesemia [14] may also impair muscle performance to provoke incipient fatigue. In direct contrast to the malnourished thin patients, the physician is commonly faced with obese patients, in whom ventilatory muscle strength has been reported to be reduced by 30 % [15]. Work of breathing is also increased due to elastic loading and the predilection for hypoventilation and ventilatory failure is therefore clear.

c. Collagen Vascular Disease. Polymyositis significantly reduces respiratory muscle strength below 50 % of predicted. Gibson et al. [16] noted that also in systemis lupus erythematosus the diaphragm failed to perform normally as measured by P_{di} and maximal inspiratory and expiratory pressures (MIP & MEP). As with to other collagen diseases, sclerodermia is well known to cause myositis and involves the diaphragm and intercostal muscles [17].

d. Neuromuscular Diseases. Respiratory muscle weakness is well documented in pathologies such as poliomelitis, kyfoscoliosis, Duchenne dystrophy, myastenia gravis and others. Chronic respiratory weakness is characterized by a reduction in pressure-gencrating capacity affecting the ability to inflate the lungs and to produce effective cough. Loss of strength is probably the major factor increasing the tidal/maximal pleural pressure ratio but also reductions in lung and chest wall compliance, distortion of the chest wall (*i.e.* scoliosis) and muscle stiffening often increase the tidal demands on the respiratory muscles. Of these diseases the most devastating presentations of acute ventilatory failure are represented by acute inflammatory polyneuritis [18] (Guillain-Barre'-Landry syndrome) and botulism [19] (through reduction of neuromuscular transmission by impaired acetylcholine release).

e. Endocrinopathy. Hypothyroidism may impair ventilatory pump function as reflected in a reduced vital capacity and maximal inspiratory pressure [20]. The skeletal myopathies seen for example in Cushing's syndrome and acromegaly could also affect the strength of respiratory muscles on a chronic basis [21].

f. Healthy Individuals. Healthy people never approach the diaphragm fatigue threshold, except for two conditions: a) during "extreme" physical exercise, such as marathon running [22] but not during shorter competitions [23] and b) during the expulsive period of labour [24].

g. Drugs. Several drugs (xanthines, beta2-agonists) have been shown to potentiate the inotropic properties of the respiratory muscles, however their effects are still controversial [25-28]. Fluorinated and non-fluorinated corticosteroids at high doses, among the most commonly used pharmaceutical preparations, may produce significant impairment of the contractile and histochemical properties of the respiratory muscles leading to severe weakness [29, 30].

h. Chronic Obstructive Pulmonary Disease (COPD). This disease is characterized by increased resistance to airflow, air trapping and hyperinflation of the lungs [31, 32]. The increased resistance to airflow increases the work of breathing and energy requirements. Hyperinflation puts the respiratory muscles at mechanical disadvantage, as lung volume increases the muscles are passively shortened by their own elasticity rather than by active contraction. Thus, COPD not only makes it harder to breathe but aslo impairs the capacity of the respiratory muscles to handle the added loads. The occurence of respiratory muscle fatigue have been shown to occur acutely in these patients [2]. Nonetheless, it is surprising that almost all studies have been performed in a laboratory setting, the subjects being asked to modify their natural breathing pattern or to breathe against high inspiratory resistance. Only indirect evidence of acute respiratory muscle fatigue has therefore been described in "natural" conditions such as disconnection from mechanical ventilation [33] and asthmatic attack [34]. Evidence of "chronic" respiratory muscle fatigue has never been demonstrated and its existance is still controversial. Indeed Similowski et al. [35] showed that diaphragm function in stable eucapnic COPD is not as seriously compromised as was originally thought, since at very high lung volumes the diaphragm of these patients can generate substantially more pressure than the normal diaphragm a higher fraction of which is available to inflate the lungs.

References

1. Bellemare F, Grassino A (1982) Effect of pressure and timing of contraction on human diaphragm fatigue. J Appl Physiol 53:1190-1195
2. Bellemare F, Grassino A (1983) Force reserve of the diaphragm in patients with chronic obstructive pulmonary disease. J Appl Physiol 55:8-15
3. Black LF, Hyatt RE (1971) Maximal static respiratory pressures in generalized neuromuscular disease. Am Rev Respir Dis 103:641-650
4. NHLBI workshop summary (1990) Respiratory muscle fatigue. Am Rev Respir Dis 142:474-480
5. Monod H, Scherrer J (1965) The work capacity of a synergic muscular group. Ergonomics 8:329-337
6. Tzelepis G, McCool FD, Leith DE, Hoppin FG (1988) Increased lung volume limits endurance of inspiratory muscles. J Appl Physiol 64:1796-1802
7. Zocchi L, Fitting JW, Majani U, Fracchia C, Rampulla C, Grassino A (1993) Effect of pressure and timing of contraction on human rib cage muscle fatigue. Am Rev Respir Dis 147:857- 864
8. Asmussen E (1979) Muscle fatigue. Med Sci Sports 11:313-321
9. Aubier M, Trippenbach T, Roussos C (1981) Respiratory muscle fatigue during cardiogenic shock. J Appl Physiol 51:499-508
10. Nava S, Bellemare F (1989) Cardiocirculatory failure and apnea in shock. J Appl Physiol 66:184
11. Field S, Kelly SM, Macklem PT (1982) The oxygen cost of breathing in patients with cardiorespiratory disease. Am Rev Respir Dis 126:9-13
12. Braun NMT, Keim NL, Dixon RM, et al (1984) The prevalence and determinants of nutritional changes in chronic obstructive pulmonary disease. Chest 86:558-563

13. Newman JH, Neff TA, Ziporin P (1977) Acute respiratory failure associated with hypophosphatemia. N Engl J Med 296:1101-1102
14. Dhingta S, Solven F, Wilson A, et al (1984) Hypomagnesemia and respiratory muscle power. Am Rev Respir Dis 129:497-498
15. Arora NS, Rochester DF (1979) Respiratory muscle function in obesity and obesity hypoventilation syndrome. Clin Res 27:394 (abstract)
16. Gipson GJ, Edmonds JP, Huges GRV (1977) Diaphragm function and lung involvement in systematic lupus erythematosus. Am J Med 63:926-932
17. Clements PJ, Furst DE, Campion DS (1978) Muscle disease in progressive systemic sclerosis. Arthritis Rheum 21:62-71
18. Hewer RL, Hilton PJ, Crampton Smith A et al (1968) Acute polyneuritis requiring artificial ventilation. Q J Med 147:479-491
19. Schmidt-Nowara W, Sumet JW, Rosano PA (1983) Early and late pulmonary complications of botulism. Arch Intern Med 143:451-456
20. Massumi RA, Winnacker JL (1964) Severe depression of respiratory centre in myxedema. Am J Med 36:876-882
21. Braun NMT, Arora NS, Rochester DF (1983) Respiratory muscle and pulmonary function in polymyositis and other proximal myopathies. Thorax 38:616-623
22. Loke J, Mahler DA, Virgulto JA (1982) Respiratory muscle fatigue after marathon running. J Appl Physiol 52:821-824
23. Nava S, Zanotti E, Rampulla C, Rossi A (1992) Respiratory muscle fatigue does not limit exercise performance during short endurance run. J Sport Med Phys Fitness 32:39-44
24. Nava S, Zanotti E, Ambrosino N, Fracchia C, Scarabelli C, Rampulla C (1992) Evidence of acute diaphragmatic fatigue in a "natural" condition. The diaphragm during labor. Am Rev Respir Dis 146:1226-1230
25. Murciano D, Aubier M, Viires N, Mal H, Pariente R (1987) Effects of theophylline and enprofylline on diaphragmatic contractility. J Appl Physiol 63:51-57
26. Levy RD, Nava S, Gibbons L, Bellemare F (1990) Aminophylline and human diaphragm strength in vivo. J Appl Physiol 68:2591-2596
27. Javaheri S, Smith JT, Thomas JP, Guilfoile TD, Donovan EF (1988) Albuterol has no effect on diaphragmatic fatigue in humans. Am Rev Respir Dis 137:197-201
28. Nava S, Crotti P, Gurrieri G, Fracchia C, Rampulla C (1992) Effect of a B_2 agonist (broxaterol) on respiratory muscle strength and endurance in patients with COPD with irreversible airway obstruction. Chest 101:133-140
29. Nava S, Gayan-Ramirez G, Bisschop A, Dom R, de Bock V, Decramer M (1994) Acute-steroid induced myopathy in rats. Am J Respir Crit Care Med 149(4):A273
30. Williams TJ, O'Hehir RE, Czarny D, Horne M, Bowes G (1988) Acute myopathy in severe acute asthma treated with intravenously administered corticosteroids. Am Rev Respir Dis 137:460-463
31. Agostoni E, Rahn H (1960) Abdominal and thoracic pressures at different lung volumes. J Appl Physiol 15:1087-1092
32. Hubmayr RD, Litchy WJ, Gay PC, Nelson SB (1989) Transdiaphragmatic twitch pressure: effects of lung volume and chest wall shape. Am Rev Respir Dis 139:647-652
33. Cohen CA, Zagelbaum G, Gross D et al (1982) Clinical manifestations of inspiratory muscle fatigue. Am J Med 73:308-316
34. Nava S, Bruschi C (1993) Respiratory muscles and asthma. Eur Respir Rev 3(14):448-451
35. Similowski T, Sheng Yan, Gauthier AP, Macklem PT, Bellemare F (1991) Contractile properties of the human diaphragm during chronic hyperinflation. N Engl J Med 325:917-923

Chapter 4

Static and dynamic behaviour of the respiratory system

E. D'ANGELO

Introduction

In this chapter only the most fundamental aspects of respiratory mechanics in normal humans are considered; detailed accounts can be found elsewhere in the literature [1-6]. The first section deals with the pressures exerted by the passive respiratory system and the respiratory muscles under static conditions and the second the pressures which develop with the breathing movements (dynamics).

Statics

Volume-pressure relations of the relaxed respiratory system

Total respiratory system

The static behaviour of the respiratory system, like that of its component parts, is studied by determining and analyzing the volume-pressure relation. During relaxation of the respiratory muscles the net pressure developed at any given lung volume by the respiratory system under static conditions ($P_{st,rs}$) results from the forces exerted by its elastic elements and equals the difference between alveolar pressure (P_A) with airway openings closed, or mouth pressure with the glottis open, and body surface pressure (P_{bs}). Conversely, (P_A-P_{bs}) indicates the pressure that the respiratory muscles must exert to maintain that lung volume with open airways, *i.e.* to exactly balance the elastic forces of the respiratory system. This applies, however, only if the shape of the respiratory system is the same whether the respiratory muscles are active or not. For a given volume, the elastic energy, and hence the elastic pressure, is minimum for the configuration occurring during relaxation, and is increased whenever that configuration is changed. The extra pressure required to distort the respiratory system and its relation to the kind and entity of distortion is largely unknown. It appears, however, that during rest or moderately increased ventilation departures from the relaxed configuration are usually modest [4].

The volume-pressure curve of the relaxed respiratory system is sigmoidal. In the middle volume range the relation is almost linear with a slope, the compliance of the respiratory system (C_{rs}), which is 2 % of the vital capacity (VC) per 1 cm

H_2O, or 0.1 L/cm H_2O. Approaching the volume extremes, *i.e.* above 85 % and below 15 % VC, C_{rs} rapidly falls off. The volume at $P_A = P_{bs}$ is the resting volume of the respiratory system: during quiet breathing it usually corresponds to the lung volume at the end of a spontaneous expiration, which is the definition of the functional residual capacity (FRC). The measurement of lung volume and mouth pressure does not pose any major technical problem; but voluntary relaxation is difficult to obtain. Also the assumption by Heaf and Prime [7] that the muscles are relaxed at the end of expiration during spontaneous breathing at atmospheric and moderately increased airway pressure, may not be valid. Indeed, recent evidence suggests that tonic respiratory muscle activity is always present in awake subjects [5]. Certainly the volume-pressure relation obtained in the paralyzed subject reflects only the elastic forces that develop in the respiratory system. Its comparison with that in the awake subject requires, however, some caution because the effects on the volume-pressure characteristics of the respiratory system produced by muscular paralysis in combination with general anesthesia cannot be explained only by loss of tonic activity of the respiratory muscles [8].

Lung and chest wall

A mechanical analogue of the chest wall (W) and lung (L) under static conditions is provided by two parallel springs: thus the volume changes of the chest wall (ΔV_w) and the lung (ΔV_L) should be the same (except for shifts of blood) and equal to that of the respiratory system ($\Delta V_{rs} = \Delta V_w = \Delta V_L$), whereas the algebraic sum of the pressure exerted by each part equals the pressure of the respiratory system ($P_{st,rs} = P_{st,w}+P_{st,L}$). It follows that the reciprocal of the compliance of the respiratory system equals the sum of the reciprocals of the lung and chest wall,

$$1/C_{rs} = 1/C_L+1/C_w$$

and since the elastance (E) is the reciprocal of C.

$$E_{rs} = E_L+E_w$$

Because $P_{st,rs}$ is the difference between alveolar and body surface pressure, when the latter is atmospheric $P_A = P_{st,w}+P_{st,l}$. Because $P_{st,w}$ indicates pressures exerted by the relaxed chest wall, when the respiratory muscles contract at fixed lung volumes.

$$P_A = P_{st,w}+P_{st,L}+P_{mus}$$

The pressure exerted by the lung is the difference between alveolar and pleural surface pressure, $P_{st,L} = P_A\text{-}P_{pl}$; that exerted by the chest wall is the difference between pleural surface and body surface pressure, $P_{st,w} = P_{pl}\text{-}P_{bs}$. Thus, during relaxation $P_{pl} = P_{st,w}$; when the muscles contract at constant lung volume $P_{pl} = P_{st,w}+P_{mus}$ and $P_{pl} = P_A\text{-}P_{st,L}$; when the subject actively holds a given lung volume with airway and glottis open $P_{pl} = -P_{st,L}$.

The volume-pressure relations of the lung and chest wall are curvilinear: the former increases its curvature with increasing lung volume, the opposite being true for the latter. The fall in C_{rs} at high lung volumes is therefore due to the decrease of C_L, that at low lung volume to the decrease of C_w. In the tidal volume range the volume-pressure relations of both the lung and chest wall are nearly linear and C_L and C_w are about the same, amounting to 4 % VC per 1 cm H_2O, or 0.2 l/cm H_2O. In normal young subjects the resting volume of the lung, *i.e.* that occurring when $P_{st,L} = P_{bs}$, is close to residual volume (RV) and the lung recoils inward over nearly all the VC. Hence, the resting volume of the respiratory system is reached when the inward recoil of the lung is balanced by the outward recoil of the chest wall; $P_{st,w}+P_{st,L} = 0$. This volume depends on posture, being 40, 22 and 13 % VC in erect, supine, and head-down subjects respectively [1]. Indeed, while the volume-pressure relation of the lung is largely independent of posture, gravity markedly affects the volume-pressure relation of the chest wall, mainly through its effects on the abdomen [3]. Thus the resting volume of the chest wall, *i.e.* that occurring when $P_{pl} = P_{bs}$, amounts to 55 and 30 % VC in the erect and supine posture respectively [1]. Above this volume the chest wall recoils inwards, below it recoils outwards.

Assessment of the volume-pressure relationships of the lung and chest wall involves the measurement of P_{pl}. In humans P_{pl} is usually estimated from esophageal pressure (P_{es}) measurements. The interpretation of this measure requires, however, some caution, because of both technical and theoretical problems [9, 10]. Although in the volume-pressure diagrams P_{pl} is expressed for analytical purposes as a single value represented by P_{es}, under physiological conditions pleural surface pressure varies at different sites due to the effects of gravity on the lung and chest wall, the different natural shapes of these two structures and the changes in shape caused by the action of the respiratory muscles; more importantly, changes in P_{pl} with changing volume can be non uniform in various instances [11].

Static volume-pressure relationships are usually represented by single lines, as if there were a unique relationship between static pressures and lung volumes. These pressures differ, however, depending on the volume and time history of the respiratory system. Static pressure tend to be lower if a given lung volume is reached on deflation, higher if on inflation. Thus static curves obtained by changing lung volume in steps from RV to total lung capacity (TLC) and then back to RV are loops rather then single lines. These loops are called hysteresis loops and reflect the failure of a structure to react identically upon application and withdrawal of a forcing agent. They also represent energy lost from the system. Hysteresis occurs both in the lung and chest wall: in the former it is attributed to surface properties and alveolar recruitment-derecruitment [12], in the latter it seems related to muscles and ligaments [13, 14]. Hysteresis in the respiratory system is commonly ascribed to both viscoelasticity, *i.e.* a rate-dependent phenomenon, and on plasticity, *i.e.* a rate-independent phenomenon. This relates partly to the definition chosen to qualify static conditions, and partly to the technical difficulties encountered in order to satisfy that definition, particularly in *in vivo* studies. Indeed only plasticity should be held responsible for true static hysteresis, which, in a mechanical analogue, would occur only in the presence of dry friction. Moreover, only the energy spent to overcome static and dynamic friction is totally lost, whereas part of that spent to stretch a viscoelastic element can be recovered (see below). There is no information concerning pressure dissipation due to tissue plasticity in humans; however, it has been suggested that this work component should be very small in the tidal volume range [15].

Volume-pressure relation of the respiratory system during static muscular efforts

Alveolar pressure, relative to that occurring during relaxation at that lung volume, decreases and increases, during inspiratory and expiratory maximum static efforts respectively. These changes in PA are taken to represent the net pressure exerted by the inspiratory and expiratory muscles. They do not necessarily represent the maximum that the respiratory muscles can exert because antagonistic muscles may be active, especially during the efforts performed close to the volume extremes, particularly expiratory. Moreover, because of the concomitant distortion of the chest wall, only part of the muscular force developed during the efforts results in PA changes.

The expiratory pressures are larger the larger the lung volume at which the effort is performed, whereas the opposite is true for the inspiratory pressures. Thus in normal adults, the inspiratory muscle pressure decreases from about 120 cm H_2O near RV to about 50 cm H_2O at TLC; corresponding values of expiratory muscle pressure are about 50 and 200 cm H_2O [1, 5]. This behaviour reflects primarily the force-length relation of the muscles, though the mechanical characteristics of the passive structures, the action of antagonist muscles and the reflex inhibition caused by the effort itself are also involved. Indeed the length of the inspiratory muscles decreases with the lung volume and the opposite occurs for the expiratory muscles. Finally, the pressures exerted by the respiratory muscles depend on age and sex. The decrease of maximum pressures with age, the lower maximum pressures in women and the variability of these pressures among subjects parallel observations for maximum strength of other skeletal muscles. They also depend on the subject's activity; with appropriate training programs maximum pressures can increase up to 55 % [16].

Dynamics

Driving and opposing pressures

The potential range of driving pressures available to produce the breathing movements is given by the relationships between lung volume and changes in PA from relaxation values during maximal voluntary static inspiratory and expiratory efforts, respectively (see above). In theory, the maximal mechanical work potentially available for a breathing cycle is given by the area subtended by those curves which amount to 20-30 calories for male adults. However, this potential work is never achieved during the actual breathing movements, mainly because of the intrinsic muscle property expressed by the force-velocity relationship [17]. Other mechanisms also contribute to limit the maximal external work per breath, such as the speed of activation of the respiratory muscles and gas compressibility [18], as well as distortion of the chest wall which becomes probably substantial at high levels of ventilation [19].

The opposing pressures arise from several factors which include: (*a*) elastic forces within the lung and chest wall; (*b*) viscous forces due to flow of gas along the airways and lung and chest wall tissues; (*c*) viscoelastic forces due to stress adaptation units within the tissues of the lung and chest wall; (*d*) plastoelastic forces, as reflected by differences in static elastic recoil pressure of the lung and chest wall at inflation and deflation; (*e*) inertial forces; (*f*) compressibility of thoracic gas; and (*g*) distortion of the respiratory system from the configuration during muscular relaxation. Among these factors items (*a*)-(*c*) provide the relevant pressures that oppose the driving force under most physiological conditions. Item (*a*) has been dealt with above here.

Viscous forces

Rohrer [20] provided indirect estimates of the airway resistance (R_{aw}) by applying the laws of fluid dynamics to post-mortem measurements of the dimension of the airways. He described the following relationships which are known as Rohrer's equations:

$$P_{res} = K_1\dot{V} + K_2\dot{V}^2 \quad \text{and} \quad R_{aw} = K_1 + K_2\dot{V}$$

where P_{res} represents the pressure dissipation within the airways due to gas flow ($\dot{V}$) and K_1 and K_2 are constants. Though the physical meaning assigned by Rohrer to these constants are no longer accepted, these equations are still used because they provide a close empirical description of experimental results. Values for K_1 and K_2 vary considerably among different reports depending on the experimental procedure and conditions: indicative values in normal seated subjects are 1.2 cm $H_2O \cdot l^{-1} \cdot s$ and 0.3 cm $H_2O \cdot l^{-2} \cdot s^2$ during mouth breathing, and 1.8 cm $H_2O \cdot l^{-1} \cdot s$ and 3 cm $H_2O \cdot l^{-2} \cdot s^2$ when breathing through the nose [2].

Direct measurements of R_{aw} are obtained by means of the interrupter method [21] and the body plethysmographic method [22]. Using the latter technique Briscoe and Dubois [23] found that in seated subject breathing through the mouth, airway conductance (G_{aw}), *i.e.* the reciprocal of R_{aw}, is approximately proportional to lung volume; $G_{aw} = -0.23+0.28V$ (V in liters). The dependency of R_{aw} on volume reflects changes in dimensions of the conducting airways caused by the volume dependent changes in lung recoil. The technique, however, has the disadvantage that almost all body plethysmographs are designed to be used only at rest in the seated position. Moreover, some degree of cooperation from the subject is necessary. These limitations have recently lead to a revival of the interrupter technique which can be readily applied in different body postures both at rest and during increased ventilation, as well as in mechanically ventilated subjects.

With the interrupter method the resistance is obtained as the ratio of the immediate change in mouth pressure (P_{ao}) following a brief airway occlusion performed during the breathing cycle and the airflow immediately preceding the occlusion. The rapid change in P_{ao} following occlusion is the resistive pressure existing prior to airflow interruption. If this pressure change is thought to represent the pressure difference between the mouth and the alveoli prior to airflow interruption, then the interrupter resistance (R_{int}) would correspond to airway resistance ($R_{int} = R_{aw} = P_{res}/\dot{V}$). On the other hand, Mead and Whittenberger [24] suggested, on theoretical grounds, that total interrupter resistance ($R_{int,rs}$) should include a chest wall component ($R_{int,w}$) as well as a lung component ($R_{int,L}$) reflecting mainly R_{aw}. Partitioning of $R_{int,rs}$ into its two components has been recently performed in mechanically ventilated normal anesthetized paralyzed subjects: at flows between 0.24 and 1.12 L s^{-1} average values for $R_{int,L}$ and $R_{int,w}$ were 1.2 and 0.4 cmH_2O s L^{-1}, respectively, the latter being independent of volume and flow [25]. The value of $R_{int,L}$ does not include the resistance of the upper airways because the measurements of $R_{int,rs}$ were based on tracheal pressure; hence, $R_{int,L}$ of intact normal subjects should contribute substantially more than 30 % of $R_{int,rs}$ ($R_{int,rs} = R_{int,L}+R_{int,w}$). This is supported by the results of Liistro et al. [26] who in normal subjects found that the values $R_{int,rs}$ were close to those of R_{aw} measured with the body plethysmographic technique. Finally, $R_{int,L}$ could include a component due to lung tissues, whereby $R_{int,L}>R_{aw}$, although animal studies have shown that viscous resistance of pulmonary tissues does not contribute appreciably to $R_{int,L}$ [27].

Values of chest wall "resistance" reported in the literature for normal subjects (~1 cmH_2O s l^{-1}) [2] are higher than those of $R_{int,w}$ reported above because they include substantial contributions from viscoelastic forces [28]. Such contributions do not represent "true" flow-resistance, though they are included in the "lumped" measurements of total chest wall (R_w) and pulmonary (R_L) resistance (see below). The mechanical analogue of $R_{int,w}$ or $R_{int,L}$ can be therefore represented by a dashpot placed in parallel to the spring which simulates the pure elastic properties (E_{st}) of the corresponding structure.

Viscoelastic forces

The viscoelastic behaviour of lung tissue has often been recognized [29], but only recently has a substantial role in respiratory dynamics been attributed to the viscoelastic properties of the respiratory system. Pressures applied to the viscoelastic elements (P_{visc}) cannot be directly measured, but can be obtained from the slow decay of pressure occurring when flow is suddenly stopped and volume kept fixed until a constant pressure, taken to represent static presssure, is reached. This phenomenon, which is commonly referred to as stress relaxation, is the basis of the rapid airway occlusion method that has been used to assess the viscoelastic pressures of the respiratory system, lung and chest wall in normal anesthetized paralyzed subjects, as well as the viscous (P_{res}) and static recoil pressures (P_{st}) [15, 28, 30, 31].

The simplest mechanical analogue of a viscolelastic element is represented by a Maxwell body, *i.e.* a spring (E_{visc}) and a dashpot (R_{visc}) arranged serially. In spite of the complexity and the large number of elements included in the lung and chest wall, a single Maxwell body can adequately reproduce the patterns of stress relaxation of the lung and chest wall observed in normal anesthetized paralyzed subjects, thus allowing the assessment of the viscoelastic parameters E_{visc} and R_{visc}. For volumes up to 1 litre above FRC and flows in the range 0.24-1.2 l/s, average values (±SD) of these parameters obtained in 18 normal anesthetized paralyzed subjects were 3.2±1.1 cm H_2O l^{-1} and 3.4±1 cm H_2O s l^{-1} for the lung, and 1.7±0.4 cm H_2O l^{-1} and 2.1±0.6 cm H_2O s l^{-1} for the chest wall [28]. Hence the viscoelastic time constants ($\tau_{visc} = R_{visc}/E_{visc}$) of lung (1.1±0.4 s) and chest wall tissues (1.3±0.3 s) are essentially the same and considerably longer than the standard time constant of the respiratory system ($\tau_{rs} = R_{int,rs}/E_{st,rs}$), which, in the tidal volume range, amounts to 0.15-0.3 s. Once the values of viscoelastic parameters are known and the system is assumed to be linear, Pve is computed by solving the differential equation:

$$dP_{visc}/dt = -P_{visc}/\tau_{visc}+R_{visc}\ dV/dt.$$

The solution of this equation can be written as the product of two factors: the first has the dimension of pressure ($R_{visc}V_T/T$; where V_T is tidal volume and T is duration of the breathing phase), the second is dimensionless, depends on the ratio τ_{visc}/T, and varies with the pattern of flow.

Viscoelastic forces have important effects on expiration. Since the elastic energy stored in the viscoelastic elements of the lung and chest wall is greater with rapid than with slow inspirations, lung deflation should be faster following rapid inflation. Thus, during increased ventilation some of the requirements for increased expiratory flow rates are intrinsically met by the viscoelastic forces. Augmentation of the expiratory driving pressure through viscoelastic mechanisms can explain the observation that in paralyzed subjects lung deflation is slower if the expiration is preceded by an end-inspiratory hold [30]. In fact, during the end-inspiratory hold the effective elastic recoil pressures of the lung and chest wall should decrease progressively due to stress relaxation. Moreover, the viscoelastic forces, by increasing the effective lung recoil, should decrease airway resistance, in addition to increasing the expiratory driving pressure. Indeed in normal humans the maximal flows during forced vital capacity manoeuvers are greater when the manoeuver is performed following a rapid inspiration to TLC with a concomitant increase in effective PL and without an end-inspiratory pause to avoid pressure dissipation into $R_{visc,L}$, than after a slow inspiration or a rapid inspiration followed by an end-inspiratory pause, this occurring also in the volume range where maximal flows are effort independent [32]. Finally, because of viscoelastic behaviour, the decrease of lung volume during passive expiration follows a double-exponential function [33], instead of the mono-exponential function that describes the deflation of a simple RC model characterized by a single time constant. This model provides the rationale of various methods of measurement of respiratory mechanics [34, 35]; the results obtained with these methods are therefore open to criticism. On the other hand, the constants in the double-exponential function are related to the mechanical parameters E_{st}, R_{int}, E_{visc} and R_{visc} in a complex manner; as a consequence respiratory mechanics cannot be easily assessed during passive expiration.

Time dependency of elastance and resistance

Otis et al. [36] proposed a single-compartment model of the respiratory system which consisted of a constant elastance (E) served by a pathway of constant flow resistance (R). It is based on the assumption that the mechanical properties of the respiratory system, as well as its component parts, are independent of lung volume and flow and that inertial factors are negligible. They recognized that time-constant inequality within the lung could confer time-dependency of pulmonary elastance and resistance, but in normal subjects the impact of time-constant inequality appears to be negligible. Accordingly, the single-compartment model is represented by a single first-order differential equation:

$$P(t) = EV(t) + R\dot{V}(t)$$

where $P(t)$ is the forcing pressure that produces volume displacement V(t) from the relaxation volume and $\dot{V}(t)$ is instantaneous flow. A similar equation forms the basis of the "elastic subtraction method" [37] for determining effective resistance (R) and dynamic elastance (Edyn), and, in a variety of ways, it has been and still is commonly used [38]. However, measurements obtained with these methods include substantial viscoelastic contributions, depending on respiratory frequency (f) and duration of inspiration [28, 30]; they provide "lumped" values of resistance ($R = R_{int}+\Delta R$) and elastance ($E_{dyn} = E_{st}+\Delta E$) which are highly time-dependent. During sinusoidal breathing, the contribution of viscoelastic properties to dynamic elastance and effective resistance should change with f according to the following functions [28]:

$$\Delta E = \omega^2 \tau_{visc}^2 E_{visc}/(1 + \omega^2 \tau_{visc}^2) \quad \text{and}$$
$$\Delta R = R_{visc}/(1 + \omega^2 \tau_{visc}^2)$$

where ω is angular frequency ($2\pi f$). Hence, both $E_{dyn,L}$ and $E_{dyn,w}$ should increase with increasing f, tending to $E_{st}+E_{visc}$, whereas R_L and R_w should decrease, approaching the corresponding value of R_{int}. Using the values of the viscoelastic parameters (see above) obtained in normal anesthetized paralyzed subjects [28], it appears that $E_{dyn,L}$ and $E_{dyn,w}$ approach plateau values at frequency of about 0.5 Hz. At these frequencies, on average, $E_{dyn,L}$ is about 38 % higher than $E_{st,L}$ while the corresponding increase for the chest wall is about 26 %. On the other hand, both ΔR_L and ΔR_w become negligible at $f > 0.5$ Hz.

Time-dependency of pulmonary and chest wall elastance and resistance has been also described using forced oscillation techniques by several investigators in awake, relaxed normal humans [39-41], as well as in spontaneously breathing subjects (*cfr.*42). As noted above, R_L and R_w at high frequencies should reflect $R_{int,L}$ and $R_{int,w}$, respectively. Indeed, values of R_w obtained in normal awake subjects with the forced oscillation technique at f above 2 Hz (40, *cfr.*42) are close to the values of $R_{int,w}$ obtained in normal anesthetized paralyzed subjects [25].

References

1. Agostoni E, Mead J (1964) Statics of the respiratory system. In: Fenn WO, Rahn H (eds) Handbook of Physiology, Section 3, Respiration. vol. I, chapt.13. American Physiological Society, Washington D.C., pp 387-409
2. Mead J, Agostoni E (1964) Dynamics of breathing. In: Fenn WO, Rahn H (eds) Handbook of Physiology, Section 3, Respiration. vol. I, chapt.14. American Physiological Society, Washington D.C., pp 411-427
3. Agostoni E, D'Angelo E (1985) Statics of the chest wall. In: Roussos C, Macklem PT (eds) The Thorax, M Dekker, New York, pp 259-295
4. Mead J, Smith JC, Loring SH (1985)Volume displacements of the chest wall and their mechanical significance. In: Roussos C, Macklem PT (eds) The Thorax, M Dekker, New York, pp 369-392
5. Agostoni E, Hyatt R (1986) Static behavior of the respiratory system. In: Macklem PT, Mead J (eds) Handbook of Physiology. The Respiratory System, Mechanics of Breathing, Section 3, vol. III, chapt. 9. American Physiological Society, Bethesda, pp 113-130
6. Rodarte JR, Rehder K (1986) Dynamics of Respiration. In: Macklem PT, Mead J (eds) Handbook of Physiology. The Respiratory System, Mechanics of breathing. Section 3, vol.III. American Physiological Society, Washington D.C., pp131-144
7. Heaf PJD, Prime FJ (1956) The compliance of the thorax in normal human subjects. Clin Sci 15:319-327.
8. Rehder K, Marsh HM (1986) Respiratory mechanics during anesthesia and mechanical ventilation. In: Macklem PT, Mead J (eds) Handbook of Physiology. The Respiratory System, Mechanics of Breathing. Section 3, vol. III, chapt. 43. American Physiological Society, Bethesda, pp 737-752
9. Milic-Emili J (1984) Measurements of pressures in respiratory physiology. In: Otis AB (ed) Techniques in Life Sciences, vol. P4/II, Elsevier, Amsterdam, pp 412:1-22
10. D'Angelo E (1984) Techniques for studying the mechanics of the pleural space. In: AB Otis (ed) Techniques in Life Sciences, vol. P4/II Elsevier, Amsterdam, pp 415:1-32
11. Agostoni E (1986) Mechanics of the pleural space. In: Macklem PT, Mead J (eds) Handbook of Physiology. The Respiratory System, Mechanics of Breathing. Section 3, vol. III, chapt. 30, American Physiological Society, Bethesda, pp 531-560
12. Gil J, Weibel ER (1972) Morphological study of pressure-volume hysteresis in rat lungs fixed by vascular perfusion. Respir Physiol 15:190-213
13. Buchthal F, Rosenfalck P (1957) Elastic properties of striated muscles. In: Remington JW (ed) Tissue Elasticity. American Physiological Society, Washington DC, pp 73-93
14. Rodarte JR, Burgher W, Hyatt RE, Rehder K (1977) Lung recoil and gas trapping during oxygen breathing at low lung volumes. J Appl Physiol 43:138-143
15. Jonson B, Beydon L, Brauer K, Manson C, Valid S, Grytzell H (1993) Mechanics of respiratory system in healthy anesthetized humans with emphasis on viscolestaic properties. J Appl Physiol 75:132-140

16. Leith DE, Bradley M (1976) Ventilatory muscle strength and endurance training. J Appl Physiol 41:508-516
17. Agostoni E, Fenn WO (1960) Velocity of muscle shortening as a limiting factor in respiratory air flow. J Appl Physiol 15:349-353
18. Jaeger MJ, Otis AB (1964) Effects of compressibility of alveolar gas on dynamics and work of breathing. J Appl Physiol 19:83-91
19. Goldman MD, Grimby G, Mead J (1976) Mechanical work of breathing derived from rib cage and abdominal V-P partitioning. J Appl Physiol 41:752-763
20. Rohrer F (1915) Der Stromungswiderstand in den menschlichen Atemwegen und der Einfluß der unregelmässigen Verzweigung des Bronchialsystems auf den Atmungsverlaud verschiedenen Lungenbezirken. Arch Gesamte Physiol Mens Tiere 162:225-299
21. Neergaard K von, Wirz K (1927) Die Messung der Stromungswiederstände in der Atemwege des Menschen, insbesondere bein Asthma und Emphysema. Zeitschrift für Klinische Medizin 195:51-82
22. DuBois AB, Botelho SY, Comroe JH jr (1956) A new method for measuring airway resistance in man using a body plethysmograph: values in normal subjects and in patients with respiratory disease. J Clin Invest 35:322-326
23. Briscoe WA, DuBois AB (1958) The relationship between airway resistance, airway conductance and lung volume in subjects of different age and body size. J Clin Invest 37:1279-1285
24. Mead J, Whittenberger JL (1954) Evaluation of airway interruption technique as a method for measuring pulmonary air-flow resistance. J Appl Physiol 6:408-416
25. D'Angelo E, Prandi E, Tavola M, Calderini E, Milic-Emili J (1994) Chest wall interrupter resistance in anesthetized paralyzed humans. J Appl Physiol 77
26. Liistro GD, Stanescu D, Rodenstein D, Veriter C (1989) Reassessment of the interruption technique for measuring flow resistance in humans. J Appl Physiol 67:933-937
27. Bates JHT, Baconnier P, Milic-Emili J (1988) A theoretical analysis of interrupter technique for measuring respiratory mechanics. J Appl Physiol 64:2204-2214
28. D'Angelo E, Robatto FM, Calderini E, et al (1991) Pulmonary and chest wall mechanics in anesthetized paralyzed humans. J Appl Physiol 70:2602-2610
29. Hoppin FG, Stothert JC, Greaves IA, Lai YL, Hilderbrandt J (1986) Lung recoil: elastic and rheological properties. In: Macklem PT, Mead J (eds) Handbook of Physiology. The Respiratory System, Mechanics of Breathing. Section 3, vol. III, chapt. 3. American Physiological Society, Bethesda, pp 195-216
30. D'Angelo E, Calderini E, Torri G, Robatto F, Bono D, Milic-Emili J (1989) Respiratory mechanics in anesthetized-paralyzed humans: effects of flow, volume and time. J Appl Physiol 67:2556-2564
31. D'Angelo E, Calderini E, Tavola M, Bono D, Milic-Emili J (1992) Effect of PEEP on respiratory mechanics in anesthetized paralyzed humans. J Appl Physiol 73:1736-1742
32. D'Angelo E, Prandi E, Milic-Emili J. Dependence of maximal flow-volume curves on time-course of preceding inspiration. J Appl Physiol 75:1155-1159
33. Chelucci GL, Brunet F, Dall'Ava-Santucci J et al (1991) A single-compartment model cannot describe passive expiration in intubated, paralysed humans. Eur Respir J4:458-464
34. McIlroy MB, Tierney DF, Nadel JA (1963) A new method of measurement of compliance and resistance of lungs and thorax. J Appl Physiol 18:424-427
35. Zin WA, Pengelly LD, Milic-Emili J (1982) Single-breath method for measurement of respiratory system mechanics in anesthetized animals. J Appl Physiol 52:1266-1271
36. Otis AB, McKerrow CB, Bartlett RA et al (1956) Mechanical factors in distribution of pulmonary ventilation. J Appl Physiol 8:427-443

37. Mead J, Whittenberger JL (1953) Physical properties of human lungs measured during spontaneous respiration. J Appl Physiol 5:779-796
38. Peslin R, Felicio da Silva J, Chabot F, Duvivier C (1992) Respiratory mechanics studied by multiple linear regression in unsedated ventilated patients. Eur Respir J 5:871-878
39. Hantos Z, Daroczy B, Suki B, Galgoczy G, Csendes T (1986) Forced oscillatory impedance of the respiratory system at low frequencies. J Appl Physiol 60: 123-132
40. Barnas GM, Yoshiro K, Loring STL, Mead J (1987) Impedance and relative displacements of relaxed chest wall up to 4 Hz. J Appl Physiol 62:71-81
41. Barnas GM, Yoshiro K, Stamenovic D, Kikuchi Y, Loring SH, Mead J (1989) Chest wall impedance partitioned into rib-cage and diaphragm-abdominal pathways. J Appl Physiol 66:350-359
42. Grimby G, Takishima T, Graham W, Macklem P, Mead J (1968) Frequency dependence of flow resistance in patients with obstructive lung disease. J Clin Invest 47:1455-1465

Chapter 5

Lung tissue mechanics

F.M. ROBATTO

Introduction

The basic aspects of lung mechanics were first described in 1820 when Carson [1] published his work on the elasticity of the lung. He demonstrated that lungs collapse because they are elastic and that lung elastic forces are volume dependent. In 1921 Von Neergaard [2] described the other important factor in generating lung recoil, surface tension.

Lung pressure-volume relationship

It was Fenn [3] who first pointed out that the study of respiratory system mechanics can be done by the analysis of its pressure-volume (P-V) characteristics. Whereas obtaining the P-V curve of an isolated lung is easy, it may be difficult in humans for theoretical and technical reasons. The P-V curve obtained in an isolated lung inflated with air up to total lung capacity (TLC) from a completely degassed condition can be divided into 4 segments. The first, nearly flat, segment is characterised by the very high (20-25 cm H_2O) pressure necessary to pop up the atelactasic airways and alveoli. When this critical opening pressure is reached the emptying of the distended into the just opened alveoli causes lung pressure to decrease in spite of an increasing lung volume. The P-V relationship is nearly linear up to 60-70 % TLC. Thereafter the lung becomes more and more rigid because of both surface phenomena and increasing stiffness of elastic network. As proposed by Setnikar and Meschia [4] the elastin and collagen fibres embodied in lung connective tissue could act as an independent but parallel network: elastin fibres can be lengthened out more than 100 % and could be the stress-bearing elements at low to intermediate lung volumes; collagen fibres, on the other hand, are quite rigid and are stressed only at high lung volumes. Their function may be that of preventing overdistension of the lung.

The P-V characteristics of the lung cannot be described with a single parameter. However, lung elastic properties are often represented by the slope of the quasi rectilinear segment of the P-V curve, *i.e.* the lung compliance (C_L). In humans C_L is about 0.2 l/cm H_2O. As the P-V curve tends to be similar when the volume is normalized to some reference volume, such as the volume at TLC, both between or within species, C_L is often referred to as specific compliance:

$$sC_L = \frac{(dV/dP)}{V_{30}}$$

where V_{30} is the volume at 30 cm H_2O conventionally taken as TLC. In spite of the utility of C_L, it does not give any information about the alinearity of the P-V relationship. To describe the upper part of lung's P-V curves a single exponential function of the form $V=A-B^{-KP}$ has been used where A is the asymptote, B is the volume decrement below A at P=0 and K describes the shape of the relation, being smaller the stiffer the lung.

Lung hysteresis and surface forces

If an inflated lung is allowed to deflate, the deflation limb does not follow the inflation one, this phenomenon is known as lung hysteresis. The presence of an area (A) inside the curves indicates that the work done to inflate the lung is larger than that recovered during deflation: A is an index of the energy loss per cycle. Lung hysteresis can be due to both static and quasi-static phenomena. It has been shown in quasi static conditions [5] that A is a constant (k) of the rectangle that surrounds the loop: $A = k\, V_T\, dP$.

The V_t dP area represents the maximum energy dissipation per cycle possible for the system, and k is therefore the fraction of that maximum that is actually dissipated. The values of k could range from 0, corresponding to a conservative, perfectly elastic system, to 1, corresponding to a dissipative, perfectly plastic system.

A is inversely related to compliance and frequency. Indeed during sinusoidal forcing of isolated lung it can be demonstrated that $A = \int_0^{\pi/2\omega} P_{res}\, \dot{V} dt$, where $\dot{V}$ is istantaneous flow, P_{res} is the pressure drop between the alveoli and the pleura and ω is the angular frequency ($2\pi f$). Since lung tissue resistance (R_{tis}) is given by $P_{res}/\ \dot{V}$ it follows that $R_{tis} = (2/\pi^2)\ k\ /\ (C_L\ f)$, where f is the cycling frequency. Recently, Fredberg and Stamenovic [6] have advanced the hypothesis that elastic and dissipative processes within the tissues are coupled at the level of the stress bearing elements (structural damping hypothesis). They introduced a coefficient η, called hysteresivity, defined as

$$\eta = \omega\, R_{tis}\ /\ E_{dyn}$$

where E_{dyn} is dynamic elastance. It appears that h is similar between different lung tissue components, lung structures and species. According to the structural damping hypothesis, any factor affecting E_{dyn} causes R_{tis} to respond in the same direction and to a similar degree. It has been demonstrated [7] that when lungs are challenged with a bronchoconstrictor agent the larger part of the fractional change in R_{tis} is accounted for by the fractional change in E_{dyn} and only the lesser part by the fractional change in h. This has been taken as evidence [6, 7] that a coupling of elastic and dissipative processes captures some unifying attribute of underlying mechanism, whatever it would be. It should be noted that k is related to η by this simple algebrical equation:

$$\eta = [(\pi/4k)^2-1]^{-1/2}$$

If A were only a dynamic phenomenon related to stress adaptation then A would be zero when the system is in "true" static condition. There is evidence that if lungs are cycled with a relatively small tidal volume (15 ml/kg body weight) starting from a volume around 30 % TLC (*i.e.* close to functional residual capacity) static lung hysteresis is negligible [8, 9]. Static lung hysteresis would be evident only when lungs are ventilated from residual volume (RV) up to TLC [8]. Related to quasi-static hysteresis is the phenomenon of stress adaptation, *i.e.* the change in pressure observed when a lung inflation is suddenly interrupted at a given lung volume and that lung volume is held constant. Under these circumstances the pressure inside the lung starts to decrease in a quasi exponential manner, the major changes occurring in the first few seconds. Stress relaxation is present independently of gas or liquid filling although it is much larger in the former case. It is difficult to determine which structures account for hysteresis and stress adaptation. Obviously, due to the differences noted above between gas and liquid filling, the presence of a gas-liquid interface accounts for most of them. When the lung is ventilated with gas starting from low lung volumes part of the static hysteresis could be attributable to opening and closing of airways and alveoli (see below). In the liquid filled lung hysteresis can be due to energy losses in the connective tissue as well as in the interstitial fluid. "Network" phenomena represent one more possibility: fibres that are poorly organised when the lung is collapsed become more ordered when the lung inflates and then need energy to return to their original arrangement.

As previously noted, the gas-liquid interface is the major factor responsible for hysteresis and stress adaptation. The force present at such an interface, known as surface tension, contributes substantially to lung recoil, as in the liquid filled lung not only hysteresis is reduced but also the inflating pressure is smaller for each given volume. Surface tension tends to reduce alveolar diameter: if this is not allowed, it causes a pressure inside the alveolus given by Laplace law: $P = 2T/r$, where T is the tension of the alveolar wall and r is the radius of curvature of the alveolus. The presence of surface phenomena makes lung parenchyma intrinsically instable, because the smaller alveoli would tend to empty into the larger ones. In normal lungs this is prevented by the presence of a "surfactant", *i.e.* a substance that lowers surface tension. The lung surfactant is a dipalmitoyl lecytine produced by II° order pneumocytes and has the ability to lower surface tension in a volume dependent manner. Roughly, surface tension (γ) varies with volume according to the following equation [10]:

$$\gamma = Ps \; \frac{\Delta V}{\Delta A}$$

where Ps is the pressure difference between air and liquid deflation curves, ΔV is volume decrement on deflation and ΔA is the corresponding change in alveolar surface area.

The presence of surface tension in the terminal units of the lung may be responsible for volume dependent asymmetry of lung espansion and for volume dependent changes of the alveolus-alveolar duct configuration. The issue of whether lung expansion is uniform or not, has been addressed by several authors. Macroscopically, Ardila et al. [11] demonstrated that lung expansion is symmetrical well below the lobar level, the linear dimensions changing uniformly as the cube root of volume. Microscopically, however, experimental results are contradictory. For example, D'Angelo [12] demonstrated that subpleural alveoli, as well as those in deeper zones, expand symmetrically for volumes between 35 % and 100 % TLC, whereas Gil et al. [13] showed that this is the case in liquid filled but not in air filled lungs. It is presently unclear how the various forces are distributed at subacinar level; it seems, however, that surface tension may alter the configuration of the alveolus-alveolar duct system, especially at intermediate lung volumes.

Airway closure

In a degassed lung the volume recovered during the first deflation is always less than the volume present in the lung at the end of the first maximal inflation. Some gas is trapped inside the lung and cannot be removed applying a negative pressure at the airway opening. This is a consequence of airway closure [14]. As discussed earlier, surface tension tends to collapse alveoli and small non cartilagineal airways. Lung surfactant helps to prevent closure but other mechanisms are involved, the most important being the so called "mechanical interdependence". Each unit forming the lung is not free to move, but is conditioned in its movements by the tethering action of the surrounding structures that are mechanically connected to it. If an alveolus tends to collapse, it distends the structures next to it and this opposes to the collapse itself. This is a powerful stabilising effect. The smaller non cartilagineal airways may require radial traction to remain open. When transpulmonary pressure approaches zero, radial tension also approaches zero, and the airways will collapse. Of course, the presence of liquid in the airways and/or the absence of surfactant make closure more probable. Applying a negative pressure at airway opening, the gas trapped beyond the occlusion point cannot be removed. Alveolar collapse, also known as atelectasis, cannot therefore be produced by applying a negative pressure. Atelectasis is usually due to the absorption of the gas distal to the occluded airway. It is possible that alveoli have some intrinsic "resistance to collapse" [15] whose structural basis is not clear and that, like the airways, they require radial tension to remain open. There is evidence [16] that airway closure occurs normally in humans especially in the dependent regions because of the smaller radial traction due to the relatively smaller volume. To reopen closed airways as well as atelectatic alveoli it is usually sufficient to inflate the lung up to a pressure of about 30 cm H_2O. For the airways, howeve, the critical opening pressure seems to be much smaller, in the range of 5-15 cm H_2O. Airways opening pressure can be inferred by the shape of the pressure volume curves that, during inflation, may show an upward inflection or "knee".

Lung modelling

The model most commonly utilised in the study of lung mechanics is that of a single alveolus, represented by a spherical elastic balloon connected to a pipe. The pressure across the wall of this balloon is given by Laplace law and tension in the wall (T) corresponds to tissue and interfacial tensions in the lungs. Lungs are considered as built by a whole bunch of such structures, each acting independently from the others and whose mechanical characteristics add up to determine lungs mechanics.

The balloon-pipe model has its mechanical analogue in a spring, representing lung elastance, connected in parallel to a dashpot. The equation of motion of such a system is:

$$P_{tr}(t) = R\,\dot{V}(t) + E_{dyn}\,V(t)$$

where P_{tr} is tracheal pressure, R is total lung resistance, $\dot{V}$ and V are instantaneous tracheal flow and volume. If the model should exhibit viscoelastic behaviour, then R would be given by the sum of airway resistance and ΔR, and E_{dyn} by the sum of static elastance and ΔE. ΔR and ΔE represent the contribution of viscoelastic behaviour to effective resistance and dynamic elastance, respectively. Both ΔR and ΔE are frequency dependent: with increasing frequency the former decreases from R_2 to 0 whereas the latter increases from 0 to E_2. When P_{tr} is substituted by alveolar pressure (P_A) the equation of motion becomes:

$$P_A(t) = R_{tis}\,\dot{V}(t) + E_{dyn}\,V(t)$$

where tissue resistance (R_{tis}) corresponds to ΔR, if the newtonian viscous resistance of lung tissue were negligible, and E_{dyn} to $E_{st}+\Delta E$, as noted above. Mount [17] in 1955 first described a reduction of the dynamic work per breath with increasing breathing frequency. He proposed a four parameters viscoelastic model to account for the time dependence of the elastic and resistive properties. This model consists of a parallel arrangement of a spring (E_1), representing static lung elastance, a dashpot (R_1), representing R_{aw}, and a spring-dashpot element (E_2 and R_2 respectively) (Maxwell body). The Maxwell body and its corresponding time constant ($\tau_2 = R_2 / E_2$) accounts for the viscoelastic properties of the lung. If the frequency of breathing were infinite, E_{dyn} would be the sum of E_1 and E_2 because the last would not have the time to discharge into the dashpot. Conversely, should the frequency of respiration be very low, E_{dyn} would be very close to E_{st} because E_2 cannot be distended for the presence of the dashpot. It is now recognised that viscoelastic forces contribute substantially to lung dynamics. In experiments performed in anaesthetised paralysed normal humans [18] ventilated with tidal volumes in the resting range, viscoelastic parameters have been evaluated as: R_2 3.44±0.97 cm H_2O l^{-1} s, E_2 3.21±1.14 cm H_2O/l and τ_2 1.13±0.36 s. In this study plastoelastic behaviour was not taken into consideration, which seems admittable because static hysteresis is present only when large ventilatory volumes are delivered.

The pressure exerted by the viscoelastic element can be calculated by the following differential equation:

$$\tau_2 \frac{dP_2}{dt} + P_2 = R_2 \frac{dV}{dt}$$

where P_2 is the pressure across the viscoelastic element, dV/dt is istantaneous flow and R_2 is the resistance of the dashpot in the Maxwell body. The solutions of this differential equation vary with the pattern of inspiration and can be written as follows:

$$P_2 = \frac{R_2 V}{T_I} \cdot F$$

where T_I is inspiratory time. The first factor (R_2V/T_I) has the dimension of a pressure and is common to any inspiratory pattern. F is a dimensionless function that is unique for each pattern of inspiration. From the above equations it is possible to calculate the work per breath done to overcome viscoelastic forces (W_{visc}).

References

1. Carson J (1820) On the elasticity of the lungs. Philos Trans R Soc; Part 1:29-44
2. Von Neergaard K (1929) Neue Auffassungen, ber einen Grundbegriff der Atemmechanik. Die Retraktionskraft der Lunge, abhängig von der Oberflachenspannme in den Alveolen. Z Gesamte Exp Med 66:373-394
3. Fenn WO (1951) Mechanics of respiration. Am J Med 10:77-91
4. Setnikar I, Meschia G (1953) Proprietà elastiche del polmone e di modelli meccanici. Arch Fisiol 52:288-302
5. Hildebrandt J (1969) Pressure-volume data of cat lung interpreted by a plastoelastic, linear viscoelastic model. J Appl Physiol 28:365-372
6. Fredberg JJ, Stamenovic D (1989) On the imperfect elasticity of lung tissue. J Appl Physiol 67:2408-2419
7. Ludwig MS, Robatto FM, Simard S, Stamenovic D, Fredberg JJ (1992) Lung tissue resistance during contractile stimulation: structural damping decomposition. J Appl Physiol 72:1332-1337
8. Robatto FM, Romero PV, Fredberg JJ, Ludwig MS (1991) Contribution of quasi static hysteresis to the dynamic alveolar pressure-volume loop. J Appl Physiol 70:708-714
9. Setnikar I (1955) Meccanica Respiratoria. In: Macri L (ed), Aggiornamenti di Fisiologia. Firenze, vol. 3:4
10. Brown ES, Johnson RP, Clements JA (1959) Pulmonary surface tension. J Appl Physiol 14:717-720
11. Ardila R, Horie T, Hildebrandt J (1974) Macroscopic isotropy of lung expansion.

Respir Physiol 20:105-115
12. D'Angelo E (1972) Local alveolar size and transpulmonary pressure in situ and in isolated lungs. Respir Physiol 14:251-266
13. Gil J, Bachofen H, Gehr P, Weibel ER (1979) Alveolar volume-surface area relation in air- and saline-filled lungs fixed by vascular perfusion. J Appl Physiol 47:990.1001
14. Greaves IA, Hildebrandt J, Hoppin FG (1986) Micromechanics of the lung. In: Fishman AP, Geiger SR Macklem PT, Mead J, (eds) Handbook of Physiology. The Respiratory System. Mechanics of Breathing. Section 3, vol. III, pt. 1, chapt. 14. American Physiological Society, Bethesda, pp 217-231
15. Cavagna GA, Stemmler EJ, DuBois AB (1967) Alveolar resistance to atelectasis. J Appl Physiol 22:441-452
16. Burger EJ Jr, Macklem P (1968) Airway closure: demonstration by breathing 100 % O_2 at low lung volumes and by N_2 washout. J Appl Physiol 25:139-148
17. Mount LE (1955) The ventilation flow-resistance and compliance of rat lungs. J Physiol 127:157-167
18. D'Angelo E, Robatto FM, Calderini E et al. (1991) Pulmonary and chest wall mechanics in anesthetized, paralyzed humans. J Appl Physiol 70:2602-2610

Chapter 6

Elasticity, viscosity and plasticity in lung parenchyma

P.V. Romero, C. Cañete, J. Lopez Aguilar, F.J. Romero

Introduction

Mechanical modelling of lung parenchymal behaviour has tried to define some of its characteristic features by using different combinations of basic rheological elements, arranged in multiple ways. Springs, dashpots and dry frictions are usually combined to describe mechanical lung properties. Static and dynamic properties of lung parenchyma point to the behaviour of the elastic storage and the frictional dissipation of energy, respectively, under different conditions of breathing frequency, lung volume, tidal volume or special manoeuvres (flow interruption, forced oscillation, etc.). The object of modelling lung mechanical behaviour is to determine, as far as possible, the relative significance of different rheologic phenomena and to find the simplest way for a global determination of lung mechanics.

A short description of some elementary rheological concepts may be helpful to understand the meaning of more complex models found in the literature.

Elasticity

Most materials behave elastically or nearly so under small stresses: an immediate elastic strain response is obtained upon loading. The strain stays constant as long as the stress is fixed and disappears immediately upon removal of the load. The main characteristic of elastic strain is reversibility.

An elementary intuitive concept of elasticity is the physical behaviour of a spring when stretched or compressed from a relaxed length (Fig. 1a). A force, proportional to the length change, has to be applied. The proportion of force to length change depends on the intrinsic characteristics of the spring (material, number and size of spires, etc.). In a purely elastic spring the energy applied is fully restored when the force is released and the spring comes back to its resting length. Work done to stretch or compress a spring is stored as a potential energy (U). Elasticity is physically characterized by the so called Young's modulus, or relation of stress (force or pressure) to strain (change in length or volume generally related to the initial length or volume). The inverse magnitude of elasticity is known as compliance, or rate of change in length or volume by unit change in force or pressure. If several elastic elements are mechanically arranged in paral-

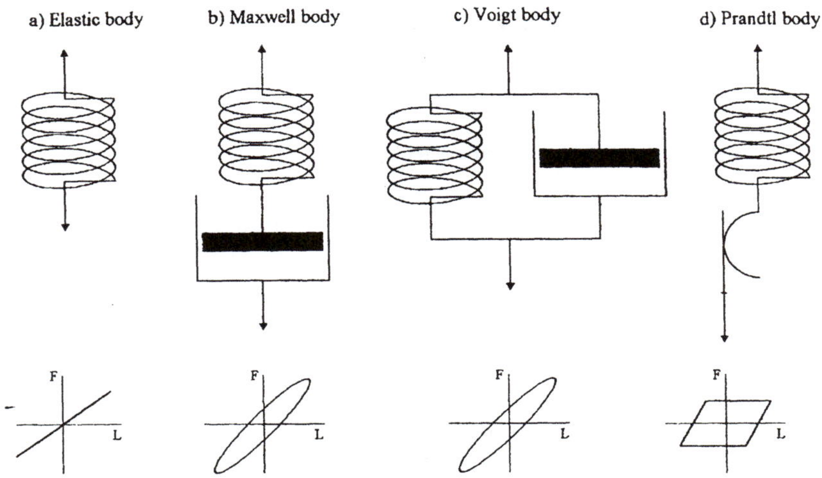

Fig. 1. Schematical representation of the basic elements usually employed in pulmonary rheology. Springs, dashpots and static frictions are used to represent elastic, viscous and plastic behaviours respectively

lel the total elasticity is the sum of the elasticity of each element. Therefore, if several elastic elements are placed in series, the inverse of total elastance or compliance is the sum of the elementary compliances.

Viscosity

When a fluid is compelled to flow a shearing force is developed that opposes the sliding of the fluid layers. Viscous behaviour means dissipation of energy in a moving fluid or viscous solid in motion. To define viscosity we can imagine two planes, an infinitesimal distance (ds) apart, in a viscous fluid that is flowing horizontally in parallel layers (Fig. 2). A given layer of fluid will exert a tangential, or shearing, force of magnitude F on the adjacent fluid layer, tending to speed it up. At the same time, this fluid layer is acted on by a retarding force of equal magnitude. The shearing force F is proportional to the area A of the layer, and therefore F/A is the shearing stress. The shearing stress is a function of the time rate of change of shearing strain dø/dt in many viscous fluids:

$$\frac{F}{A} \mu \cdot \frac{d\phi}{dt}$$

where μ is a constant of proportionality called the coefficient of viscosity. Fluids obeying this law are called Newtonian, or true, fluids. Viscous behaviour is usually expressed as a dashpot in graphical representation of rheological models. In non Newtonian fluids, like very viscous liquids, gels and soft biological tissues, the

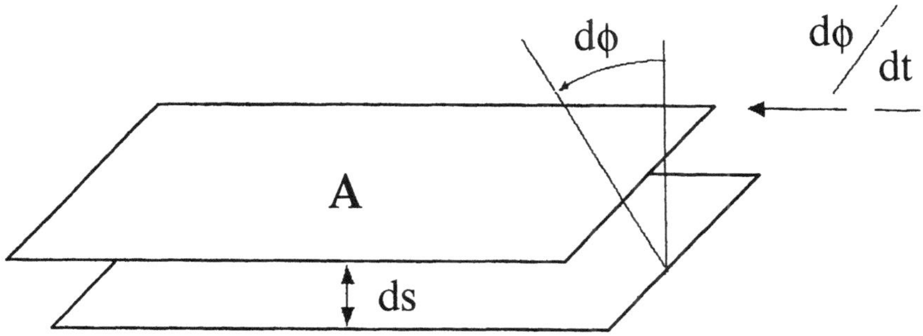

$$\frac{F}{A} = \mu \frac{d\phi}{dt}$$

Fig. 2. A two planes representation of a purely viscous fluid flowing in parallel layers. Stress is directly proportional to the rate of strain

relationship between shearing stress and strain is more complex and viscosity (μ) usually varies with shearing stress or rate of change of shearing strain.

Viscoelasticity

Some materials exhibit elastic action upon loading (if loading is fast enough), then a slow and continuous increase of strain at a decreasing rate is observed if stress is kept constant. When stress is removed a continuously decreasing strain follows a sudden inmediate elastic recovery. Such materials are significantly influenced by the rate of straining or stressing and are called viscoelastic. Time is a very important factor in the behaviour of viscoelastic materials. The time-dependent behaviour of materials under a quasistatic state may be studied by means of several types of experiments: creep, stress relaxation and frequency response to forced oscillations are common.

Relaxation processes. In a first approach viscoelastic behaviour can be introduced by means of the combination of a viscous element (dashpot) and an elastic element (spring) placed in series (Maxwell body, figure 1b) or in parallel (Voigt body, figure 1c). If a Maxwell body undergoes a sudden or step change in length, energy is stored in the spring (Fig. 3). Then energy is transferred from the elastic spring to the dashpot which moves and dissipates progressively the stored energy, without change in total length. As the spring progressively shortens tension decreases with time, this phenomenon is known as stress relaxation. The decrease of tension with time is exponential having a time constant equal to

$$\tau = \mu/\varepsilon$$

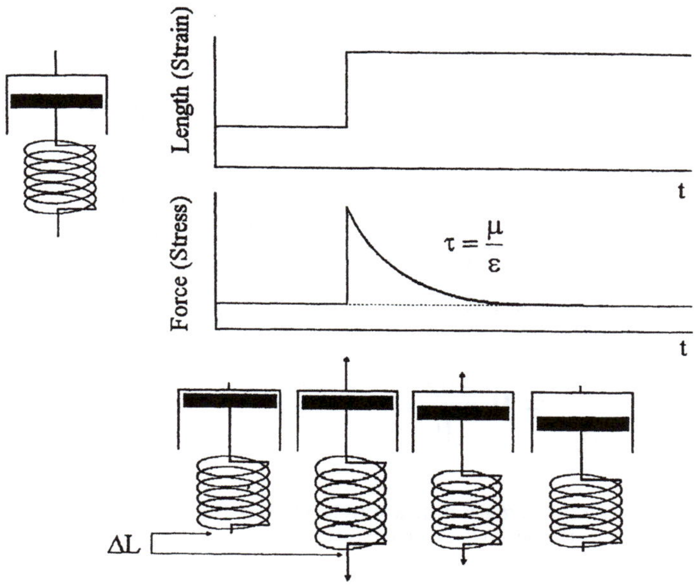

Fig. 3. Schematic drawing showing stress relaxation in terms of a Maxwell element suddenly stretched at a fixed displacement from its resting length. Interaction between elastic and viscous elements generates an exponential decrease of tension with time

where μ is the viscous coefficient of the dashpot and ε is the elastic (Young's) modulus of the spring. In terms of lung tissue behaviour μ would represent tissue viscous resistance (R_{tis}). In lung mechanics stress adaptation is the transient change of pressure seen when the lung is held at a given volume after inflation or deflation to that volume; pressure falls after inflation (stress relaxation) and rises after deflation (stress recovery) in quasi exponential fashion, the major changes occurring in the first few seconds. Creep is the equivalent phenomenon when the lung is held at a constant pressure, volume increases after inflation and decreases after deflation.

Plasticity

The quality of a material that allows it to permanently change its shape when a force is applied is known as its plasticity. In a pure plastic material a restoring force of the same magnitude should be applied anew to recover the previous shape (Fig. 1c). Energy expended in plastic deformations has striking similarities with dry friction in solid bodies. Plasticity is another form of dissipative energy in the motion of a plastic body. A static or yield force should be applied before the plastic material begins to distort, this force is equivalent to the static friction coefficient of a dry friction. For applied forces smaller than the prescribed yield force the unit will not displace; when displacements do occur, the sliding unit opposes a force independent of the rate or extent of the displacement. The mechanical analogue of this behaviour is often represented by a dry (Coulomb) sliding unit. The displacement of the sliding unit depicts plastic deformation and the force exerted on the unit represents stress. The combination of an elastic (spring) plus a Coulomb unit istitutes a plastoelastic element, the most basic being the Prandtl body (Fig. 1d). Many materials exhibit a yield point (usually characterized by a critical stress value) beyond which the mechanical behaviour is radically different from that involved below yield. Thus many materials behave viscoelastically below yield and plastoelastically after yield.

Hysteresis

An event closely related to stress adaptation and creep is seen during volume cycling of lung and is known as hysteresis. If a system composed of an elastic and a dissipative element (Fig. 1b, c) is cycled, so that it is periodically stretched and released, we observe that force during stretching is higher than during relaxation at the same length; the stress strain plot describes a loop. This loss of force is due to the dissipative process whatever its nature. Hysteresis always indicates an out-of-phase behaviour in the system.

Linear equation of motion

A material is said to be linearly viscoelastic if the stress is proportional to the strain at a given time and the linear superposition principle holds. Linear behaviour implies that the sum of strain outputs resulting from each component of stress input is the same as the strain output resulting from the combined stress input. Even though the rheological behaviour of lung tissue is clearly nonlinear, a linear approach is usually employed, provided that the amplitudes of changes represent a small fraction of maximal volume (total lung capacity, TLC), and both tidal amplitude and lung volume do not change appreciably during different manoeuvres. Lung tissue is then considered to be composed of two basic elements: a tissue elastance or rate of change of pressure in phase with the volume change, and a dissipative process called tissue resistance (or viscance) that accounts for pressure changes in phase with the rate of volume change with time or flow. If frequency is low enough and flows are small, inertia does not play a significant role in the mechanical behaviour of lung. Then the classic equation of motion implies that the pressure difference across lung tissue is related to lung volume change by an equation of the form:

$$\Delta P = (P_{Alv}\text{-}P_{pl}) = E_{tis} \bullet V + R_{tis} \bullet (dV/dt)$$

applicable during quiet breathing. The term ΔP refers to the pressure difference expressed across lung tissue from alveolar gas to pleural space (P_{Alv}-P_{pl}). V is lung volume and (dV/dt) is the rate of volume change or flow. In the case of periodic forcing the above equation can be reexpressed in terms of real (pressure in phase with volume change, or elastic) and imaginary (pressure out of phase with volume change, or dissipative) parts

$$\Delta P = (E_{tis} + j \cdot w \cdot R_{tis}) \cdot V$$

where j is the unit imaginary number (indicating out-of-phase behaviour) and ω is circular frequency, 2πf. Any tracing of periodic changes in pressure and volume may be transformed into empirically determined values of E_{tis} and R_{tis}. Although the equation of motion is usually employed by overlooking any model assumption, in fact it describes the behaviour of a viscoelastic model composed of an elastic and a resistive element mechanically acting in parallel (Voigt body).

Biological correlates of rheological properties in lung parenchyma

Lung elasticity

Two main structures account for the elastic behaviour of lung parenchyma: tissue fibres and the alveolar lining. Mechanical interaction makes it difficult to separate their relative contribution to the global elastic behaviour. Classically the role of the tissue component has been characterized by the saline-filled lung preparation, lung strip behaving similarly. Transpulmonary pressure reflects only tensile forces in the fibrous structures of the parenchyma because of the elimination of interfacial tension when air is replaced by isotonic saline. Elastic recoil pressure is decreased for a given volume and the volume-pressure curve in saline filled lung is therefore displaced to the left and is more sharply curved than the "air" VP curve, showing marked stiffening at high lung volumes (Fig. 4). According to Setnikar and Meschia [1] this peculiar behaviour of the "saline" lung would signify that two parallel systems exist in lung tissue, one highly extensible and the other much less so. They surmised that these systems were elastin and collagen. With two types of fibre acting in parallel, elastin would account for the properties over most of the volume range and collagen would account for the decreased compliance at high lung volumes. This simple model would predict a biphasic length-tension relationship with an abrupt decrease in compliance near maximal lung volumes. Actually, the length-tension loop is smoothly curved over its entire range, and uniaxial deformation of lung strips does not allow us to distinguish two different elastic behaviours (Fig. 5).

A network behaviour can account for this smoothing. It has been shown that the more organized and aligned the collagen, the less extensible is the tissue [2]. Network phenomena at a microscopic level, involving changes of angle between adjacent primary elements and recruitment within the composite structure, are

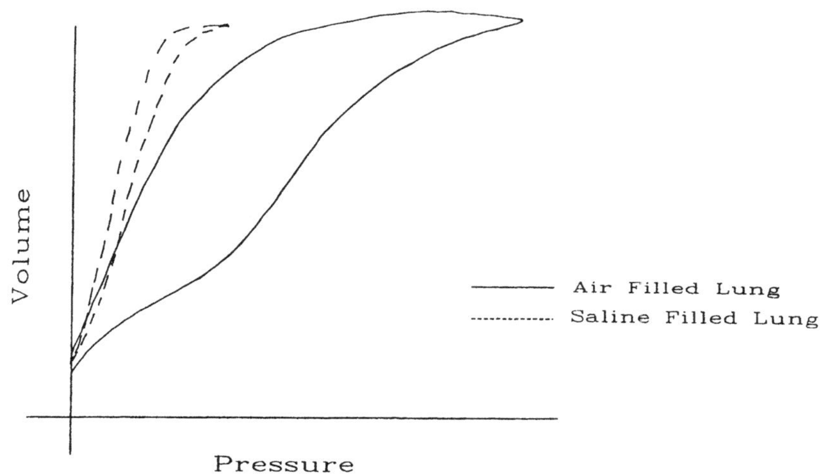

Fig. 4. Pressure volume curves from air and saline filled excised lungs

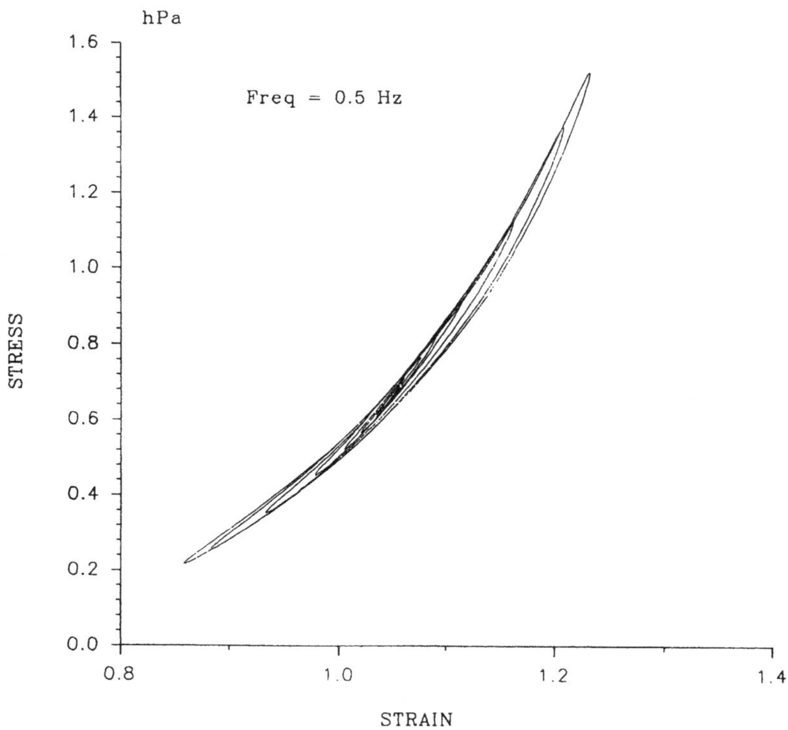

Fig. 5. Stress strain nested loops obtained from a rabbit lung strip submitted to an uniaxial forced oscillation of increasing amplitude and fixed frequency

responsible for the greater extensibility of less organized tissues [3]. In vitro destruction of elastin by the enzyme elastase raises the compliance in the low and mid-volume range but affects neither volume nor compliance at high transpulmonary pressures [4]. Destruction of collagen by collagenase increases compliance at high lung volumes without a major change at low lung volumes. It seems that elastin and collagen act functionally as independent networks.

As can be noted by comparing pressure-volume curves from air- and saline-filled lungs, the major determinant of lung recoil is derived from the interface between air and the lung lining layer. Differences in pressure are greater the higher the lung volume showing a prominent hysteresis [5]. This systematic volume-dependence of the surface-tension effects has been attributed to a prominent surface-area dependency and hysteresis of surface tension (g). The interface stores energy during inflation in two ways: a) by an increase in interfacial tension when the area of the alveolar wall increases, and b) by an increase in surface area itself. Therefore a major assumption underlying all the foregoing analysis is the equivalence between fluid- and air- filled states. The saline-filled lung presumably only has forces due to tissue elements. In the air-filled lung, however, the tissue network is distorted from the saline-filled configuration because the mechanical arrangement of interfacial tension respective of the tissue elastic elements. Surface forces have been probably overestimated resopective to tissue forces by that fact [6, 7].

The pressure-volume behaviour of lung parenchyma can be rapidly and reversibly changed by several interventions known to affect smooth muscle, vagal stimulation, aerosolized or intravenous histamine or methacholine, atropine and isoproterenol [8-10]. Three types of contractile elements have been thought to participate: smooth muscle of small airways, smooth muscle in alveolar ducts, and interstitial contractile cells. They also participate in determining the "elastic state of lung parenchyma" that accordingly would be more adaptable that it was thought until recently [9, 10].

Lung viscosity

Air-liquid interface seems to be also the primary source of hysteresis in the air-filled lung. Indeed, the hysteresis in the air-filled state is much greater than in the saline-filled state [11]. The surface tension-surface area hysteresis seems responsible for this effect. Mechanisms related to surface component of viscosity may relate to molecular rearrangements within the surface film, exchanges between the air-liquid interface and the subfase, and viscous sliding of surfactant on alveolar surfaces [12]. Energy losses in the solid connective tissue elements and in the semisolid or fluid intracellular and interstitial matrices account for hysteresis seen in the saline filled lung. Mechanisms related to tissue component of viscosity are sliding and friction between layers in the interstitial space as well as sliding of solid elements in the matrix. Internal molecular forces, specially low energy interactions, can act like friction elements in opposing to distortion of structural molecules [13, 14]. This seems to be the case for hydrogen bridges, bipolar interactions and actomyosin bridges until a critical (breaking force) is reached.

Lung plasticity

Plastic or plastoelastic deformations could take place at the microstructural level. Plastic hysteresis reflects thermodynamic irreversibilities resulting from mechanisms such as dry friction between microstructural elements, dislocation of these elements, or mechanical, chemical and phase changes of the microstructure [15-17]. The following processes have been identified to have this behaviour:

1. attachment/detachment of cross bridges in the contractile elements;
2. adsorption/desorption of surface-active molecules in the alveolar surface film;
3. movement of the collagen and elastic fibre network;
4. recruitment/derecruitment of alveoli;
5. folding and unfolding of alveolar septal pleats;
6. mechanical shear of cellular and fibrilar contents.

Basic mechanisms underlying plastic behaviours are mainly three: those that imply the expenditure of an energy to reach a new steady configuration (4 and 5). Those that imply the brokening of intermolecular low energy bridges (2, 3 and 6) and finally those implying a change of the configurational shape of large structural molecules (glycoproteins, collagen), detachment of actomyosin bridges or structural changes in polymers at interstitial matrix, all requiring a greater energy expenditure (1 and 3). However, in all the processes before mentioned there exist also rate-dependent features that can be interpreted as viscoelasticity [17].

Rheological modelling of lung parenchyma

In a first approximation, close to the classical monoalveolar model of lung mechanics, lung parenchyma can be considered as a pure viscoelastic body, having at least one elastic and one viscous elements, accounting for elasticity and dissipation respectively. Both elements need to be arranged in series, because a step deformation is normally feasible without appreciable friction. Maxwell body is therefore more adequate than any viscoelastic body having an elastance and a resistance placed in parallel. As previously exposed Maxwell body behaviour can account for stress relaxation and stress recovery, and by consequent for hysteretic behaviour. Frequency dependence of resistance (Fig. 6 a, b) is also accounted for by the viscoelastic model. The behaviour of Maxwell element and the stress relaxation time constant, account for the fequency dependence: as frequency of oscillation increases, the lesser the motion of the dissipative element and so the lower the hysteresis and viceversa. However, Maxwell body cannot account for static elastance, a well known characteristic of lung mechanical behaviour. When lung tissue is suddenly stretched it relaxes with time asymptotically to a value of pressure that depends on the strain or added volume. It means that an elastic element in parallel should be added to Maxwell element to limit relaxation of lung until a new position of equilibrium is reached and predetermined by the intrinsic elasticity of this new component. This ensemble (a Maxwell body plus an elastic element

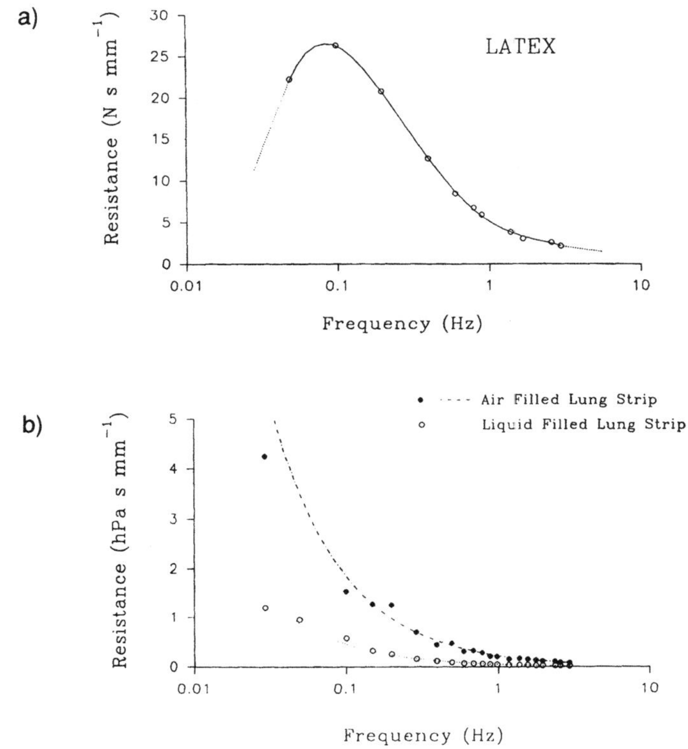

Fig. 6. Frequency dependence of resistance (dissipative behaviour) in viscoelastic material (Latex) and two rat lung strips. Lung strips were filled either with air or saline. Samples were uniaxially loaded and oscillated at fixed amplitude and increasing frequency

in parallel) composes the so called Kelvin body in biorheology (Fig. 7) and it has been suggested to account for the basic rheological properties of lung parenchyma in linear modelling [18, 13, 19, 24]. Elements in the model does not preclude any predetermined relationship with histologic or anatomic elements, except in differentiating resistive and elastic processes at the level of the stress bearing elements.

Elastance and resistance can be obtained by a multivariant adjustment of the above linear equation of motion to experimental data. Variation of both R_{tis} and E_{tis} with angular frequency is predicted by this model (Kelvin body) in function of its constitutive components, having the following expressions

$$R_{tis}(\omega) = \mu/(1+\omega^2\tau_2)$$
$$E_{tis}(\omega) = [\varepsilon_1 \cdot \varepsilon_2{}^2+(\varepsilon_1+\varepsilon_2) \cdot \omega^2 \cdot \mu^2]/(\varepsilon_2{}^2+\omega^2 \cdot \mu^2)$$

where μ is the viscous (dashpot) element, ε_1 and ε_2 are the parallel and series elastic (spring) elements respectively, and ω is the angular frequency, $2\pi f$, and $\tau = \mu/\varepsilon_2$ is the time constant of the linear viscoelastic or Maxwell element.

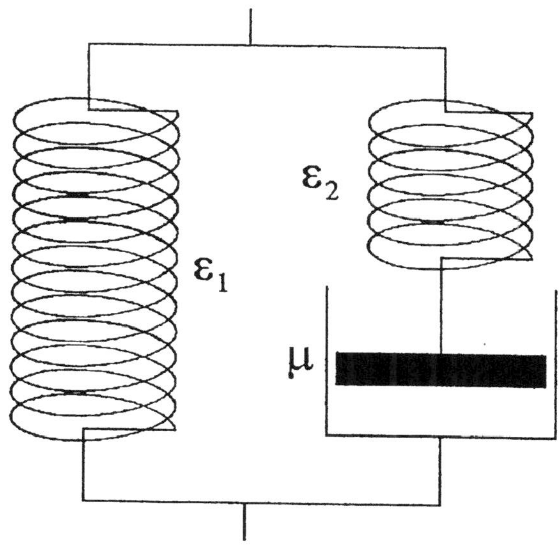

Fig. 7. Schematic representation of Kelvin body

Let us consider briefly the behaviour of this viscoelastic model. It has the merit of predicting a decrease of tissue resistance with the increase of frequency as well as the dependence of dynamic elastance on resistance. Therefore it assumes a linear inverse relationship between R_{tis}, as measured by adjusting the equation of motion, and the square magnitude of angular frequency:

$$1/R_{tis} = a + b\,\omega^2$$

where $a = 1/\mu$ and $b = \tau_2/\mu$. This is not the case, however, when experimental studies are addressed to determine resistive behaviour of lung parenchyma at low frequencies, the relationship of R_{tis} with frequency being near hyperbolic [21-23] (Fig. 6 b). Stress relaxation is described by this model in terms of exponential decay of pressure with time. However it has been shown that pressure tends to decrease with the logarithm of time [21]. Still Kelvin body has the merit to describe mechanics of lung parenchyma as the combination of two parallel systems: an elastic network and a coupled viscoelastic system, giving a first conceptual approach to lung tissue modelling.

A more advanced step in modelling lung parenchyma as a viscoelastic body is to assume a model representing a linear viscoelastic material possessing a continuous spectrum of time constants (Fig. 8). The mechanical analogue known as the generalized Maxwell body is composed by a parallel array of spring-dashpot units modified to include a parallel spring to account for asymptotic (static) elastance. This model allows to adjust for frequency dependence of elastance and resistance as well as for stress relaxation. In this model elastance increases almost

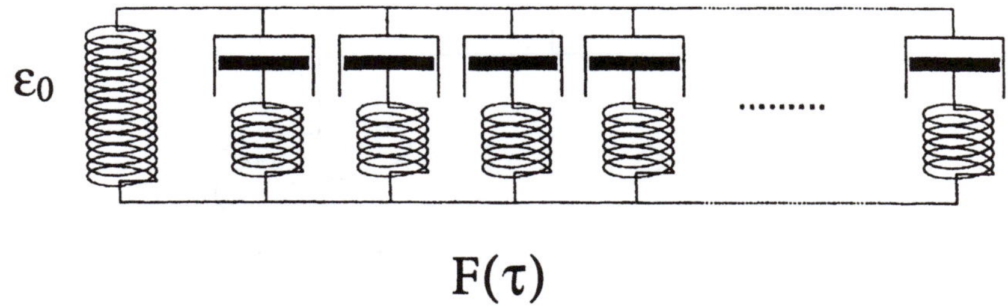

Fig. 8. Schematic representation of generalized Maxwell body

linearly with log ω, whereas R_{ti} changes nearly with 1/ω in a given interval defined by the function of distribution of time constants F(τ) [17]. It is a more accurate definition of lung mechanical behaviour in the frequency domain, but a too complex model to be used in practice.

More complex viscoelastic models generally refer to the non linear viscoelastic theory proposed by Y.C.B. Fung [6], and have been invoked to explain the non linear behaviour of resistance and elastance with changes in amplitude and lung volume. In general these models are phenomenological and lacking of a clear physical correlate [24, 25]. Consequently they remain in the scope of speculation and their use is very restricted to the description of experimental findings.

Several features are systematically observed when lung parenchyma is carefully studied, and suggest a plastoelastic mechanism more or less coupled to the viscoelastic bchaviour. These features include the decrease of dynamic elastance and resistance with increasing amplitude of forcing, stress relaxation being more pronounced during loading than during unloading as well as some features still described by the linear viscoelastic theory like the hyperbolic relationship between lung resistance and frequency. A critical fact is that viscoelastic models predict the resistance to be zero at both infinite and zero frequencies, so an inflection point should exist at low frequencies (Fig. 6a). Experimental studies performed at very low frequencies have shown that tissue resistance increases hyperbolically with frequency and no inflection has been found. In general these characteristics can be more or less described by the nonlinear viscoelastic theory without including plasticity [27]. Nonetheless plasticity is a well known property of lung parenchyma, that can be observed in definite situations as inflation after total deflation or alveolar recruitment during inflation from residual volume. Incorporatin plasticity to global models of lung behaviour is not unreasonable. However plastoelastic behaviour by itself cannot account for the global mechanical behaviour of lung parenchyma.

Systems composed by viscous (dashpots), elastic (springs) and plastic (dry friction) elements are called viscoplastic. In his pioneer work J. Hildebrandt [21, 22] proposed a particular viscoplastic analogue composed by a generalized Maxwell body (Fig. 8) in series with a generalized Prandtl body (Fig. 9c). The latter would be composed by an infinite number of units, each composed by a dry sliding unit in series with a spring (Prandtl body, Fig. 9a), and in parallel with an elastic element. The plastoelastic system of Fig. 9c is assumed to represent a material possessing a continuous distribution of yield forces. Hildebrand [22] assumed that the number of units sliding (n) at a time (t) depends on the level of the force, P, applied to the compartment at that time, according to the power law $n = a \cdot P^b$, where a and b are nonnegative constants. The larger is b the larger the number of the sliding units for a given stress. For any b>0 this system displays nonlinear behaviour even for the smaller amplitudes; some sliding units always will have exceeded their yield stress. In fact, there is an increasing evidence in favour of considering plastoelasticity as responsible of an appreciable portion of the energy dissipation in tissues depending on the tissue system in question.

Biomechanical modelling of lung parenchyma should account for frequency and amplitude dependence of mechanical behaviour as well as for nonlinearity. Viscoelastic linear models account fairly well for frequency dependence of elastance and viscance, especially if they include a continuous distribution of time constants. The simple Kelvin body can be used as an approach to explain the basic mechanism of tissue rheology, but it lacks of precision. By definition amplitude dependence cannot be accounted for by any linear viscoelastic process. Alternative viscoelastic models are based in the non linear viscoelastic theory have been described for several biological tissues as well as for respiratory tissues and account fairly well for both frequency and amplitude dependence. They do not assume any precise biophysical configuration or interactions at the microstructural level. Plastoelastic processes are present in lung parenchyma, especially at the alveolar surface but also inside the tissue. Therefore, it has to be taken into account in any rheological modelling of the lung. Probably as B. Suki and J. Bates [26] pointed out, the question of nonlinear viscoelasticity versus

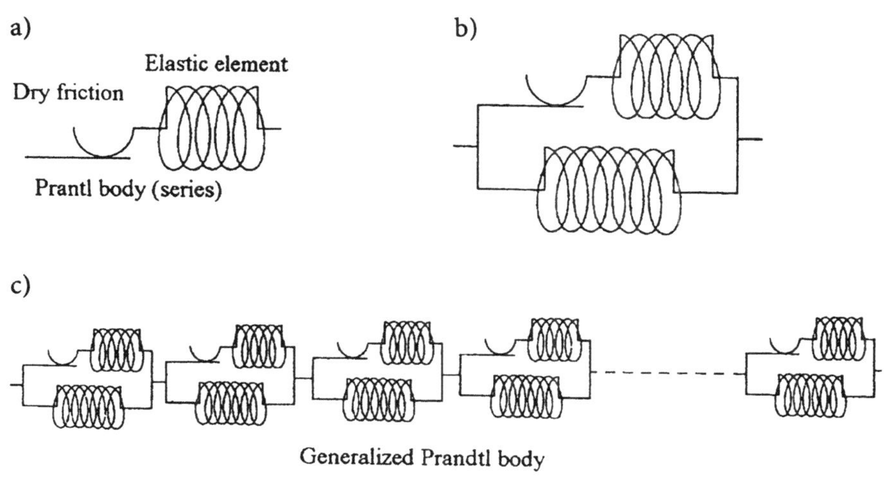

Fig. 9. Several plastoelastic configurations combine spring and dry friction elements

plastoelasticity is one of mathematical convenience rather than a matter of fundamental importance.

Hysteresivity and the structural damping theory

Recently Fredberg and Stamenovic [5] introduced the concept of structural damping by postulating that elasticity and resistivity within the tissues are coupled at the level of the stress bearing elements, whatever they may be. This theory is built from the previous studies by Bachofen and Hildebrandt [2, 3] and states a single postulate; the coupling of elastic and dissipative process at the level of the stress bearing element.

In 1971 Bachofen and Hildebrandt [18] studied the out-of-phase pressure to volume behaviour of lung parenchyma, and concluded empirically that the ratio of hysteresis loop to the global elastic work done by the system remained constant or with very insignificant changes when frequency or amplitude were modified in an operating range. The shape coefficient (K) was characterized as:

$$K = A/(\Delta P \cdot V_t)$$

Where A is the area of the pressure volume loop, equivalent to the amount of work dissipated by cycle. ΔP is the amplitude of pressure swing and V_T is the tidal volume. The product $\Delta P \cdot V_t$ is the area of the box enclosing the pressure-volume loop. The constant ratio K means essentially that dissipative work is a constant fraction of the total work stored in the system at the end of an inspiratory cycle. The constant K can vary between 0 (a perfectly elastic system) and 1 (a purely dissipative viscoplastic system). K values in lung parenchyma from different species oscillate around 0.11.

Fredberg and Stamenovic [5] interpreted this energetic behaviour as an optimal coupling between elastic and dissipative processes at the level of the stress bearing element, through a constant called hysteresivity (h). The linear motion equation states that driving pressure is determined by the sum of two pressures: an elastic pressure in phase with volume and a resistive pressure in phase with flow. The structural damping hypothesis states that resistance and elastance being coupled, the linear equation of motion can be rewritten as:

$$P = (E_{dyn} + j \cdot h \cdot E_{dyn}) \cdot V$$

or simply

$$P = E_{dyn} \cdot V \cdot (1 + j \cdot h)$$

where $h = \omega \cdot R_{tis}/E_{tis}$

Hysteresivity is defined as the ratio of tissue resistance to dynamic elastance multiplied by angular frequency. Referred to tissue energetics, hysteresivity represents the ratio between the energy dissipated by cycle (W) to the stored potential energy at maximal volume (U), and so it can be expressed as $h = W/(2 \cdot p \cdot U)$.

The structural damping theory has the advantage of not precluding any special kind of arrangement between elastic, viscous and plastic elements in lung parenchyma, but defines hysteresivity as a constant reflecting the intrinsic coupling between elastic and dissipative processes whatever their nature.

References

1. Setnikar I, Meschia G (1952) Proprietà elastiche del polmone e di modelli meccaniche. Arch Fisiol 52:288
2. Alfrey T Jr (1948) Mechanical behaviour of high polymers. Interscience, New York
3. Fredberg JJ, Stamenovic D (1989) On the imperfect elasticity of lung tissue. J Appl Physiol 67:2408-2419
4. Moretto A, Dallaire M, Romero PV, Ludwig M (1993) Effect of elastase on oscillation mechanics of lung parenchymal strip. Amer Rev Respir Dis 147 [Suppl]: A970
5. Hoppin FG Jr, Hildebrandt J (1977) Mechanical properties of the lung, in J.B. West, Bioengineering aspects of the lung. Marcel Dekker Inc, New York, pp 83-162
6. Fung YCB (1981) Biomechanics. Mechanical properties of living tissues. Springer Verlag, New York
7. Goerk J, Clements JA (1986) Alveolar surface tension and lung surfactant. In: Fishman AP, Macklem PT, Mead J, Geiger SR (eds) Handbook of Physiology. The Respiratory System. Mechanics of Breathing. Section 3, vol. III, pt. 1, chapt. 16. American Physiological Society, Bethesda, pp 247-261
8. Romero PV, Robatto FM, Simard S, Ludwig MS (1992) Lung tissue behaviour during methacholine challenge in rabbits in vivo. J Appl Physiol 73:207-212
9. Ingenito EP, Davison B, Fredberg JJ (1993) Tissue resistance in the guinea pig at baseline and during methacholine constriction. J Appl Physiol 75:2541-2548
10. Romero PV, Ludwig MS (1991) Maximal methacholin-induced constriction in rabbit lung: interaction between airways and tissues. J Appl Physiol 46:1251-1262
11. Bachofen H, Hildebrandt J, Bachofen M (1970) Pressure-volume curves of air- and liquid-filled excised lungs: surface tension in situ. J Appl Physiol 29:422-431
12. Hoppin FG Jr, Stothert JS Jr, Greaves IA, Lai YL, Hildebrand J (1986) Lung recoil: elastic and rheological properties. In: Handbook of Physiology. The Respiratory System. Mechanics of Breathing. Section 3, vol. III, pt. 1, chapt. 13. American Physiological Society, Bethesda 195-215
13. Bates JHT (1993) Understanding lung tissue mechanics in terms of mathematical models. Monaldi Arch Chest Dis 48:2 134-139
14. Sato J, Davey LK, Shardonowsky F, Bates JHT (1991) Low frequency respiratory system resistance in the normal dog during mechanical ventilation. J Appl Physiol 70:1536-1543
15. Shardonowsky FR, McDonough JM, Grunsten MM (1993) Effects of positive end-expiratory pressure on lung tissue mechanics in rabbits. J Appl Physiol 75:2506-2513
16. Stamenovic D, Glass GM, Barnas GM, Fredberg JJ (1990) Viscoplasticity of respiratory tissues. J Appl Physiol 69:973-988
17. Stamenovic D, Lutchen KR, Barnas GM (1993) Alternative model of respiratory tissue viscoplasticity. J Appl Physiol 75:1062-1069

18. Bachofen H, Hildebrandt J (1971) Area analysis of pressure-volume hysteresis in mammalian lungs. J Appl Physiol 30:493-97
19. Lorino AM, Harf A (1993) Techniques for measuring respiratory mechanics: an analytic approach with a viscoelastic model. J Appl Physiol 74:2373-79
20. Nicolai T, Lanteri CJ, Sly P (1993) Inherent coupling of elastic and dissipative behaviour of the lung through a viscoelastic time constant. J Appl Physiol 74:2358-64
21. Hildebrandt J (1969) Comparison of mathematical models for cat lung and viscoelastic balloon derived by Laplace transform methods from pressure-volume data. Bull Math Biophys 31:651-67
22. Hildebrandt J (1970) Pressure-volume data of cat lung interpreted by a plastoelastic, linear viscoelastic model. J Appl Physiol 28:365-72
23. Vetterman J, Warner DO, Brichant JF (1989) Halotane decreases both tissue and airways resistance in excised canine lungs. J Appl Physiol 66:2689-703
24. Bates JHT, Shardonowsky F, Stewart DE (1989) The low frequency dependence of respiratory system resistance and elastance in normal dogs. Respir Physiol 78:369-382
25. Navajas D, Maksym GN, Bates JHT (1993) Viscoelastic nonlinearity of lung tissue (Abstract) Eur J Respir Dis 6[Suppl 17]: 405s
26. Suki B, Bates JHT (1991) A nonlinear viscoelastic model of lung tissue mechanics. J Appl Physiol 71:826-33
27. Suki B (1993) Nonlinear phenomena in respiratory mechanical measurements. J Appl Physiol 74:2574-84

Chapter 7

Viscoelastic model and airway occlusion

V. ANTONAGLIA, A. GROP, F. BELTRAME, U. LUCANGELO, A. GULLO

Introduction

During mechanical ventilation, the *rapid airway occlusion method* [1-3] and the "single-breath" method [4-8] are probably the most commonly employed techniques for measuring the respiratory mechanics.

In anaesthetized humans, the mechanical behaviour of the respiratory system during passive lung emptying has been assessed by the latter method.

Using the technique of rapid airway occlusion during constant flow inflation it has been possible to determine the static mechanical properties and the newtonian airways and chest wall resistance of the respiratory system and the viscoelastic constants which in turn allow assessment of the time-dependent behaviour of the lung and chest wall [9-13].

In fact, this method has been used particularly to test the linear viscoelastic model proposed by Bates et al. [14] in response to volume inputs.

The mechanical behaviour of the lung and the chest wall can be described from nonlinear viscoelastic [15] and viscoplastoelastic models [16], when the whole pulmonary volume range and the frequency-dependence of energy dissipation of the transpulmonary pressure-volume loop are considered. Moreover, the viscoplastoelastic models are rarely used in vivo as the parameters obtained have been found difficult to interpret mechanically [17]. By contrast, linear viscoelastic models have been used to assess the mechanical behaviour of the respiratory system during mechanical ventilation in anesthetized humans [18, 19, 20].

These models are characterised by four mechanical elements placed in parallel and/or in series. Using the technique of rapid airway occlusion, the slow decay of pressure following the rapid end-inspiratory occlusion represents the viscoelastic behaviour during the occluded breath (stress relaxation) and/or the gas redistribution.

The constant parameter viscoelastic model which has been shown experimentally [20, 30] to be more appropriate for normal lungs is the viscoelastic model proposed by Bates et al. [14, 21].

The results of the most recent studies on anesthetized subjects [11, 12], animals [9, 10, 13, 21, 22], ARDS [23, 24] and COPD [25, 26] during mechanical ventilation have been interpreted according to this model.

The viscoelastic model

The "spring-and-dashpot" rheological model proposed by Bates [14, 21] is based on the studies of Mount [27] and Sharp et al. [28].

This model is made up of two parallel components: a dashpot, R_1 representing $R_{int,rs}$, and a Kelvin body [29]. The latter is made up of a spring (E_1) representing the static elastance of the respiratory system, $E_{st,rs}$, in parallel with a Maxwell body [29], *i.e.* a spring (E_2) and a dashpot (R_2) placed in series. E_2 and R_2 represent the viscoelastic properties of the respiratory system. The time constant of the Maxwell body, τ_2, is reflected by the R_2 / E_2 ratio. These two components are placed in parallel between two equidistant bars. One is fixed and the other is moving at a constant rate. This rate corresponds to constant flow inflation, $\dot{V}$, and at the end of inflation (T_i) the distance between them corresponds to the volume that entered the lung. This model is shown in Fig. 1.

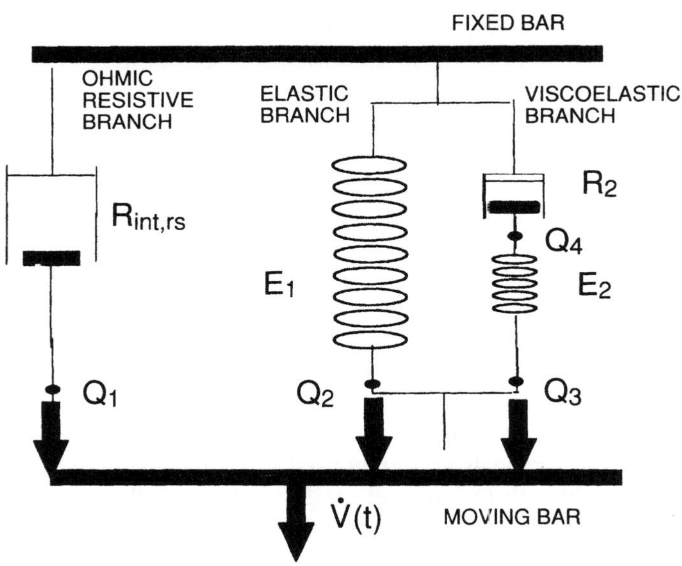

Fig. 1. The "spring-and-dashpot" rheological model during inflation

With reference to Fig. 1, if the distance between the two bars increases with $\dot{V}$, starting from the elastic equilibrium volume, points Q_1, Q_2 and Q_3 move at the same constant speed, $\dot{V}$. If we remove the bonds due to the springs and dashpots, points Q_1, Q_2 and Q_3 may be seen as the mobile seats of three different forces $F_1(t)$, $F_2(t)$ and $F_3(t)$ corresponding to the pressures of the system, i.e. the flow-resistive pressure, the elastic pressure and the viscoelastic pressure of the respiratory system respectively. These forces hinder the mobile bar's movement and their total sum, $F(t)$, presents opposite sign with respect to $F_1(t)$, $F_2(t)$ and $F_3(t)$

and corresponds to the total distending pressure of the model (Fig. 2). In our analysis this pressure is represented by the tracheal pressure, Ptr.

Ptr may be used as a substitute for mouth pressure to avoid the resistance caused by the endotracheal tube, tubing and measuring equipment.

In particular, point Q_1 in the resistive branch is dragged at the same $\dot{V}$ and the relevant dashpot reacts with a force $F_1(t)$.

Similarly, point Q_2 in the elastic branch is dragged at the same $\dot{V}$ and spring $E_{st,rs}$ applies an elastic return force $F_2(t)$ corresponding to $E_{st,rs} \cdot V(t)$.

The viscoelastic branch behaves in a different way because of the combined presence of spring E_2 and dashpot R_2. While point Q_3 is dragged at the same $\dot{V}$, point Q_4 reaches this constant speed after a longer time (when $t > 3\ \tau_2$).

During inspiration the pressures of the system cannot be distingued. This is possible with a rapid airway occlusion at the end of inspiration.

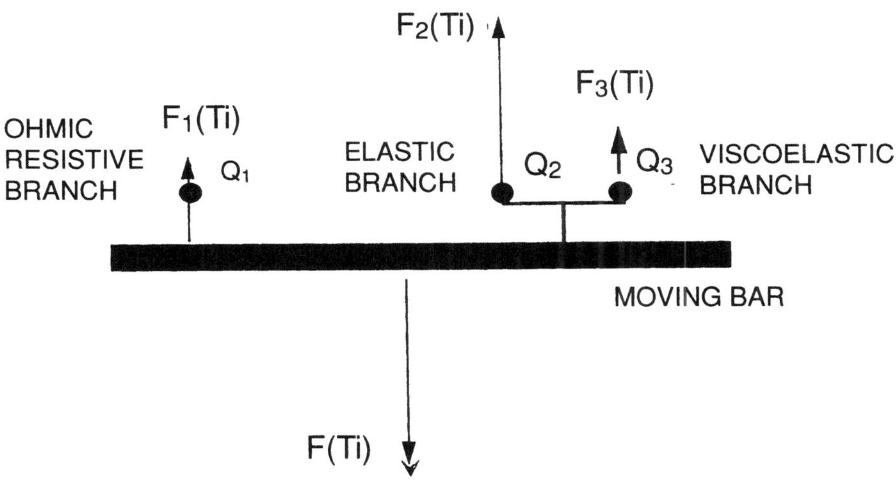

Fig. 2. Force diagram of the "spring-and-dashpot" rheological model at Ti

The model during occlusion

When the flow is suddenly interrupted and the airway occlusion prolonged, the bars of the model remain at the same distance because the inflated volume, V(t), is trapped in the lungs and airways. In particular, based on its characteristics, dashpot $R_{int,rs}$ completes its work at $t = T_i^+$ and the related pressure goes down to zero. Spring $E_{st,rs}$ is blocked between the bars and continues to apply the elastic return force $F_2(Ti)$. On the other hand, in the viscoelastic branch, Q_3 is blocked while Q_4 is moving in the same direction as prior to airway occlusion. During the occlusion the spring E_2 may go back to its equilibrium length (which corresponds to resting conditions) whereas dashpot R_2 continues to lengthen until 3 τ_2 is reached.

After occlusion a rapid drop is seen in the recorded pressure (P_{max} - P_1), which is followed by a gradual decrease in pressure to an apparent plateau value (P_2) (Fig. 3).

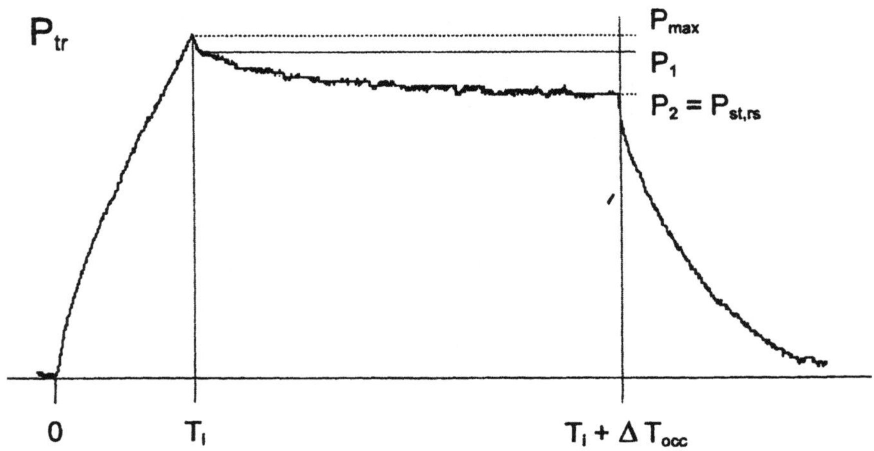

Fig. 3. Tracheal pressure (Ptr) during constant inflation flow and end-inspiratory occlusion

The initial pressure drop corresponds to the resistive pressure related to the airway distal to the measurement point. This value divided by the immediately preceeding steady flow, $\dot{V}$, provides the interrupter resistance, $R_{int,rs}$, reflecting airway resistences [30]. The force $F_1(t)$ in the resistive branch at the end of inspiration is $F_1(Ti) = R_{int,rs} \dot{V}$.

The slow decay of pressure from P_1 to P_2 represents the stress relaxation that takes into account the viscoelastic behaviour and time constant inequalities of the lung and chest wall. We can analyze the time course of the pressure decay or measure P_{diff}, *i.e.* the difference between P_1 and P_2. P_{diff} divided by the preceeding occlusion $\dot{V}$ yields the additional resistance, ΔR_{rs}.

If the occlusion time is long enough, P_2 is taken to represent the static end-inspiratory elastic recoil pressure of the respiratory system ($P_{st,rs}$).

During airway occlusion, the "spring-and-dashpot" rheological model may be drawn as in Fig. 4. The relevant force diagram is shown in Fig. 5.

In Fig. 5 at time $t = 3\ \tau_2$ after airway occlusion the additional force $F_4(t)$ applied to point Q_3 in the viscoelastic branch goes down to zero. Summarizing, the distance between the two bars remains the same, but the force applied between the bars changes until reaching a constant value at $t > 3\ \tau_2$ because of spring Est,rs remaining blocked at a fixed length as shown in Fig. 6 and Fig. 7.

As the equation of motion of the respiratory model describing nonhomogeneous lungs [18] is comparable to that of the Bates model [14, 21], it is quite impossible to discern how much stress relaxation is due to heterogeneities within the lung or to viscoelastic behaviour. In ARDS patients it was found that the hetero-

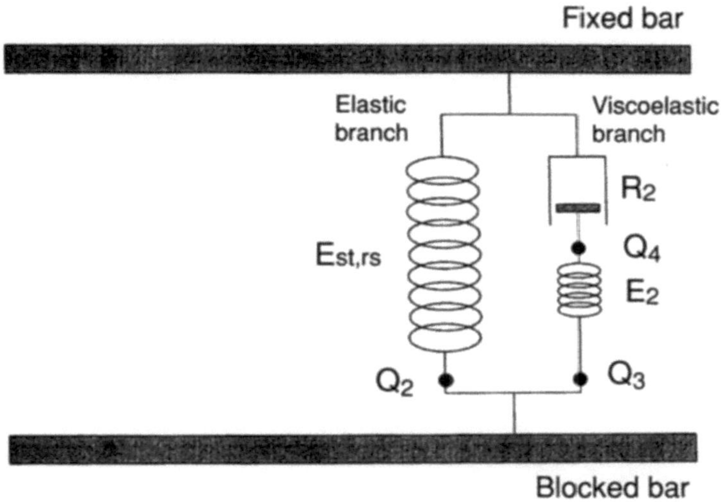

Fig. 4. The "spring-and-dashpot" rheological model during end-inspiratory occlusion (occlusion time < $3\tau_2$)

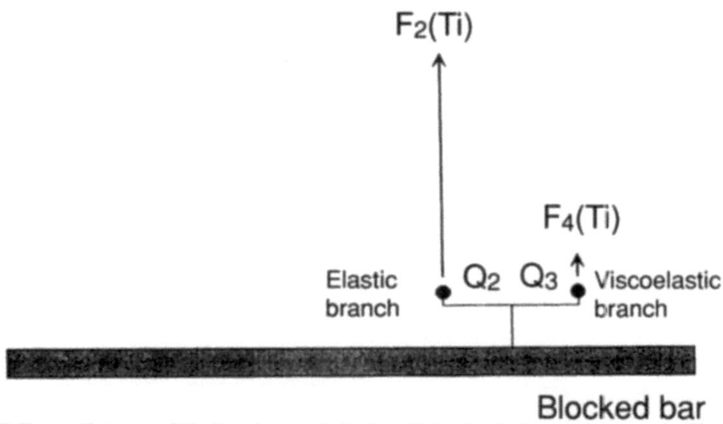

Fig. 5. Force diagram of the "spring-and-dashpot" rheological model shown in Fig. 4

geneities within the lung contributed relatively little to stress relaxation [23]. In the present analysis only the viscoelastic behaviour is taken into account and P_{diff} reflects the relaxation of the spring E_2 resulting in energy dissipation in the dashpot R_2, i.e. the viscoelastic pressure. It depends on the degree of E_2 stretch at occlusion time.

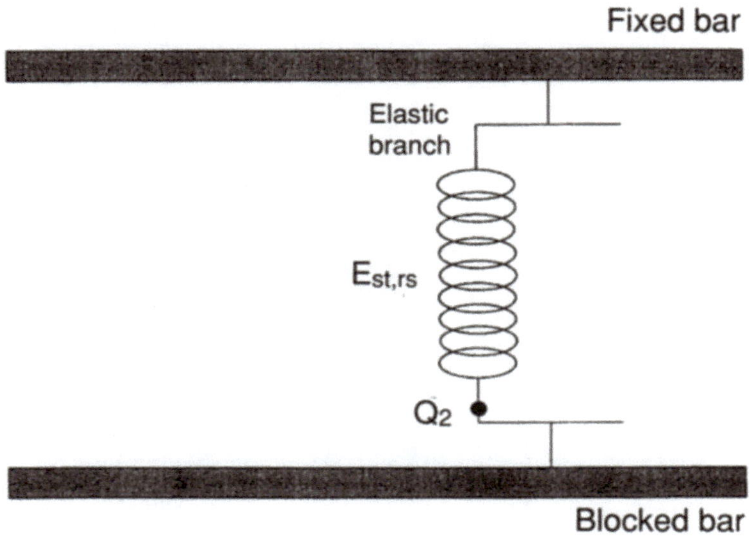

Fig. 6. The "spring-and-dashpot" rheological model during end-inspiratory occlusion (occlusion time > $3\tau_2$)

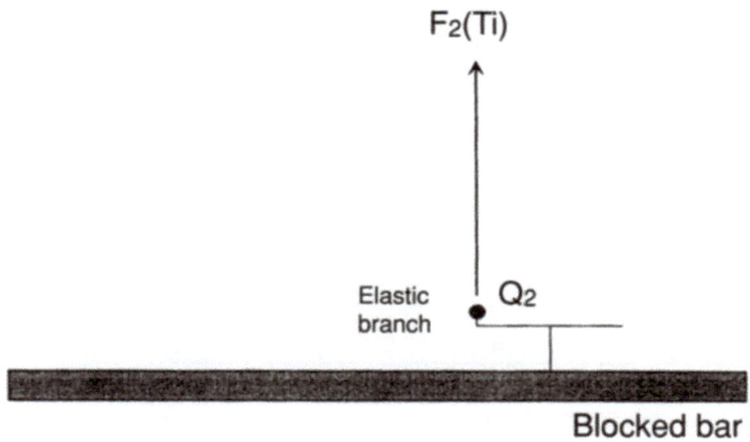

Fig. 7. Force diagram of the "spring-and-dashpot" rheological model shown in Fig. 6

Standard respiratory variables and viscoelastic constants

The technique of rapid airway occlusion during constant flow inflation allows evaluation of the standard respiratory variables and the viscoelastic constants.

At each occlusion the following standard respiratory variables were computed from the values of $P_{tr,max}$, P_1, and $P_{st,rs}$: interrupter resistance [Rint = ($P_{tr,max}$ - P_1)

/ $\dot{V}$]; viscoelastic resistance ($R_{visc} = P_1 - P_{st,rs} / \dot{V}$); respiratory system resistance [$R_{tot} = (P_{tr,max} - P_{st,rs}) / \dot{V}$]; static and dynamic elastances of the respiratory system ($E_{st,rs} = P_{st,rs} / V_t$ and $E_{dyn,rs} = P_1 / V_t$).

It has been observed [31, 26] that for time $\dot{V}$ and volume dependency of the respiratory variables, the inflation volume and $\dot{V}$ have to be standardized when comparison between respiratory variables of different subjects is required.

The viscoelastic constants were obtained by performing a series of occlusions at different lung volumes, or a series of occlusions at a fixed lung volume achieved with different inflation flows [11, 12].

The viscoelastic constants of the respiratory system were assessed by fitting the equation:

$$\Delta R_{rs} = R_2 \left(1 - e^{-T_i / \tau_2}\right) \tag{1}$$

to the experimental data, where T_i is the inspiratory time and ΔR_{rs} is the additional resistance (in our analysis corresponding to the viscoelastic resistance). Eq. (1) is the final value at $t = T_i$ of the following function

$$\Delta R_{rs,ins}(t) = R_2 \left(1 - e^{-t / \tau_2}\right) \tag{2}$$

that represents the exponential increase of additional resistance in response to a ramp of applied volume at constant-flow inflation according to the Bates analysis [14]. This exponential increase and the related viscoelastic constants are shown in Fig. 8.

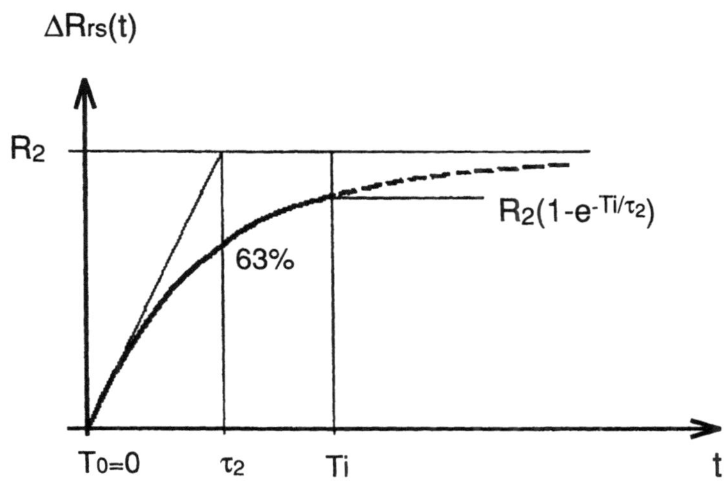

Fig. 8. Additional resistance ΔRrs(t) vs. inspiratory time T_i and the related viscoelastic constants

The average values of R_2 and E_2 obtained in healthy anesthetized paralyzed humans were 4.6 $cmH_2O\ s\ L^{-1}$ and 4.7 $cmH_2O\ L^{-1}$ for the total respiratory system using iso-flow (0.5 $L\ s^{-1}$) conditions [11]. Partitioning of the respiratory system obtained mean values of R_2 and E_2 for lung and chest wall corresponding to 3.4 $cmH_2O\ s\ L^{-1}$ and 3.2 $cmH_2O\ L^{-1}$ and 2.1 $cmH_2O\ s\ L^{-1}$ and 1.7 $cmH_2O\ L^{-1}$ respectively [12].

The estimates of the viscoelastic constants allow assessment of the contribution of viscoelastic mechanisms to the time dependency of the resistance and elastance of the respiratory system, lung and chest wall [12].

The average values of the viscoelastic constants for both lung and chest wall of mechanically ventilated patients with ARDS [23] and COPD [26] were significantly higher than those of normal subjects. This elicits a higher time dependency of the resistance and elastance of the respiratory system, lung and chest wall in these patients and implies a markedly increased viscoelastic work relative to normal subjects [12, 26].

In other studies [21, 32-34] the stress relaxation has been represented by analyzing the slow decay of the pressure as an exponential function rather than in terms of Pdif. The exponential function during occlusion represents the solution of the equation of motion of the viscoelastic element.

Jonson et al. [32] computed the viscoelastic time constant in healthy humans by exponential fitting of the P_{tr} during occlusions and fitting the equation of motion of the Maxwell element to P, V and $\dot{V}$ data obtained during several inspiratory and expiratory pauses. In this method constant flow is not necessary.

In experimental studies the tissue viscoelastic behavior has been represented as stress adaptation or as tissue viscance (R_{tis}) calculated from alveolar pressure (P_A) recordings [20, 35]. In dogs, Bates et al. [21] took into account the stress relaxation as an exponential pressure decrease during occlusion to calculate the viscoelastic time constant and the stress recovery of the occlusion performed immediately after the beginning of the expiration to calculate E_2. Hantos et al. [36] calculated values of E_2 and R_2 by measuring pulmonary impedance by low-frequency oscillations in open-chest dogs. Nicolai et al. [33] calculated R_{tis} by fitting the single-compartment model of the respiratory system to the P_A, V and $\dot{V}$ data during quasi-sinusoidal ventilation. The viscoelastic time constant was obtained by exponential fitting of the occlusion-pressure and, consequently, from R_{tis} and τ_2, R_2.

The clinical application of methods to determine the viscoelastic constants is very complex and time-consuming. Recently a single breath method has been described to easily calculate the viscoelastic constants by analyzing the decay of the P_{tr} curve after a single rapid end inspiratory airway occlusion during baseline ventilation [37].

In conclusion, although the rapid airway occlusion analysis is limited to inspiration and does not include the contribution of plastoelastic phenomena present during cycling breathing [38], it does consent easy evaluation of the mechanical properties of the respiratory system and the time-dependent behaviour of lung and chest wall.

References

1. Mead J, Whittenberger JL (1954) Evaluation of airway interruption technique as a method for measuring pulmonary airflow resistance. J Appl Physiol 6:408-416
2. Bates JHT, Rossi A, Milic-Emili J (1985) Analysis of the behaviour of the respiratory system with constant inspiratory flow. J Appl Physiol 58:1840-1848
3. Bates JHT, Baconnier P and Milic-Emili J (1988) A theoretical analysis of interrupter technique for measuring respiratory mechanics. J Appl Physiol 64:2204-2214
4. Zin WA, Pengelly L, Milic-Emili J (1982) Single breath method for measurement of respiratory mechanics in anesthetized animals. J Appl Physiol: Respirat Environ Exercise Physiol 52:1266-1277
5. Behrakis P, Higgs B, Baydur A, Zin WA, Milic-Emili J (1983) Respiratory mechanics during halothane anesthesia and anesthesia-paralysis in humans. J Appl Physiol: Respirat Environ Exercise Physiol 55:1085-1092
6. Bates JHT, Decramer M, Chartrand D, Zin W, Boddener A, Milic-Emili J (1985) Volume-time profile during relaxed expiration in the normal dog. J Appl Physiol 59:732-737
7. Chelucci G, Brunet F, DallíAva-Santucci J, Dhainaut J, Paccaly D, Armaganidis A, Milic-Emili J, Lockhart A (1991) A single-compartment model cannot describe passive expiration in intubated, paralysed humans. Eur Respir J 4:458-464
8. Guttmann J, Eberhard L, Fabry B, Bertschmann W, Zeravik J, Adolph M, Eckart J, Wolff G (1995) Time constant/volume relationship of passive expiration in mechanically ventilated ARDS patients. Eur Respir J 8:114-120
9. Kochi T, Okubo S, Zin A, Milic-Emili J (1988) Flow and volume dependence of pulmonary mechanics in anaesthetized cats. J Appl Physiol 64:441-450
10. Ludwig MS, Dreshaj I, Solway J, Munoz A, Ingram RH (1987) Partitioning of pulmonary resistance during constriction in the dog: effect of volume history. J Appl Physiol 62:807-815
11. D'Angelo E, Calderini E, Torri G, Robatto FM, Bono D, Milic-Emili J (1989) Respiratory mechanics in anesthetized paralyzed humans: effects of flow, volume, and time. J Appl Physiol 67:2556-2564
12. D'Angelo E, Robatto FM, Calderini E, Tavola M, Bono D, Torri G, Milic-Emili J (1991) Pulmonary and chest wall mechanics in anesthetized paralyzed humans. J Appl Physiol 70:2602-2610
13. Similovski T, Levy P, Corbeil C, Albala M, Pariente R, Derenne JP, Bates JHT, Jonson B, Milic-Emili J (1989) Viscoelastic behaviour of lung and chest wall in dogs determined by flow interruption. J Appl Physiol 67:2219-2229
14. Bates JHT, Brown K, Kochi T (1987) Identifying a model of respiratory mechanics using the interrupter technique. Proceedings of the Ninth American Conference, Engineering Medical Biology Society, pp 1802-1803
15. Suki B, Bates JHT (1991) A nonlinear viscoelastic model of lung tissue mechanics. J Appl Physiol 71:826-833
16. Hildebrandt J (1970) Pressure-volume data of cat lung interpreted by a plastoelastic, linear viscoelastic model. J Appl Physiol 28:365-372
17. Navajas DR, Farre J, Cannet J, Roger M, Sanchis J (1990) Respiratory imput impedance in anasthetized paralyzed patients. J Appl Physiol 69:1372-1379
18. Otis AB, McKerrow CB, Bartlett RA, Mead J, McIlroy MB, Selverstone NJ, Radford EP (1956) Mechanical factors in distribution of pulmonary ventilation. J Appl Physiol 8:427-443

19. Mead J, Whittenberger JL (1954) Evaluation of airway interruption technique as a method for measuring pulmonary airwflow resistance. J Appl Physiol 6:408-416
20. Ludwig MS, Dreshaj I, Solway J, Munoz A, Ingram RH (1987) Partitioning of pulmonary resistance during constriction in the dog: effect of volume history. J Appl Physiol 62:807-815
21. Bates JHT, Brown K, Kochi T (1989) Respiratory mechanics in the normal dog determined by expiratory flow interruption. J Appl Physiol 67:2276-2285
22. Kochi T, Okubo S, Zin WA, Milic-Emili J (1988) Chest wall and respiratory system mechanics in cats: effects of flow and volume. J Appl Physiol 64:2636-2646
23. Eissa NT, Ranieri VM, Corbeil C, Chassé M, Robatto FM, Braidy J, Milic-Emili J (1991) Analysis of behaviour of the respiratory system in ARDS patients: effect of the flow, volume and time. J Appl Physiol 70 6:2719-2729
24. Tantucci C, Corbeil C, Chassé M, et al (1992) Flow and volume dependece of respiratory system flow resistance in ARDS patients. Am Rev Respir Dis 145:355-360
25. Tantucci C, Corbeil C, Chassé M et al (1991) Flow resistance in COPD patients in acute respiratory failure: effects of flow and volume. Am Rev Respir Dis 144:384-389
26. Guérin C, Coussa M-L, Eissa NT, Corbeil C, Chassé M, Braidy J, Matar N, Milic-Emili J (1993) Lung and chest wall mechanics in mechanically ventilated patients. J Appl Physiol 74:1570-1580
27. Mount LE (1955) The ventilation flow-resistance and compliance of rat lungs. J Physiol 127:157-167
28. Sharp JT, Johnson N, Goldberg NB, Van Lith P (1967) Hysteresis and stress adaptation in the human respiratory system. J Appl Physiol 23:487-497
29. Reiner M (1958) Rheology. Handbook of Physics. McGraw-Hill Book Company Inc. vol 3, pp 40-49
30. Bates JHT, Ludwig MS, Sly PD, Brown K, Martin JG, Fredberg JJ (1988) Interrupted resistance clucidated by alveolar pressure measurement in open-chest normal dogs. J Appl Physiol 65:408-414
31. Tantucci C, Eissa NT, Ranieri VM et al (1992) Respiratory mechanics in ventilated patients. J Crit Care 7:251-255
32. Jonson B, Beydon L, Brauer K, Manson C, Valind S, Grytzell H (1993) Mechanics of respiratory system in healthy anesthetized humans with emphasis on viscoelastic properties. J Appl Physiol 75:132-140
33. Nicolai T, Lanteri CJ, Sly P (1993) Inherent coupling of elastic and dissipative behaviour of the lung through a viscoelastic time constant. J Appl Physiol 74:2358-2364
34. Bigos D, Perez Fontan JJ (1994) Contribution of viscoelastic stress to the rate-dependence of pulmonary dynamic elastance. Respiration Physiology 98:53-67
35. Sly PD, Lanteri CJ (1990) Differential responses of the airways and pulmonary tissues to inhaled histamine in young dogs. J Appl Physiol 68:1562-1567
36. Hantos ZB, Daroczy B, Csendes T, Suki B, Nagy S (1990) Modelling of low-frequency pulmonary impedance in dogs. J Appl Physiol 68:849-860
37. Antonaglia V, Grop A, Demanins P, Beltrame F, Lucangelo U, Gullo A, Milic-Emili J (1995) A new method for determination of viscoelastic constants of respiratory system. Int Care Med 21:129
38. Bates JHT, Milic-Emili J (1991) The flow interruption technique for measuring respiratory resistance. J Crit Care 6:227-238

Chapter 8

Breathing pattern in acute ventilatory failure

M.J. Tobin, A. Jubran, F. Laghi

Introduction

Patients modulate respiratory center output and the pattern of respiratory muscle contraction to prevent the development of acute ventilatory failure. The precise nature of these alterations is poorly understood, since it is very difficult to obtain detailed physiological measurements at the time a patient is developing acute respiratory failure. Instead, most clinical research on the neuromuscular control of breathing has been conducted in relatively stable patients [1]. Recently, investigators have taken patients who fail a trial of weaning from mechanical ventilation as a model of acute ventilatory failure, since it is possible to obtain detailed physiologic measurements in these patients and the pathophysiology is presumed to be quite similar [2].

Volume and time components

Patients who fail a trial of weaning from mechanical ventilation commonly develop hypercapnia, indicating alveolar hypoventilation. Since this is not usually accompanied by a decrease in minute ventilation [3], an increase in the physiologic deadspace-to-tidal volume ratio (V_d/V_T) is thought to be responsible for the increase in arterial carbon dioxide tension ($PaCO_2$) [1]. This explanation is supported by data of Tobin et al. [3] who found that patients who failed a weaning trial developed rapid shallow breathing, whereas patients with a successful outcome displayed no difference in breathing pattern compared with that observed during mechanical ventilation (Table 1). In the patients who failed the weaning trial a significant relationship was observed between $PaCO_2$ and tidal volume ($r = 0.84$, $p < 0.025$), whereas the correlation between $PaCO_2$ and minute ventilation was not significant (Fig. 1). Additional evidence supporting a decrease in tidal volume as the determinant of abnormal gas exchange was the lack of concomitant widening in the alveolar-arterial oxygen difference, indicating no major change in ventilation:perfusion relationships [3].

These observations were subsequently confirmed in a prospective study of 60 patients who tolerated a weaning trial and were successfully extubated and 40 patients who failed a weaning trial and required reinstitution of mechanical ventilation [4]. In this study minute ventilation was a poor predictor of weaning out-

Table 1. Breathing pattern in patients being weaned from mechanical ventilation. From [3]

	Mechanical	Weaning Trial	
	Ventilation	*Start*	*End*
Minute ventilation (L/min)			
- success group	7.11 ± 0.88	7.06 ± 0.97	7.91 ± 0.81
- failure group	7.68 ± 1.32	5.82 ± 0.53	7.31 ± 0.52
Tidal volume (ml)			
- success group	441 ± 45	398 ± 56	385 ± 51
- failure group	400 ± 61	194 ± 23	231 ± 27
Frequency (breaths/min)			
- success group	17.9 ± 1.6	20.9 ± 2.8	24.0 ± 3.0
- failure group	21.0 ± 2.0	32.3 ± 2.3	33.9 ± 2.2

Values represent mean ± SE

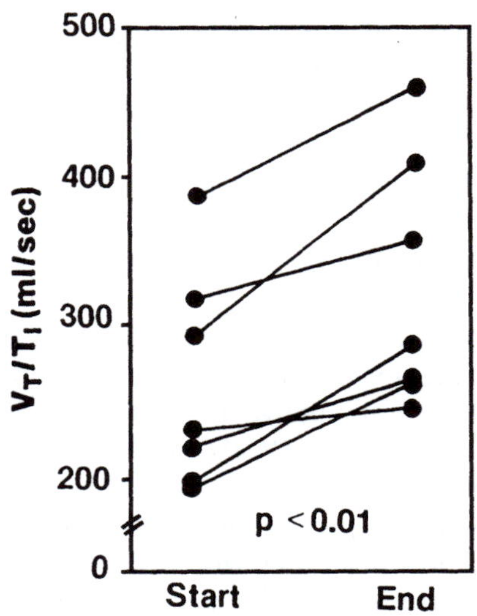

Fig. 1. Relationship between tidal volume (V_T) and respiratory frequency (f) and arterial carbon dioxide tension ($PaCO_2$) during spontaneous breathing in patients who failed a weaning trial. The equations for the regression lines are $PaCO_2$ (mm Hg) = 74.1 (V_T, ml) - 0.11 ($r = 0.84$, $p < 0.025$) and $PaCO_2$ (mm Hg) = 16.7 (f, breaths/min) + 1.13 ($r = 0.87$, $p < 0.025$). The combination of V_T and f accounted for 81 % of the variability in $PaCO_2$ [3])

come, whereas frequency (f) and tidal volume (V_t) combined as an index of rapid shallow breathing, namely the f/V_t ratio, was an accurate predictor (Fig. 2). Of the patients who had an f/V_t value greater than 100 breaths/min/L, 95 % failed a weaning trial, whereas 80 % of the patients with lower f/V_t values were success-

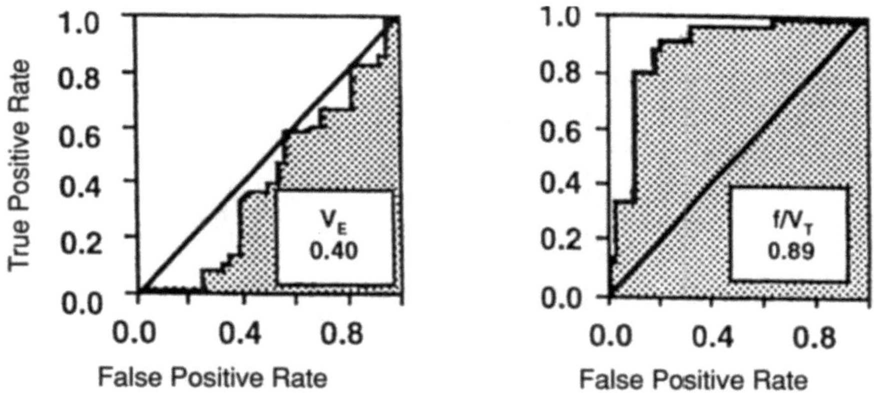

Fig. 2. Receiver-operating characteristic (ROC) curves for minute ventilation ($\dot{V}_E$) and frequency-to-tidal volume ratio (f/V_T) in patients being weaned from mechanical ventilation. The ROC curve is generated by plotting the proportion of true positive results against the proportion of false positive results for each value of a test. The curve for an arbitrary test that is expected *a priori* to have no discriminatory value appears as a diagonal line, whereas a useful test has a ROC curve that rises rapidly and reaches a plateau. The area under the curve (shaded) is expressed (in box) as a proportion of the total area of the graph. (From [4])

fully weaned. As a method of assessing pulmonary performance in critically ill patients the f/V_t ratio has a number of attractive features: it is easy to measure; it is independent of the patient's effort and cooperation; it appears to be quite accurate in predicting the ability to sustain ventilation; and, fortuitously, it has a "rounded off" threshold value (100) that is easy to remember.

An interesting observation in these studies is that the changes in frequency and tidal volume in patients who fail a trial of weaning occur immediately upon the discontinuation of mechanical ventilation (Fig. 3). The mechanism of the change in breathing pattern is unknown. The rate of lung inflation, as reflected by mean inspiratory flow (V_t/T_I), is similar in patients with a successful and unsuccessful outcome, but inspiratory time is significantly shorter in the latter group (Fig. 4) [3]. This resetting of the inspiratory off-switch results in a smaller tidal volume and faster frequency. Several factors may play a role in the activation of inspiratory-inhibiting reflexes in these patients. Stimulation of irritant or J receptors in laboratory animals characteristically produces rapid shallow breathing. It has been suggested that diaphragmatic fatigue may be responsible for the rapid shallow breathing [5, 6]. Mador and Tobin [7] investigated this question in healthy subjects in whom they induced respiratory muscle fatigue using a standard protocol of inspiratory resistive loading to task failure. Breathing pattern was recorded under resting conditions, and also during CO_2 rebreathing so as to obtain values over a wide range. The change in breathing pattern following induction of fatigue was quantitated by constructing a Hey plot [8], where an increase in the slope of the minute ventilation-tidal volume relationship signifies

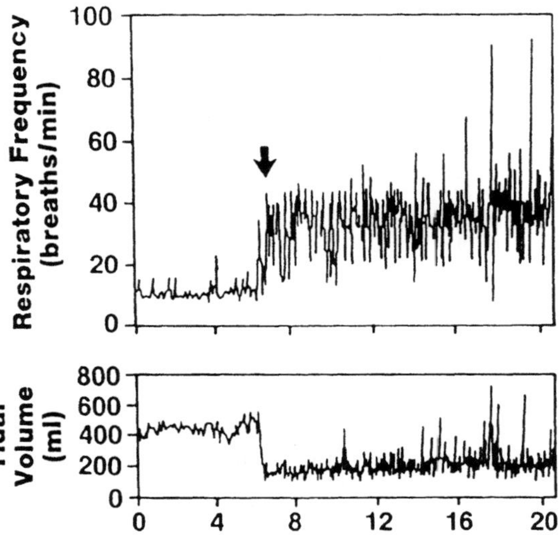

Fig. 3. A time-series, breath-by-breath plot of respiratory frequency and tidal volume in a patient who failed a weaning trial. The arrow indicates the point of resuming spontaneous breathing following discontinuation of ventilator support. Rapid, shallow breathing developed almost immediately, suggesting the prompt establishment of a new steady state. Although it has been considered that rapid, shallow breathing may reflect the presence of respiratory muscle fatigue, its almost instantaneous development without subsequent progression is difficult to reconcile with the development of respiratory muscle fatigue. (From [3])

the development of rapid shallow breathing (Fig. 5). Induction of fatigue actually caused a significant *decrease* in the slope: 27 ± 47 min^{-1} (mean ± SE) before fatigue and 19.0 ± 3.5 min^{-1} with fatigue, indicating that fatigue does not induce rapid shallow breathing. An understanding of the mechanism of rapid shallow breathing in patients who fail a weaning trial awaits further investigation.

Respiratory drive can be evaluated on a breath-by-breath basis by measuring mean inspiratory flow (V_t/T_I) [9, 10]. However, V_t/T_I is an inherently insensitive index of respiratory drive in patients with pulmonary disease, since derangements in lung function may interfere with the mechanical transformation of neural activity, leading to an underestimation of respiratory drive. Nevertheless, an increased V_t/T_I in such patients indicates elevated respiratory drive, albeit its degree may be underestimated. In a study of patients who failed a weaning trial [3] none had a value of V_t/T_I that fell below the 95 % confidence limit in normal subjects [11]. Moreover, the patients displayed an increase in V_t/T_I between the beginning and the end of the trial (Fig. 6). This indicates that impaired respiratory center output was not the primary cause of weaning failure in these patients.

Unlike conventional methods of evaluating respiratory center performance, such as the ventilatory response to carbon dioxide or airway occlusion pressure ($P_{0.1}$) [9, 10, 12, 13], breathing pattern analysis has the advantage of providing information on respiratory timing. Patients at risk of ventilatory failure can

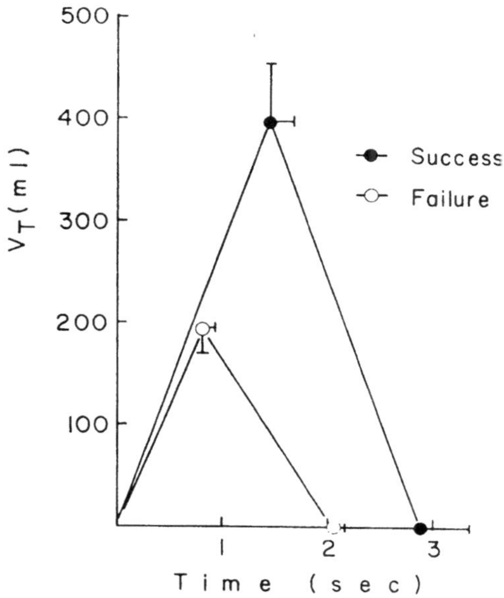

Fig. 4. The mean respiratory cycle during spontaneous breathing in 10 patients who tolerated a trial of weaning from mechanical ventilation and were extubated (success group) and in 7 patients who developed acute respiratory distress and required the reinstitution of ventilator support (failure group). Bars represent 1 SE. (From [3])

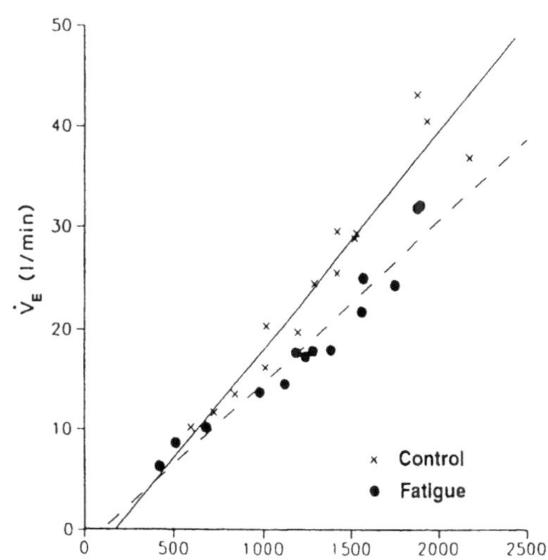

Fig. 5. The tidal volume:minute ventilation relationship (V_T: $\dot{V}_E$, Hey plot) following induction of respiratory muscle fatigue (closed symbols, interrupted line) compared with the control, non-fatigue state (crossed symbols, solid line) in a representative subject. Following the development of fatigue, the subject's breathing became slower and deeper. (From [7])

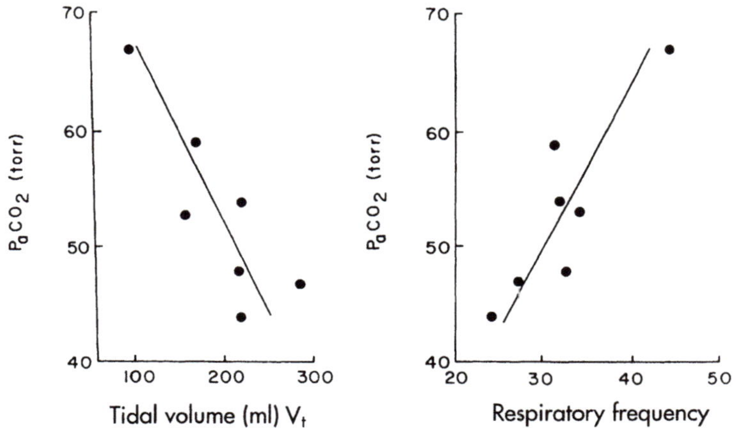

Fig. 6. Measurements of mean inspiratory flow (V_T/T_I) at the beginning and end of a trial of spontaneous breathing in patients who required the reinstitution of mechanical ventilation. (From [3])

decrease inspiratory muscle load by reducing the respiratory duty cycle (i.e., fractional inspiratory time, T_I/T_{TOT}). However, in a study of patients being weaned from mechanical ventilation T_I/T_{TOT} was similar in the successful and unsuccessful outcome groups [3], and it did not change over the course of the trial. Moreover, patients did not decrease respiratory frequency as ventilatory failure progressed. Thus, the respiratory centers continued to "push" the respiratory muscles by increasing drive, with no reduction in the frequency of contractions or in duty cycle [3].

Rib cage-abdominal motion

During normal breathing the rib cage and abdomen expand on inspiration and decrease back to the resting position during expiration. Since the rate of excursion is virtually the same for the two compartments, an X-Y plot of rib cage-abdominal motion shows the formation of a closed or a very slightly open loop [14]. Abnormal motion can be separated into three major types: [1] asynchrony, in which the two compartments continue to move in the same overall direction but the rate of motion differs, causing a widened loop to form on the X-Y plot; [2] paradox, in which one compartment moves in an opposite direction to the overall tidal volume signal, resulting in a negative slope on the X-Y plot; and [3] an increase in the breath-to-breath variation in the relative contribution of the rib cage and the abdomen to tidal volume, representing recruitment and derecruitment of the accessory intercostal muscles and diaphragm [5, 6, 10].

There has been considerable interest in the study of rib cage-abdominal motion in patients at risk of ventilatory failure. Using uncalibrated magnetometers, Ashutosh, Gilbert and colleagues [15, 16] noted that patients displaying asynchronous movements had an increased risk of ventilatory failure necessitating mechanical ventilation and a poor prognosis. Subsequently, it was suggested that abdominal paradox is virtually pathognomonic of diaphragmatic fatigue if diaphragmatic paralysis and inversion are excluded [5, 6, 17]. This interpretation was largely based on a study of 12 patients exhibiting difficulties during weaning from mechanical ventilation [5]. Seven of the patients had a power spectral shift in their diaphragmatic electromyographic (EMG) signal which was interpreted as indicating fatigue. Six of the seven patients displaying EMG changes also exhibited paradoxic motion of the abdomen. This was accompanied by "respiratory alternans" (phasic alternation in the contribution of the rib cage and abdomen to tidal volume) in four patients and six patients developed an increase in respiratory frequency; however, the degree of elevation in frequency is not clear, and no comment was made with regard to tidal volume. None of these signs were observed in the patients who did not develop EMG changes. The authors considered that these changes in breathing pattern permit a diagnosis of respiratory muscle fatigue to be made with reasonable certainty [6]. However, certain factors need to be considered before accepting this interpretation. All of the patients, including those without EMG changes and an abnormal breathing pattern, were returned to mechanical ventilation within 40 min, thus limiting the clinical significance of these findings. In addition, a shift in the EMG power spectrum has not been shown to bear a relationship to the form of fatigue that is physiologically important (i.e., low-frequency fatigue), and its physiological basis remains unknown [18]. Moreover, no attempt was made to separate the effect of respiratory load from muscle fatigue in these patients [5].

In a departure from the descriptive character of most previous studies employing Konno-Mead plots, Tobin and colleagues [19] computed several indices that provide quantitative assessment of the amount of asynchrony, paradox, and breath-to-breath variability in compartmental contribution to tidal volume. By calculating these indices from a series of breaths at fixed periods in time, it is possible to obtain a measure of the degree of inter- and intrasubject variability and thereby avoid the bias that might result with subjective selection of a few breaths. If abdominal paradox truly signifies respiratory muscle fatigue, its presence should be a good predictor of an unsuccessful weaning outcome, since, by definition, patients with fatigue cannot sustain spontaneous ventilation. In a study of patients during weaning, those who failed the weaning trial displayed significantly greater asynchrony and paradox of the rib cage and abdomen, as a group, than patients with a successful outcome [19]. However, considerable overlap in the extent of asynchrony and paradox was observed between individual patients in the two study groups (Fig. 7). Patients who failed the weaning trial also displayed greater breath-to-breath variability in the relative contribution of the rib cage and abdomen to tidal volume, quantitated in terms of the standard deviation of the rib cage/tidal volume ratio (Fig. 8) [19]. On post-hoc analysis a standard deviation of 10 % was observed in 6 of 7 (86 %) patients who failed the weaning trial, compared with only 2 of the 10 (20 %) patients who were success-

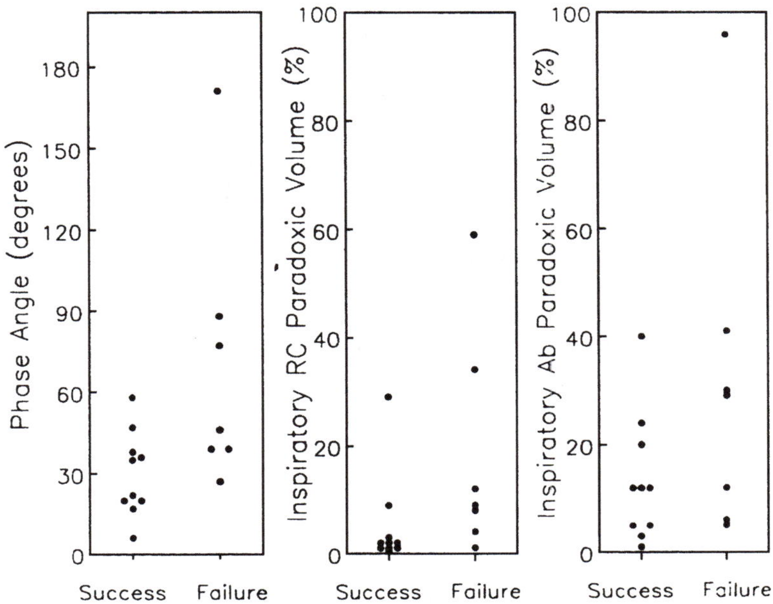

Fig. 7. Quantitative assessment of rib cage (RC)-abdominal (Ab) motion using the Konno-Mead method of analysis in 10 patients who were successfully weaned from mechanical ventilation and in 7 patients who failed a weaning trial. Each point represented the average value of four time blocks of spontaneous breathing during a weaning trial in each patient. Note the considerable overlap of values between patients of the success and failure groups. (From [19])

fully weaned ($p < 0.05$) (Fig. 9). This breath-to-breath variation in compartmental contribution suggests recruitment and derecruitment of different muscle groups, which may be an important mechanism of postponing the onset of fatigue [20].

As in the case of rapid shallow breathing, patients who failed a weaning trial developed abnormal chest motion immediately upon discontinuation of ventilator support and it showed no progression during the remainder of the trial [19]. Conceptually, it is difficult to reconcile this pattern of immediate worsening of rib cage-abdominal motion without subsequent progression with the development of respiratory muscle fatigue. The role of respiratory muscle fatigue as a determinant of abnormal rib cage-abdominal motion was investigated in healthy volunteers breathing against inspiratory resistive loads and employing an experimental design that permitted the separation of the effect of loading from fatigue [21]. While breathing against a load of sufficient magnitude to induce respiratory muscle fatigue it was noted that [1] subjects developed paradoxic motion during the first minute of loading (at which point there is load but no fatigue), [2] abnormal motion did not progress between the beginning and end of the fatigue run (load was the same throughout the run, but fatigue was present only at the end), and [3] abnormal motion disappeared immediately upon removal of the load (at

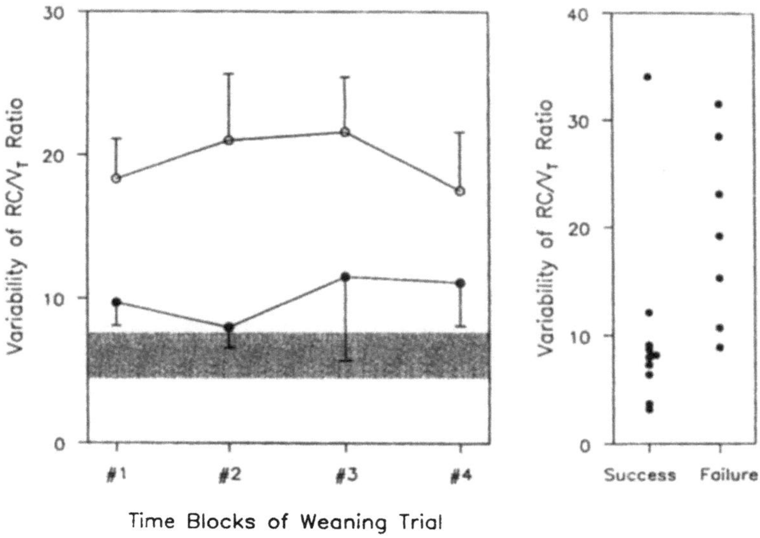

Fig. 8. *Left panel*: Sequential changes in the standard deviation of the rib cage-to-tidal volume ratio (RC/V_T) during four consecutive blocks of spontaneous breathing in 10 patients who were successfully weaned from mechanical ventilation (closed symbols) and in 7 patients who failed a weaning trial (open symbols). The shaded area represents the 95 % confidence limits of the mean value in 17 healthy subjects. The failure group displayed greater variability in the RC/V_T ratio than the success group ($p < 0.001$). Bars represent 1 SE. *Right panel*: Values of the standard deviation of the RC/V_T ratio in individual patients. Each point represents the average value of the four time blocks in each patient. A standard deviation of ≥ 10 % was observed in 6 of the patients in the failure group versus 2 of those in the success group ($p < 0.05$). (From [19])

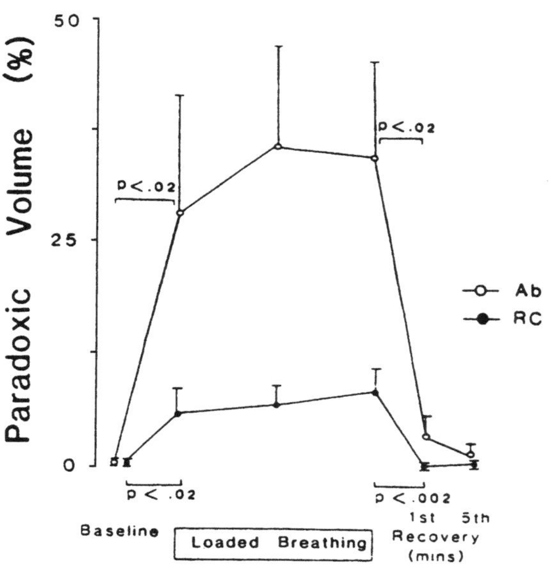

Fig. 9. Effects of breathing against a fatiguing resistive load on the inspiratory paradoxic volume of the rib cage (RC) and abdomen (Ab). Values depicted are those at baseline, first, middle and penultimate minute of the "fatigue run" and the first and fifth minute of recovery. Values are mean ± standard error for six subjects. Paradoxic volumes increased during the first minute of loaded breathing, did not progress during the loaded breathing run and returned to baseline immediately following discontinuation of the load. (From [21])

which point fatigue remained but there was no increased load) (Fig. 10). In addition, significant rib cage-abdominal asynchrony and paradox were observed in subjects breathing against lower nonfatiguing loads. Thus, it is clear that respiratory muscle fatigue is neither a sufficient nor a necessary condition for the development of rib cage-abdominal asynchrony or paradox, and that the abnormal motion is primarily determined by load rather than muscle fatigue *per se* [21].

Another possible cause of abnormal rib cage-abdominal motion is the presence of hyperinflation, since patients with chronic obstructive pulmonary disease commonly display both hyperinflation and abnormal rib cage-abdominal motion [22-24]. In addition, hyperinflation is known to have numerous adverse effects on respiratory muscle function [25]. The effect of graded levels of hyperinflation on rib cage-abdominal motion has been systematically investigated in

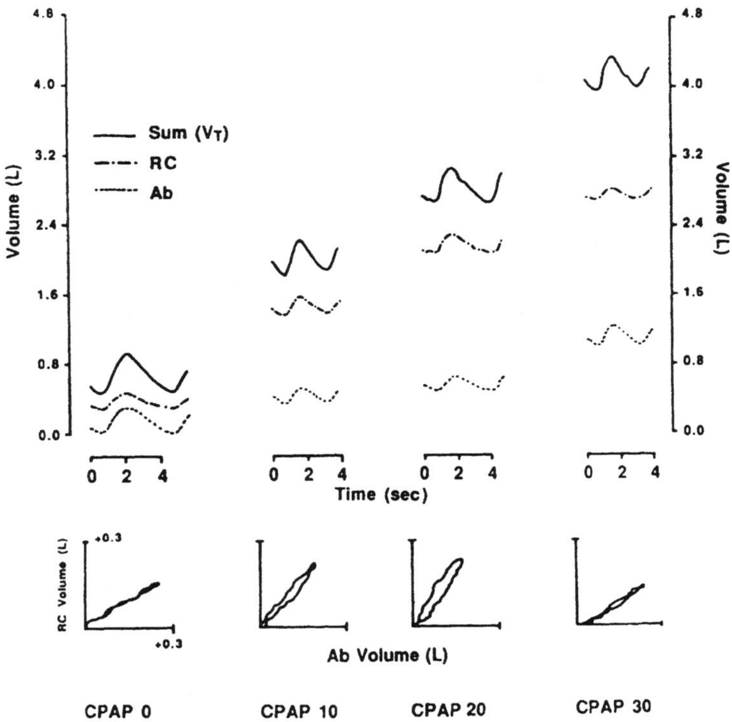

Fig. 10. Analog tracing of the sum (V_T), rib cage (RC) and abdominal (Ab) signals during the application of various levels of continuous positive airway pressure (CPAP) in a representative subject. The terminal portion of the preceding breath and the initiation of the subsequent breath are also shown. For clarity the baselines of the individual analog signals at a CPAP of 0 cm H_2O have been arbitrarily adjusted to provide visual separation of the signals, but the proportional increases at the subsequent levels of CPAP are accurately represented. The respective Konno-Mead plots of the RC-Ab relationship are displayed below each of the breaths. Clinically significant RC-Ab asynchrony or paradox did not occur, despite an increase in end-expiratory lung volume of 3.5 liters at a CPAP level of 30 cm H_2O. (From [26])

healthy subjects [26]. Despite increasing the ratio of functional residual capacity to predicted total lung capacity from 0.38 to 0.74 - comparable to the ratio observed in patients with chronic obstructive pulmonary disease - only a very slight, and clinically insignificant, increase in abdominal paradox was observed (Fig. 11). Thus, the primary mechanism of abnormal chest wall motion in patients with chronic obstructive pulmonary disease is likely to be increased airway resistance [21] and hyperinflation makes only a minor contribution.

In summary, studies of the pattern of breathing in patients who fail a trial of weaning from mechanical ventilation provide a unique opportunity to acquire a better understanding of the pathophysiologic mechanisms involved in acute ventilatory failure.

References

1. Sorli J, Grassino A, Lorange G, Milic-Emili J (1978) Control of breathing in patients with chronic obstructive pulmonary disease. Clin Sci Mol Med 54:295-304
2. Tobin MJ, Alex CG. Discontinuation of mechanical ventilation. In: Tobin MJ (ed). Principles and Practice of Mechanical Ventilation. McGraw-Hill, New York, pp 1177-1206
3. Tobin MJ, Perez W, Guenther SM, et al (1986) The pattern of breathing during successful and unsuccessful trials of weaning from mechanical ventilation. Am Rev Respir Dis 134:1111-1118
4. Yang K, Tobin MJ (1991) A prospective study of indexes predicting outcome of trials of weaning from mechanical ventilation. N Engl J Med 324:1445-1450
5. Cohen C, Zagelbaum G, Gross D, Roussos C, Macklem PT (1982) Clinical manifestations of inspiratory muscle fatigue. Am J Med 73:308-316
6. Roussos C, Macklem PT (1982) The respiratory muscles. N Engl J Med 307:786-797
7. Mador MJ, Tobin MJ (1992) The effect of inspiratory muscle fatigue on breathing pattern and ventilatory response to CO_2. J Physiol 455:17-32
8. Hey EN, Lloyd BB, Cunningham DJC, Jukes CC, Bolton DPG (1966) Effects of various respiratory stimuli on the depth and frequency of breathing in man. Respir Physiol 1:193-205
9. Milic-Emili J (1982) Recent advances in clinical assessment of control of breathing. Lung 160:1-17
10. Tobin MJ, Laghi F, Walsh JM (1994) Monitoring of respiratory neuromuscular function. In: Tobin MJ (ed). Principles and Practice of Mechanical Ventilation. McGraw-Hill, New York, pp 945-966
11. Tobin MJ, Chadha TS, Jenouri G, Birch SJ, Gazeroglu HB, Sackner MA (1983) Breathing patterns: Part 1. Normal subjects. Chest 84:202-205
12. Lopata M, Lourenco RV (1980) Evaluation of respiratory control. Clin Chest Med 1:33-45
13. Whitelaw WA, Derenne JP, Milic-Emili J (1975) Occlusion pressure as a measure of respiratory center output in conscious man. Respir Physiol 23:181-199
14. Konno K, Mead J (1967) Measurement of the separate volume changes of ribcage and abdomen during breathing. J Appl Physiol 22:407-422
15. Ashutosh K, Gilbert R, Auchincloss JH, Peppi D (1975) Asynchronous breathing movements in patients with chronic obstructive pulmonary disease. Chest 67:553-557

16. Gilbert R, Ashutosh K, Auchincloss JH, Rana S, Peppi D (1977) Prospective study of controlled oxygen therapy. Chest 71:456-462
17. Grassino A, Macklem PT (1984) Respiratory muscle fatigue and ventilatory failure. Ann Rev Med 35:625-647
18. Moxham J, Edwards HT, Aubier M, DeTroyer A, Farkas G, Macklem PT, Roussos C (1982) Changes in EMG power spectrum (high-to-low) with force fatigue in humans. J Appl Physiol 53:1094-1099
19. Tobin MJ, Guenther SM, Perez W et al (1987) Konno-Mead analysis of ribcage-abdominal motion during successful and unsuccessful trials of weaning from mechanical ventilation. Am Rev Respir Dis 135:1320-1328
20. Roussos C, Fixley M, Gross D, Macklem PT (1979) Fatigue of inspiratory muscles and their synergic behaviour. J Appl Physiol 46:897-904
21. Tobin MJ, Perez W, Guenther SM et al (1987) Does ribcage abdominal paradox signify respiratory muscle fatigue? J Appl Physiol 63:851-860
22. Sharp JT, Goldberg NB, Druz WS, Fishman HC, Danon J (1977) Thoracoabdominal motion in chronic obstructive pulmonary disease. Am Rev Respir Dis 115:47-56
23. Gilmartin JJ, Gibson GJ (1984) Abnormalities of chest wall motion in patients with chronic airflow obstruction. Thorax 39:264-271
24. Rochester DF (1991) Ventilatory failure: an overview. In: Marini JJ, Roussos C (eds)Ventilatory failure. Springer-Verlag, New York, pp 1-17
25. Tobin MJ (1988) Respiratory muscles in disease. Clin Chest Med 9:263-266
26. Jubran A, Tobin MJ (1992) The effect of hyperinflation on rib cage-abdominal motion. Am Rev Respir Dis 146:1378-1382

Chapter 9

Respiratory mechanics in COPD

J. MILIC-EMILI

Introduction

In 1954 McIlroy and Christie [1] observed that the mechanical work of breathing was increased in stable COPD patients and attributed this to increased airway and "viscous" resistance of the lung. In later studies it was suggested that in COPD patients there is an increase of work of breathing also as a result of (*a*) time constant inequality within the lung which causes an increase of effective dynamic pulmonary elastance and flow resistance [2], and (*b*) intrinsic PEEP ($PEEP_i$) [3].

Though the work of breathing has been long recognized as a useful global measure of the abnormalities in respiratory mechanics, only recently comprehensive measurements have been made in patients with severe COPD [3-5]. The inspiratory work of the respiratory system ($W_{I,rs}$) and its components in 10 mechanically ventilated sedated paralyzed COPD patients with acute respiratory failure, ARF [5] are shown in Fig. 1 together with the corresponding values obtained in 18 anesthetized paralyzed normal subjects [6]. The measurements were obtained during constant-flow inflation with a tidal volume of 0.73 l, a frequency of 12.5 bpm and an inspiratory duration of 0.92 s. $W_{I,rs}$ was two-fold greater in COPD patients that in normal subjects, the difference reflecting an increase of both static ($W_{st,rs}$) and dynamic ($W_{dyn,rs}$) work. The latter was due to an increase in airway resistive work (W_{aw}) and in the additional work done on the lung (ΔW_L) as a result of pressure dissipations caused by time constant inequality and viscoelastic behaviour of pulmonary tissue [2, 4, 5]. The dynamic work due to the tissues of the chest wall (ΔWw) was similar in COPD patients to that of normal subjects. The increase in $W_{st,rs}$ in the COPD patients was due entirely to the work due to $PEEP_i$ (W_{PEEPi}). On average, W_{PEEPi} represented 57 % of the overall increase in $W_{I,rs}$ exhibited by the COPD patients relative to normal subjects, while the corresponding values for W_{aw} and ΔW_L were 34 and 9 %, respectively.

The values of $W_{I,rs}$ in Fig. 1 do not include (*a*), the resistive work done on the endotracheal tubes which is relatively high, particularly if tubes of small size are used [5]. It should be pointed out that, for a given ventilation and breathing pattern, the work of breathing during spontaneous ventilation may be somewhat higher than during passive mechanical ventilation because during active breathing there is distortion of the chest wall from its passive (*relaxed*) configuration [7-9]. Furthermore, the data in Fig. 1 pertain to mechanical ventilation with "nor-

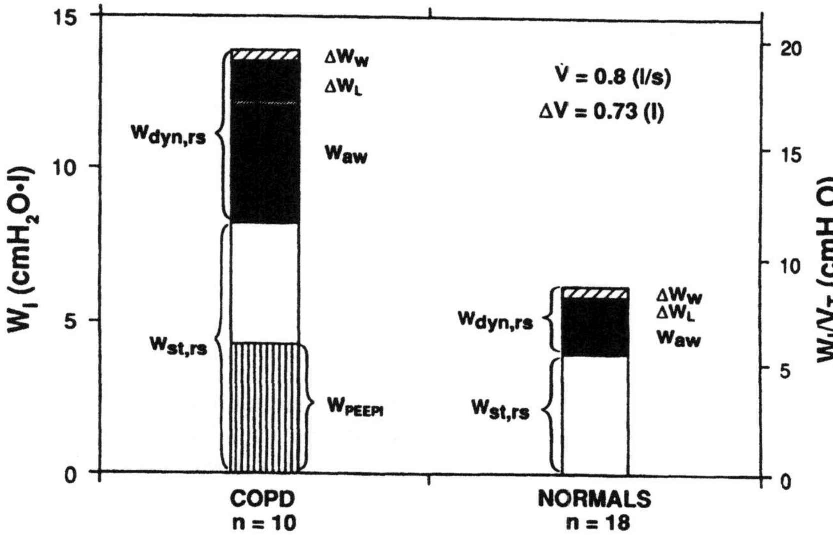

Fig. 1. Average values of inspiratory work (W_I) done of the respiratory system and its components in 10 COPD patients [5] and 18 normal anesthetized paralyzed subjects [6] with infilation flow of 0.8 l/s and tidal volume of 0.73 l. $W_{st,rs}$, total static work of respiratory system; W_{PEPPi}, static work due to intrinsic PEEP; $W_{dyn,rs}$, total dynamic work of respiratory system; W_{aw}, airway resistive work; ΔW_w, viscoelastic work of chest wall; ΔW_I, work of lung due to time constant inequality and/or viscoelasic pressure dissipations. Work per liter of inspired volume (W_I/V_T) is shown on right ordinate. (From [5])

mal" resting tidal volume whereas spontaneously breathing COPD patients with ARF usually exhibit rapid shallow breathing [3-10]. Nonetheless, the data are useful because the measurements were made under similar conditions, and hence the discrepancies between COPD patients and normal subjects are due solely to differences in respiratory mechanics. Furthermore, the COPD data in Fig. 1 pertain to patients with ARF, and hence represents extreme abnormalities of respiratory mechanics.

The right ordinate of Fig. 1 shows the total work per liter of inspired volume ($W_{I,rs}/V_T$). Since the subjects were ventilated with constant inflation flow, $W_{I,rs}/V_T$ corresponds to the mean pressure with respect to both time and volume applied during inspiration.

Static work of breathing

If $PEEP_i$ is absent and static elastance of the respiratory system ($E_{st,rs}$) is linear over the volume change considered (ΔV), the static inspiratory work per breath is given by [9]:

$$W_{I,st,rs} = 0.5\ E_{st,rs}\ \Delta V \quad (1)$$

If $PEEP_i$ is present Eq. 1 becomes:

$$W_{I,st,rs} = 0.5\ E_{st,rs}\ \Delta V + PEEP_i\ \Delta V \quad (2)$$

According to Tantucci et al. [11] and Guérin et al. [4], the values of $E_{st,rs}$ in COPD patients with ARF are similar to those of normal subjects. By contrast, Broseghini et al. [12], who studied COPD patients during the first day of mechanical ventilation, found higher values of $E_{st,rs}$ in COPD. This was probably due mainly to the fact that these patients had a more marked degree of dynamic pulmonary hyperinflation, and hence their ΔV during mechanical ventilation impinged into the flat part of their static volume-pressure (V-P) curves (*see below*).

Since in the COPD patients of Fig. 1 $E_{st,rs}$ was the same as in normal subjects, all of the increase in $W_{I,st,rs}$ was due to $PEEP_i$ (=5.7 cmH_2O), as indicated by Eq. 2. By contrast, in the COPD patients of Broseghini et al. [12] the increase in $W_{I,st,rs}$ was due both to $PEEP_i$ and increased $E_{st,rs}$. Also in these patients, however, most of the increase of static work was due to $PEEP_i$ which reflects dynamic pulmonary hyperinflation.

Pulmonary hyperinflation

In normal subjects at rest the end-expiratory lung volume (functional residual capacity, FRC) corresponds to the relaxation volume (Vr) of the respiratory system, i.e. the lung volume at which the elastic recoil pressure of the total respiratory system is zero [7] (Fig. 2). Pulmonary hyperinflation is defined as an increase of FRC above predicted normal. This may be due to increased Vr due to loss of elastic recoil of the lung (e.g. emphysema) or to *dynamic pulmonary hyperinflation* which is said to be present when the FRC exceeds Vr [13]. Dynamic hyperinflation exists whenever the duration of expiration is insufficient to allow the lungs to deflate to Vr prior to the next inspiration. This tends to occur under conditions in which expiratory flow is impeded (e.g. increased airway resistance) or when the expiratory time is shortened (eg. increased breathing frequency) [13, 14]. Expiratory flow may also be retarded by other mechanisms such as persistent contraction of the inspiratory muscles during expiration and expiratory narrowing of the glottic aperture. Most commonly, however, dynamic pulmonary hyperinflation is observed in patients who exhibit expiratory flow limitation during resting breathing.

In COPD patients with ARF expiratory flow limitation during resting breathing and the concomitant dynamic hyperinflation are almost invariably present and play a paramount role in causing respiratory failure. Accordingly, in the next sections I will review the physiologic and clinical implications of dynamic hyperinflation and outline some of the treatment strategies which are available to deal with its effects.

Effects of dynamic hyperinflation on work of breathing and mechanical performance of the inspiratory muscles

Figure 2 illustrates the static elastic work required from the inspiratory muscles for the same tidal volume inhaled from Vr and from a higher lung volume. As shown by the hatched areas, $W_{st,rs}$ increases markedly when the breath is taken at a higher lung volume. In this example the increase in $W_{I,st,rs}$ is due mainly to $PEEP_i$, though an increase in $E_{st,rs}$ (as reflected by the decreased slope of the static V-P curve at the higher lung volume) also plays a role. Clearly, during spontaneous breathing dynamic hyperinflation implies an increase of static inspiratory work, and hence in inspiratory muscle effort. Furthermore, as lung volume increases there is a concomitant decrease in effectiveness of the inspiratory muscles as pressure generators, because the inspiratory muscle fibres become shorter and their geometrical arrangement changes [7]. Thus, in COPD patients there is a vicious cycle: $W_{I,aw}$ is invariably increased due to airway obstruction which in

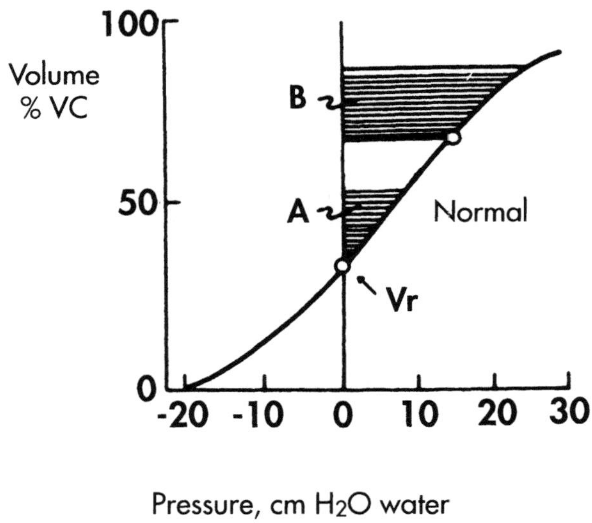

Fig. 2. Volume pressure diagram of the relaxed respiratory system showing the increase in static elastic work caused by dynamic hyperinflation. VC, vital capacity; Vr, relaxation volume of the respiratory system. *Hatched area A*, elastic work for a breath that starts from relaxation volume. *Hatched area B*, elastic work for a similar breath that starts from a volume 29 % VC higher than Vr. In case B, the intrinsic PEEP is 15 cmH_2O, as indicated by the upper circle, and W_{PEEPi} is given by $PEEP_i \cdot V_T$ tidal volume. (From [8])

turn promotes dynamic hyperinflation with a concomitant increase in elastic work and impaired mechanical performance of the inspiratory muscles. With increasing severity of airway obstruction, a critical point is eventually reached at which the inspiratory muscles become fatigued [11, 12].

Intrinsic PEEP

Under normal conditions the end-expiratory elastic recoil pressure of the respiratory system is zero (case A in Fig. 2). In this instance, as soon as the inspiratory muscles contract the alveolar pressure becomes subatmospheric and gas flows into the lungs. When breathing takes place at lung volumes higher than Vr the end-expiratory elastic recoil pressure is positive (15 cmH_2O in case B of Fig. 1). The elastic recoil pressure present at end-expiration has been termed occult PEEP [21], auto PEEP [15], or intrinsic PEEP ($PEEP_i$) [14]. When $PEEP_i$ is present the onset of inspiratory muscle activity and inspiratory flow are not synchronous: inspiratory flow starts only when the pressure developed by the inspiratory muscles exceeds $PEEP_i$ because only then does alveolar pressure become subatmospheric. In this respect, intrinsic PEEP acts as an inspiratory threshold load which increases the static elastic work of breathing. As indicated above, this places a significant burden on the inspiratory muscles which are operating under disadvantageous force-length conditions and abnormal thoracic geometry [7].

$PEEP_i$ in COPD patients with ARF

The highest values of $PEEP_i$ observed in stable COPD patients are in the order of 7-9 cmH_2O [16]. In COPD patients with ARF higher values have been reported: up to 13 cmH_2O during spontaneous breathing [3, 17, 18] and 22 cmH_2O during mechanical ventilation [12]. Such high values of $PEEP_i$ have profound consequences on the mechanics and energetics of breathing, as shown schematically in Fig. 3. Acute ventilatory failure in COPD patients is usually triggered by airway infection. As a result, there is an acute increase in airway resistance which causes increased resistive work of breathing and promotes dynamic hyperinflation. The latter is further exacerbated by the tachypnea which is invariably present in acutely ill COPD patients [7, 13]. Dynamic hyperinflation promotes an increase in the static elastic work of breathing which can be due both to $PEEP_i$ and decreased lung compliance (Fig. 2) [15]. The increase in work of breathing, in association with the impaired inspiratory muscle performance, promotes inspiratory muscle fatigue. As a result, the patient needs to be mechanically ventilated.

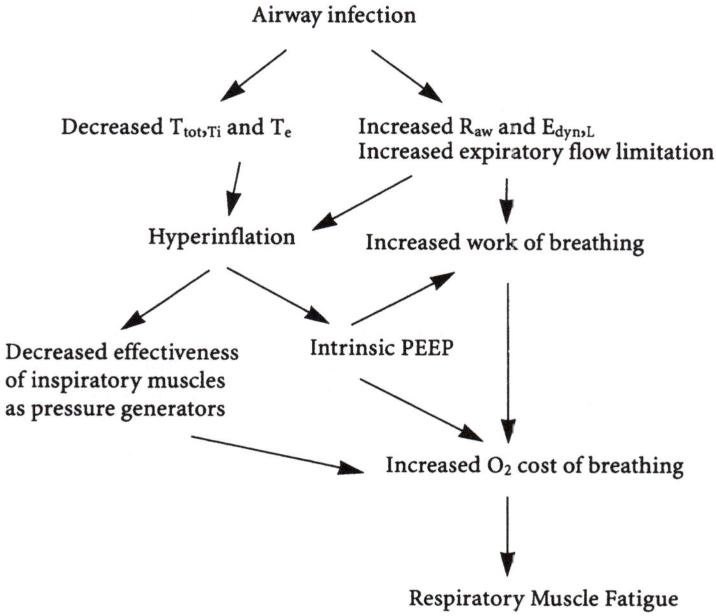

Fig. 3. Scheme of the pathophysiology causing acute ventilatory failure in COPD patients. T_{tot}, total breathing cycle duration; T_i and T_e, inspiratory and expiratory times; R_{aw}, airway resistance; $E_{dyn,L}$, dynamic lung elastance

Implications of $PEEP_i$ during mechanical ventilation

The putative role of mechanical ventilation is to reduce the activity of the inspiratory muscles to tolerable levels during patient-triggered mechanical ventilation (eg. assisted mechanical ventilation, AMV). During AMV this end is not always achieved because the pressure which has to be generated by the patient to trigger the ventilator necessarily includes $PEEP_i$. If this is high the inspiratory effort required by the patient may be excessive [19]. In contrast, during controlled mechanical ventilation all of the work of breathing is done by the ventilator. Nevertheless, $PEEP_i$ must be taken into account for correct measurement of respiratory compliance [14] and, more importantly, in terms of its adverse effects on cardiac output [15]. Patients with high levels of $PEEP_i$ are implicitly difficult to wean from mechanical ventilation and may become ventilator-dependent.

Monitoring $PEEP_i$

Fundamental in the management of the mechanically ventilated COPD patients is to monitor $PEEP_i$ [8]. Indeed, measurement of $PEEP_i$ should become a part of routine monitoring in mechanically ventilated patients, particularly those with airways obstruction. This will allow for reliable measurement and interpretation of other frequently determined cardiopulmonary variables, such as respiratory system compliance, pulmonary capillary wedge pressure, etc. The potential adverse effects of $PEEP_i$ require that, in addition, management should be specifically directed towards those factors contributing to the development of $PEEP_i$. This includes medical therapy aimed at reducing the severity of airflow obstruction as well as excessive minute ventilation due to fever, metabolic acidosis, inadequate pain relief, etc. The inspiratory flow settings should be adjusted such as to maximize the time available for passive expiration.

Strategies to reduce the inspiratory load caused by $PEEP_i$

Treatment of COPD patients with respiratory failure should be aimed toward increasing the expiratory duration as well as decreasing respiratory flow-resistance. To the extent that tachypnea is due to fever and/or airway infection, resolution of these by conventional treatment should be beneficial. Similarly, effective bronchodilator administration may be useful in reducing both flow-resistance and $PEEP_i$. A less conventional but promising approach to deal with $PEEP_i$ is the use of continuous positive pressure breathing (CPAP). Indeed, CPAP has been found to reduce the magnitude of inspiratory muscle effort and the work of breathing in stable patients with severe COPD [19]. Furthermore, CPAP has also been found to reduce the work of breathing and dyspnea in patients with severe COPD during weaning from mechanical ventilation [18]. This is related to a reduction in the inspiratory workload imposed by $PEEP_i$. In addition, CPAP administered through a face or nasal mask [20] may also be of therapeutic benefit during an acute exacerbation of severe COPD in the nonintubated patient. Conceivably, the early use of CPAP in this setting could preclude the need for intubation and mechanical ventilation in some COPD patients. Finally, it should also be noted that application of external PEEP during patient-triggered mechanical ventilation can counterbalance and reduce the inspiratory load imposed by $PEEP_i$ [19].

Detection of expiratory flow limitation during resting breathing

Patients with severe airway obstruction commonly exhibit expiratory flow limitation during resting breathing, particularly during acute exacerbations of their disease [7]. Such patients in general exhibit pronounced pulmonary hyperinflation with markedly increased work of breathing and markedly impaired inspiratory muscle function [3-5, 7]. Patients who are flow limited during mechanical ventilation are difficult to wean. Accordingly, detection of airflow limitation during quiet breathing appears to be important.

Several methods have been proposed to detect expiratory flow limitation in mechanically ventilated patients: (*a*) removal of external PEEP, if present [13]; (*b*) addition of a resistance to the expiratory circuit [13], and (*c*) application of a negative pressure of 5 cmH_2O at the airway opening during a single expiration [21]. The latter method can also be applied during spontaneous breathing [22].

Figure 4 depicts expiratory flow-volume curves obtained during passive expiration in a mechanically ventilated COPD patient with ARF (Pat. 3) and in a subject without airways obstruction (Pat. 2). In patient 2 application of negative pressure during expiration resulted in a sustained increase of expiratory flow indicating absence of expiratory flow limitation during tidal breathing. By contrast, in patient 3 application of the negative pressure resulted in no change of expiratory flow, except for a transient change immediately after application of the negative pressure which reflects displacement of gas from the expiratory line due to decompression. This lack of response to negative pressure (apart from the transient) occurs when expiratory flow limitation is present. Thus, expiratory flow limitation during resting breathing can be readily detected by analysis of expiratory flow-volume or flow-time relationships before and after application of negative pressure.

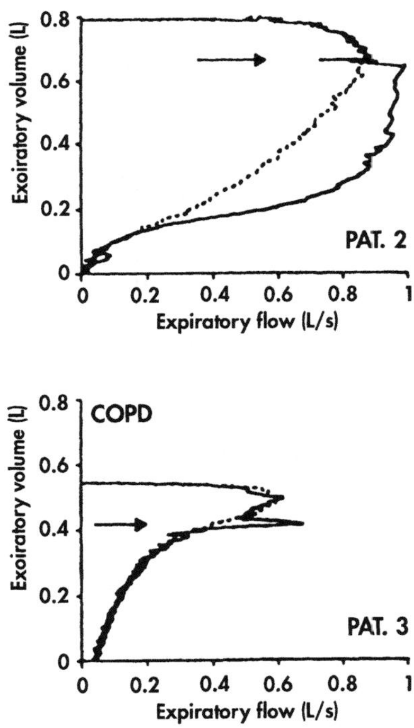

Fig. 4. Expiratory flow-volume relationships during passive expiration in a mechanically ventilated patient with COPD (*botton*) and in a patient without airway obstruction (*top*). *Broken line*: baseline expiration; *solid line*: subsequent during which a negative of -5 cm H_2O was applied at points indicated by arrows and maintained throughout the rest of expiration. (From [21])

Airway resistive work

In the COPD patients in Fig. 1 $W_{I,aw}$ was on average 3.3 times higher than in the normal subjects, the increase in $W_{I,aw}$ representing 34 % of the overall increase in $W_{I,rs}$ observed in the COPD patients.

The increase in W_{aw} in the COPD patients reflects increased airway resistance (R_{aw}) [4, 7]. According to Tantucci et al. [11] and Guerin et al. [4], at similar inflation volume and flow, R_{aw} in COPD patients with ARF is about 3.5 times higher than in normal subjects. Higher values of R_{aw} were found by Broseghini et al. [12], presumably because their patients were studied on the first day of ARF.

In COPD patients with ARF, R_{aw} exhibits more marked flow dependence than in normal subjects, as indicated by the higher values of the constant K_2 in Table 1. As for R_{aw}, at fixed inflation volume, W_{aw} (and hence $W_{aw}/\Delta V$) increases with increasing flow while at fixed inflation flow, $Waw/\Delta V$ decreases with increasing volume [5].

Table 1. Mean values (± SE) of constants K_1 and K_2 of Rohrer's equation: $R_{aw} = K_1 + K_2 \dot{V}$ of 10 COPD patients [4] and 18 normal subjects. (From [6])

	COPD	Normals
K_1, cm $H_2O \cdot l^{-1} \cdot s$	5.03 ± 0.45	1.85 ± 0.13*
K_2, cm $H_2O \cdot l^{-2} \cdot s^2$	2.69 ± 0.63	0.43 ± 0.03*

R_{aw}, airway resistance
* $P < 0.001$ between COPD and normals

The results in Fig. 1 do not include the inspiratory resistive work done on the endotracheal tubes ($W_{I,ET}$). Because the resistance offered by the endotrachel tubes in relatively high [13], $W_{I,ET}$ was also high: with endotracheal tubes of size 7 and 9 it amounted to 4.8 and 2.0 cm $H_2O \cdot l$, respectively [5]. For tube size 7, $W_{I,ET}$ was higher than W_{aw} (4.8 *vs.* 3.8 cm $H_2O \cdot l$) while for tube size 9 the opposite was true (2.0 *vs.* 3.8 cm $H_2O \cdot l$) [5]. Thus, the endotracheal tubes represent substantial respiratory loads.

Additional work

In 1955 Mount [23] assessed the dynamic pulmonary work per breathing cycle ($W_{dyn,L}$), as given by volume-pressure loops, in mechanically ventilated open-chest rats. To explain the relatively high values of $W_{dyn,L}$ found at low respiratory frequencies and the progressive decrease in dynamic pulmonary compliance ($C_{dyn,L}$) with increasing frequency, he proposed a viscoelastic model of the lung which "confers time-dependency of the elastic properties". In normal subjects, ΔW_L essentially reflects viscoelastic behaviour [6], as postulated by Mount. By contrast, in COPD patients ΔW_L should include a substantial component due to time constant inequality [2, 5]. This probably explains the higher values of ΔW_L found in the COPD patients with ARF (Fig. 1) in whom ΔW_L was on average 2.3 times higher than in normal subjects. This increase of ΔW_L, however, represented only 9 % of the overall increase in $W_{I,rs}$ observed in the COPD patients. By contrast, there was no difference in ΔW_w between COPD patients and normal subjects.

Predicably, the increase of ΔW_L in COPD patients is associated with more marked time-dependency of pulmonary elastance than in normal subjects, as shown in Fig. 5 which depicts the relationship of static and dynamic elastance of the lung ($E_{dyn,L} = 1/C_{dyn,L}$) to inspiratory flow obtained at a fixed inflation volume (ΔV=0.73 l) in 10 COPD patients with ARF [4] and 18 normal subjects [6]. While $E_{st,L}$ was independent of flow in both COPD patients and normals, $E_{dyn,L}$, increased progressively with increasing, or, more appropriately, with decreasing duration of inspiration (T_I). Indeed, at fixed inflation volume an increase in flow

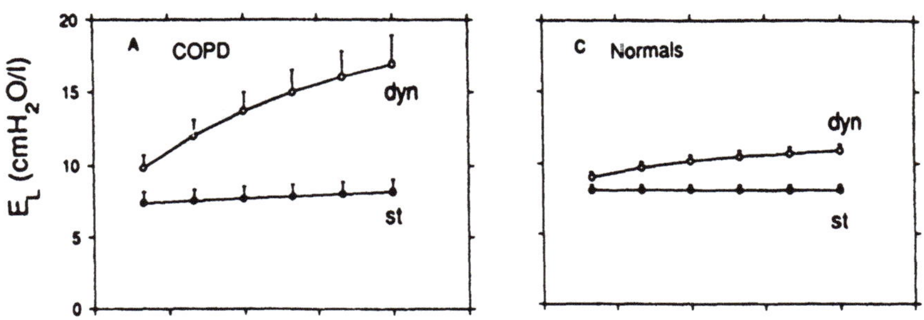

Fig. 5. Average relationship of static (*st*) and dynamic (*dyn*) elastance of the lung (E_L) to flow ($\dot{V}$) at constant inflation volume (0.73 l) of 10 COPD with ARF patients [4] (*left*) and 18 normal subjects [6] (*left*). Bars, SE when larger than symbols. (From [4])

implies a shorter duration of inspiration ($T_I = \Delta V / \dot{V}$ *where* ΔV *is constant*), and hence the data in Fig. 5 actually depict T_I-dependency of elastic properties. In COPD patients the increase in $E_{dyn,L}$ with increasing $\dot{V}$ (and hence with decreasing T_i) was greater than in normal subjects because of time constant inequality [2, 5]. In normal lungs the time-dependency of pulmonary elastance is due almost entirely to viscoelastic behaviour [6].

Figure 6 depicts the average relationships between total flow resistance (R_{rs}) and inspiratory flow obtained at fixed inflation volume (ΔV = 0.5 l) in patients with ARF and normal subjects. At all comparable flow rates R_{rs} was about threefold higher in the COPD patients. In both normals and COPD patients R_{rs} was highest at the lowest flow and decreased progressively with up to 1 l/s. At this $\dot{V}$ R_{rs} had a minimal value. This phenomenon is due to the fact that as $\dot{V}$ increased there was a greater decrease of viscoelastic resistances as compared to the con-

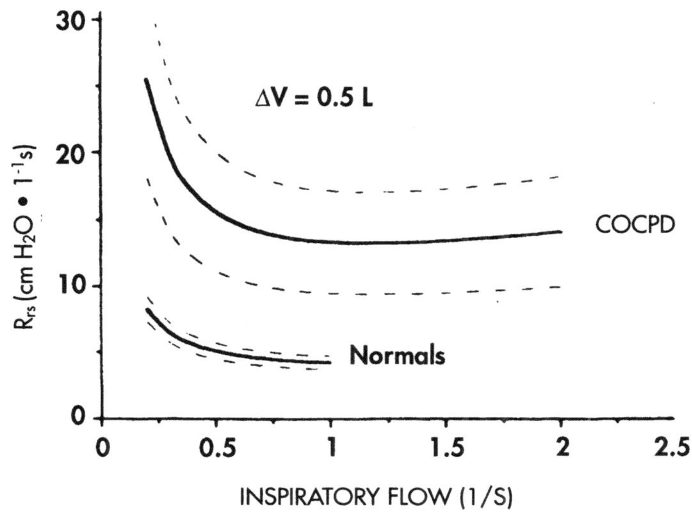

Fig. 6. Average (± SE) relationship between total resistance of respiratory system (R_{rs}) and inspiratory flow at inflation volume (ΔV) of 0.5 l in 6 sedated paralyzed COPD patients with ARF [11] and 16 normal anesthetized paralyzed subjects [6]. (From [11])

comitant increase of R_{aw} (Table 1). The initial decrease in R_{rs} with increasing flow represents a clinically important aspect because it occurs in the range of inflation flows commonly used in the ICU setting (0.5 to 1 l/s).

References

1. Mcllroy MB, Christie RV (1954) The work of breathing in emphysema. J Clin Sci 13:147-154
2. Otis AB, Mckerrow CB, Bartlett RA et al (1956) Mechanical factors in distribution of pulmonary ventilation. J Appl Physiol 8:427-443
3. Fleury B, Murciano D, Talamo C et al (1985) Work of breathing in patients with chronic obstructive pulmonary disease in acute respiratory failure. Am Rev Respir Dis 131:822-827
4. Guerin C, Coussa M-L, Eissa NT et al (1993) Lung and chest wall mechanics in mechanically ventilated COPD patients. J Appl Physiol 74:1570-1580
5. Coussa ML, Guerin C, Eissa NT et al (1993) Partitioning of work of breathing in mechanically ventilated COPD patients. J Appl Physiol 75:1711-1719
6. D'Angelo E, Robatto FM, Calderini E et al (1991) Pulmonary and chest wall mechanics in anesthetized paralyzed humans. J Appl Physiol 70:2602-2610
7. Sharp JT (1955) The chest wall and respiratory muscles in airflow limitation. In: Roussos Ch, Macklem PT (eds) The Thorax. Marcel Dekker, New York, pp 1155-1202
8. Eissa NT, Milic-Emili J (1991) Modern concepts in monitoring and management of respiratory failure. Anesthesiol Clin 9:199-218
9. Milic-Emili J (1991) Work of Breathing. In: Crystal RG, West JB (eds) The Lung: Scientific Foundations. Raven Press Ltd, New York, pp 1065-1075

10. Aubier M, Murciano D, Fournier M et al (1980) Central respiratory drive in acute respiratory failure of patients with chronic obstructive pulmonary disease. Am Rev Respir Dis 122:191-200
11. Tantucci C, Corbeil C, Chasse M et al (1991) Flow resistance in patients with chronic obstructive pulmonary disease in acute respiratory failure. Am J Respir Dis 144:384-89
12. Broseghini C, Brandolese R, Poggi R et al (1988) Respiratory mechanics during the first day of mechanical ventilation in patients with pulmonary edema and chronic airway obstruction. Am Rev Respir Dis 138:355-361
13. Gottfried SB, Rossi A, Higgs BD et al (1985) Noninvasive determination of respiratory system mechanics during mechanical ventilation for acute respiratory failure. Am Rev Respir Dis 131:414-420
14. Rossi A, Gottfried SB, Zocchi L et al (1985) Measurement of static compliance of the total respiratory system in patients with acute respiratory failure during mechanical ventilation. Am Rev Respir Dis 131:672-677
15. Pepe PE, Marini JJ (1982) Occult positive end-expiratory pressure in mechanically ventilated patients with airflow obstruction. Am Rev Respir Dis 126:166
16. Haluszka J, Chartrand DA, Grassino AE et al (1990) Intrinsic PEEP and arterial $PC0_2$ in stable patients with chronic obstructive pulmonary disease. Am Rev Respir Dis 141:1194-1197
17. Gottfried SB, Rossi A, Milic-Emili J (1986) Dynamic hyperinflation, intrinsic PEEP, and the mechanically ventilated patient. Int Care Dig 5:30-33
18. Petrof BJ, Legare M, Goldberg P et al (1990) Continuous positive airway pressure reduces work of breathing and dyspnea during weaning from mechanical ventilation in severe chronic obstructive pulmonary disease. Am Rev Respir Dis 141:281-289
19. Smith TC, Marini JJ (1988) Impact of PEEP on lung mechanics and work of breathing in severe airflow obstruction. J Appl Physiol 65:1488-1499
20. Petrof BJ, Kimoff RJ, Cheong TH et al (1989) Nasal continuous positive airway pressure reduces inspiratory muscle effort during sleep in severe chronic obstructive pulmonary disease. Am Rev Respir Dis 139:A496
21. Valta P, Campodonico R, Corbeil C et al (1994) Detection of expiratory flow limitation during mechanical ventilation. Am J Respir Crit Care Med 150:1311-1317
22. Koulouris N, Valta P, Lavoie A et al (1995) A simple technique to detect expiratory flow limitation during resting breathing. Eur Respir J 8:306-313
23. Mount LE (1955) The ventilation flow-resistance and compilation of rat lungs. J Physiol 127:157-167

Chapter 10

Work of breathing in ventilated patients

L. BROCHARD

Introduction

Assessment of respiratory muscular effort and its quantification by measuring the work of breathing is now considered an important aspect of the efficacy evaluation of assisted modes of ventilation [1, 2]. Indeed the amount of work or effort performed by the patient may vary considerably with the ventilatory settings. This has the potential of changing the global energy expenditure of the patient and may influence the duration of mechanical ventilation or outcome of weaning from ventilation.

Quantification of patient's effort or work of breathing

During spontaneous respiration the work of breathing is performed by the respiratory muscles of the patient. During controlled mechanical ventilation the work is performed by the machine. During assisted ventilation, which is used during the vast majority of episodes of mechanical ventilation, both the patient and the machine perform part of the work. The interaction between patient and ventilator plays a major role in patient's dyspnea and comfort. Assessment of the work or effort performed by the patient during assisted ventilation allows to assess the synchrony between patient and ventilator and to determine which settings act to reduce breathing workload.

The following indexes can be measured.

Work of breathing

Work is done when a force moves its point of application, it being equal to the product of force and distance moved, or to the product of the mean pressure and the change in volume [3, 4]. The work of breathing is computed as the integrated surface area enclosed in the inspiratory part of the pressure volume loop [3-5]. When the transpulmonary pressure is taken for computation, then the amount of work performed on the lungs and airways is calculated, regardless of the "engine" performing this work i.e., respiratory muscles or ventilator. The relevant pressure in assessing respiratory muscle activity is pleural pressure, estimated as esophageal minus atmospheric pressure. As in all integrals, the reference line over which integration in performed is a crucial point. For the respiratory system this reference is represented by the value of esophageal pressure over lung capacity under passive conditions, which is referred to as the chest wall compliance curve. When dynamic hyperinflation is present, the beginning of the inspiration (detected as beginning of inspiratory flow) may differ from the value of the elastic recoil pressure of the chest wall by an amount assessed as auto-positive end expiratory pressure or intrinsic-$PEEP_i$ [6]. Taking this value into account has major influence on the results of the measurement. For instance, it has been recently shown that the work needed to overcome $PEEP_i$ is in the range of 30-40 % of total work in COPD patients [7]. Work can be expressed as power of breathing (work performed per minute) or per liter of ventilation. The two expressions have different meanings.

Pressure time integral

Integration of pressure over time may give a good estimate of the force develepped by the patient, whatever the result of this effort in terms of volume displacement. The pressure time index was initially described for the diaphragm as the product of the mean transdiaphragmatic pressure, expressed as a fraction of the maximal pressure the diaphragm can develop, and the inspiratory duty cycle [8]. The same can be applied for the inspiratory muscles, using esophageal instead of transdiaphragmatic pressure. Because the maximal pressure is often not obtained or is unreliable in the critical care setting, measurement of the pressure time product or pressure time index over one minute has been proposed as the sum of integrals of esophageal pressure versus time over 60 seconds.

Simplifed methods

During airway occlusion the airway pressure swings measured at the tip of the endotracheal tube reflect the esophageal pressure swings, since lung volume does not change. The first two three breathing efforts performed immediately after occlusion may reasonably reflect the effect performed before this occlusion and could therefore be used to estimate a pressure time product per breath [9].

An inspiratory effort quotient can also be estimated in the ICU from dynamic compliance and tidal volume which allows to calculate a mean pressure per breath, the maximal inspiratory force measured after occlusion and the duty cycle [10].

Differences among these methods

There are a number of potential problems or limitations with measurement of work. As work is dissipated only in the case of displacement of gas, all isometric efforts, such as those performed during a closed demand valve or mainly resulting in chest wall distortion, do not produce work [5].

$PEEP_i$ is incorporated in the measurement of work and therefore this problem is not crucial for most measurements during assisted ventilation. During ineffective efforts however performed while the demand valve remains closed, work is obviously not appropriate to assess the amount of effort. Another potential problem with the measurement of work is it's highly dependency on inspired volume. During assisted ventilation this volume is, at least partially, passively delivered to the patient. Therefore, and especially in case of dysynchrony with a time lag between patient's effort and volume delivery by the ventilator, the amount of effort may be over estimated by assessment of work.

In part due to the above-mentioned problems, several studies have preferred measurement of the pressure time integral since it offers a way of computing the patient's effort independently of the resulting tidal volume [11]. It has been claimed that this measurement may better correlate with the oxygen cost of breathing or the oxygen consumption of the respiratory muscles [12]. This is based on very few data, however, and good correlations have also been found for the power of breathing [13]. It is logical to prefer the pressure time integral to compute patient's efforts in many situations, but comparison with the evaluation of the work of breathing should also be done, and when the results of the two methods differ an explanation should be given.

Main determinants of the inspiratory work in ventilated patients

The trigger sensitivity

The trigger sensitivity has a very reprodicible influence on the amount of work performed by the patients as shown in several studies with different modes of ventilation [14, 17]. A higher work may result from the set-up adjusted by the physician (more negative pressure to reach), from the intrinsic properties of the demand valve (long time response) or from the type of triggering device-pressure triggering or flow triggering upon an expiratory bias flow. Although some contradictory results have been published on bench studies, it has been shown that flow triggering systems offer better sensitivity and impose less work on the patients [18, 19].

The inspiratory flow rate

The peak flow rate is a major determinant of the amount of work performed during mechanical ventilation [15, 20]. During assist-control ventilation, Ward and co-workers found an inverse relationship between the amount of work performed and the peak flow rate [16]. This was also found in normal subjects with high ventilatory requirements [15]. Pressure support ventilation is an illustrative example of the importance of the peak flow rate. Indeed, the peak flow is increased when increasing the pressure support level, which decreases patient's work of breathing [13]. This is illustrated in Fig. 1.

We recently compared assisted control ventilation (ACV) and assisted pressure control ventilation (APCV), a mode in which the limited variable is pressure

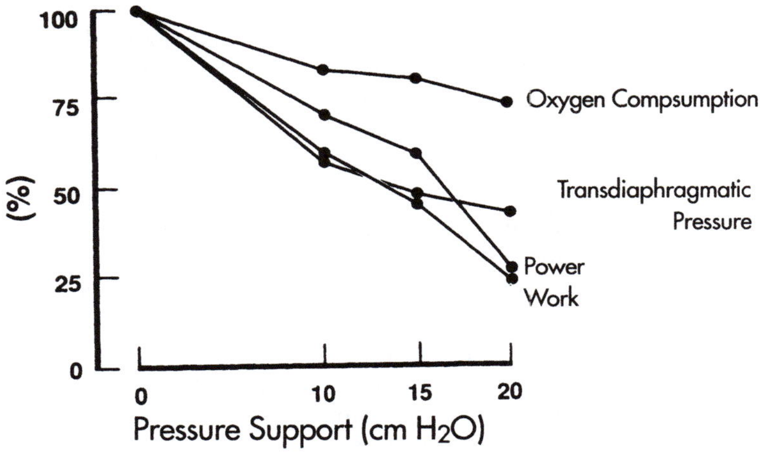

Fig. 1. Illustration of the effects of pressure support ventilation delivered at increasing levels from 0 to 20 cm H_2O to reduce the patient's work of breathing estimated from different indexes. These measurements were obtained in eight difficult-to-wean patients. (Adapted from [13])

(in contrast to ACV) and the cycling variable is time (as in ACV) [21]. When the respective settings of the two modes resulted in a large tidal volume (12 ml/kg), the amount of work or effort perfomed by the patient was small and showed no difference between the two modes. When a smaller tidal volume was used (8 ml/kg) the results were highly dependent on the peak flow setting. When a relatively low flow was used, i.e., a 1 second inspiratory time for the two modalities, then work and effort were much higher and with a square wave flow pattern than with APCV which offers a higher initial peak flow rate with a decelerating ramp. When, for the same tidal volume, the flow rate was increased in both situations, i.e., setting inspiratory time to 0.6 s for the two modalities, then differences between the two methods again became small and non significant. This suggests that when the peak flow rate, and more importantly its initial part, is lower than the patient's demand, the inspiratory drive of the patient is stimulated and the total amount of effort performed over the breath is increased.

Mechanical ventilator

The same ventilatory mode delivered with identical settings by different ventilators can result in different amounts of respiratory workload. This has been especially studied for pressure support ventilation (PSV). We found that the amount of work performed with 15 cm H_2O of PSV was twofold more with one ventilator compared to another [22]. This difference resulted probably from many factors such as: trigger sensitivity (although at PSV 0 cm H_20 no significant difference appeared), the ventilator's algorithm to deliver pressure support and particularly the rate of rise in pressure [23], the cycling criterion from inspiration to expiration and expiratory resistances which markedly differed from one ventilator to another, with the potential to induce dynamic hyperinflation, promote active expiration work or increase the sense of dyspnea.

Respiratory drive of the patient

The respiratory drive remains a major determinant of the work performed by the patient since most ventilatory modes do not adapt to an increase in the patient's demand. Proportional assist ventilation could be the exception by adapting the pressure given in proportion to the flow and volume taken by the patient [24]. There is however only limited clinical experience.

Changes in metabolic energy expenditure, cardiac output or any changes in ventilatory demand caused by many different stimulus, such as increased dead space, stimulation of irritant receptors, hypoxemia, pain or anxiety, result in a higher level of power of breathing or patient's effort.

References

1. Iotti G, Brochard L, Lemaire F (1991) Mechanical ventilation and weaning. In: Zapol W, Tinker J (eds) Care of the critically ill. J. London 2nd edition, pp 457-478
2. Kacmarek RM (1988) The role of pressure support ventilation in reducing work of breathing. Respir Care 33:99-120
3. Campbell EJM, Westlake EK, Cherniak RM (1957) Simple methods of estimating oxygen consumption and efficiency of the muscles of breathing. J Appl Physiol 11:303-312
4. Nunn JF (1972) Applied respiratory physiology with special reference to anaesthesia. Butter Work, London
5. Roussos C, Campbell EJM (1986) Respiratory muscle energetics. In: Fishman AP, Macklem PT, Mead J, Geiger SR (eds) Handbook of Physiology. The Respiratory System. Mechanics of Breathing. Section 3, vol. III, American Physiological Society, Bethesda, pp 481-509
6. Pepe PE, Marini JJ (1982) Occult positive end-expiratory pressure in mechanically ventilated patients with airflow obstruction: The auto-PEEP effect. Am Rev Respir Dis 216:166-169
7. Coussa ML, Guerin C, Eissa T, Corbeil C, Chasse M, Braidy T et al (1993) Partitioning of work of breathing in mechanically ventilated COPD patients. J Appl Physiol 74:1711-1719
8. Bellemare F, and Grassino A (1982) Effect of pressure and timing of contraction on human diaphragm fatigue. J Appl Physiol 53:1190-1195
9. Yang KL (1993) Inspiratory pressure/maximal inspiratory pressure ratio: a predictive index of weaning outcome. Int Care Med 19:204-208
10. Milic-Emili J (1986) Is weaning an art or a science? Am Rev Respir Dis 134:1107-1108
11. Marini JJ, Smith TC, Lamb VJ (1988) External work output and force generation during synchronized intermittent mechanical ventilation. Effect of machine assistance on breathing effort. Am Rev Respir Dis 138:1169-1179
12. Field S, Sanci S, Grassino A (1984) Respiratory muscle oxygen consumption estimat-

ed by the diaphragm pressure-time index. J Appl Physiol 57:44-51
13. Brochard L, Harf A, Lorino H, Lemaire F (1989) Inspiratory pressure support prevents diaphragmatic fatigue during weaning from mechanical ventilation. Am Rev Respir Dis 139:513-521
14. Brochard L, Baum T, Bedu C (1993) Les valves à la demande. Réanimation Urgences 2:97-105
15. Marini JJ, Capps JS, Culver BH (1985) The inspiratory work of breathing during assisted mechanical ventilation. Chest 87:612-618
16. Ward ME, Corbeil C, Gibbons W, Newman S, Macklem PT (1988) Optimization of respiratory muscle relaxation during mechanical ventilation. Anesthesiology 69:29-35
17. Sassoon CSH, Mahutte CK, Te TT, Simmons DH, Light RW (1988) Work of breathing and airway occlusion pressure during assist-mode mechanical ventilation. Chest 93:571-576
18. Sassoon CS, Lodia R, Rheeman H, Kuei HJ, Light RN, Mahutte CK (1992) Inspiratory muscle work of breathing during flow-by, demand-flow, and continous-flow systems in patients with chronic obstructive pulmonary disease. Am Rev Respir Dis 145:1219-1222
19. Sassoon CHS, Giron AE, Eli EA (1989) Inspiratory work of breathing on flow-by and demand-flow continuous positive airway pressure. Crit Care Med 17:1108-1114
20. Marini JJ, Rodriguez RM, Lamb V (1986) The inspiratory workload of patient-initiated mechanical ventilation. Am Rev Respir Dis 134:902-909
21. Cinnella G, Conti G, Lofaso F, Lorino H, Harf A, Lemaire F, Brochard L (1996) Effects of assisted ventilation on the work of breathing. Volume-control versus pressure-controlled ventilation. Am J Resp Crit Care Med 153:1025-1033
22. Mancebo J, Amaro P, Mollo JL, Lorino H, Lemaire F, Brochard L (1995) Comparison of the effects of pressure support ventilation delivered by three different ventilators during weaning from mechanical ventilation. Int Care Med 21:913-919
23. MacIntyre NR, Ho LI (1991) Effects of initial flow rate and breath termination criteria on pressure support ventilation. Chest 99:134-138
24. Younes M (1992) Proportional assist ventilation, a new approach to ventilatory support: theory. Am Rev Respir Dis 145:114-120

Chapter 11

Work of breathing and triggering systems

V.M. RANIERI, L. MASCIA, T. FIORE, R. GIULIANI

Introduction

The incorporation of microprocessors into the design of ventilators has produced a confounding array of products, each with its own peculiar features and modes of operation. This confusion has been compounded in the medical literature with unproved statements favouring one new device or mode of ventilation over another. We believe that physicians concerned with the ventilatory management of patients with respiratory failure must base their approach on physiologic principles and an understanding of patient-ventilator interactions [1].

According to the American Association for Respiratory Care [2] positive-pressure breaths delivered by a mechanical ventilator can be categorized by three variables: the trigger variables (initiating the breath), the limit variable (controlling gas delivery) and the cycle variable (concluding the breath). The best patient-ventilator interaction is realized when the patient's ventilatory drive, his spontaneous inspiratory flow demand, and his ratio of inspiratory time to total breath cycle (T_i/T_{tot}) are matched by these variables. In this chapter we will exam the physiology of the patient-ventilator interaction at the beginning of the breath, when the patient ventilatory drive interacts with the mechanically delivered breath through the ventilator trigger mechanism.

The trigger function is defined as the variable that is manipulated to deliver inspiratory flow [3]. This variable may be a set time, pressure or flow. Time-triggering operates when the ventilator delivers a breath according to a set frequency, independent of the patient's spontaneous effort [4]. With pressure- and flow-triggering the ventilator delivers a breath once the set pressure or flow sensitivity is attained, independent of the set frequency [4]. The following discussion on the trigger variable will be based on data obtained using one ventilator system only (Puritan-Bennett 7200ae, Puritan-Bennett Corp., Carlsbad, CA). However, when the act of initiating a breath from a ventilator is analyzed, the ventilator response algorithm should also be taken into account, remembering its important effects on the imposed work. The ventilator response algorithm may vary substantially for different ventilators, and hence data obtained with a single ventilator, while illustrative, do not reflect the broad range of possible responses.

Pressure-triggering. During pressure triggering a breath is initiated by the contraction of the patient's respiratory muscles against the occluded airway. The resulting inspiratory effort reduces the airway pressure to a pre-set negative Pao value necessary to open the inspiratory demand valve and initiate the breath. While pressure is declining the patient receives no flow from the ventilator and this period of no flow may burden the patients with additional work [5-6].

Flow-triggering (FLOW by®). Prior to the patient's inspiratory effort the ventilator delivers a level of constant flow into the patient circuit at a rate that can be set between 5 and 20 L/min. Before the patient initiates a breath the delivered flow and the returned flow are equal. As the patient begins to inhale the returned flow decreases. The ventilator recognizes this drop well before the delivered flow is consumed and cycles on to deliver the specified breath. Therefore, the initial constant flow (base flow) satisfies the patient's initial inspiratory efforts while the deficit in returned flow (flow sensitivity) causes the ventilator to cycle on either spontaneous breath (CPAP), volume assisted breaths (AMV or SIMV) or pressure assisted breaths (pressure support or pressure control ventilation) [7-9].

Several studies [5-6] have shown that ventilator systems equipped with pressure-triggering systems create an inspiratory load that may compromise the weaning process. On the other hand, a relevant reduction in work of breathing has been described when demand flow systems are replaced by continuous flow systems during continuous positive airway pressure (CPAP) ventilation [5, 10]. Effects of flow-by triggering on work of breathing have been extensively studied by Sassoon and co-workers during spontaneous mode ventilation (i.e. CPAP) [7-9]. In normal subjects [7] they found that the work of breathing was significantly less with flow-by triggered CPAP than with pressure-triggered CPAP. In patients being weaned from mechanical ventilation the same authors found that both 5 cm H_2O of flow-by triggered CPAP and pressure support ventilation decreased PTP compared to T-piece [8]. In a more recent study [9] Sassoon and co-workers compared the effects on work of breathing of flow-by CPAP with conventional continuous-flow CPAP in nine COPD patients recovering from ARF related to COPD. They found that work of breathing during flow-by CPAP is comparable to the continuous-flow CPAP and less than that with pressure-triggered CPAP. In a recent study [11] we found that flow-triggering significantly decreased inspiratory muscle effort compared to pressure-triggering also during volume and pressure-assisted breaths. These results were explained by two factors: 1) the smaller drop in P_{ao} observed with flow-triggered CPAP and 2) the increase in airway pressure above atmospheric pressure that occurs immediately after trigger sensitivity is obtained and which is maintained throughout the inspiratory cycle, acting as a small inspiratory pressure-assistance [7-9].

Recently Sassoon elegantly analyzed the triggering function in a mechanical lung model [3]. She identified two parts on the P_{ao} trace: (A) from the onset of inspiratory effort to measured trigger sensitivity and (B) from measured trigger sensitivity to maximum pressure drop (Fig. 1). Part A consists of two intervals: (1) the time for pressure within the patient circuit to decline to the true trigger threshold and (2) the response time of the pneumatic system itself once this threshold is reached. The former is determined by patient inspiratory muscle strength and drive, while the latter depends on the engineering design of the ventilator [3]. Once flow begins P_{ao} continues to decline (part B), including the time

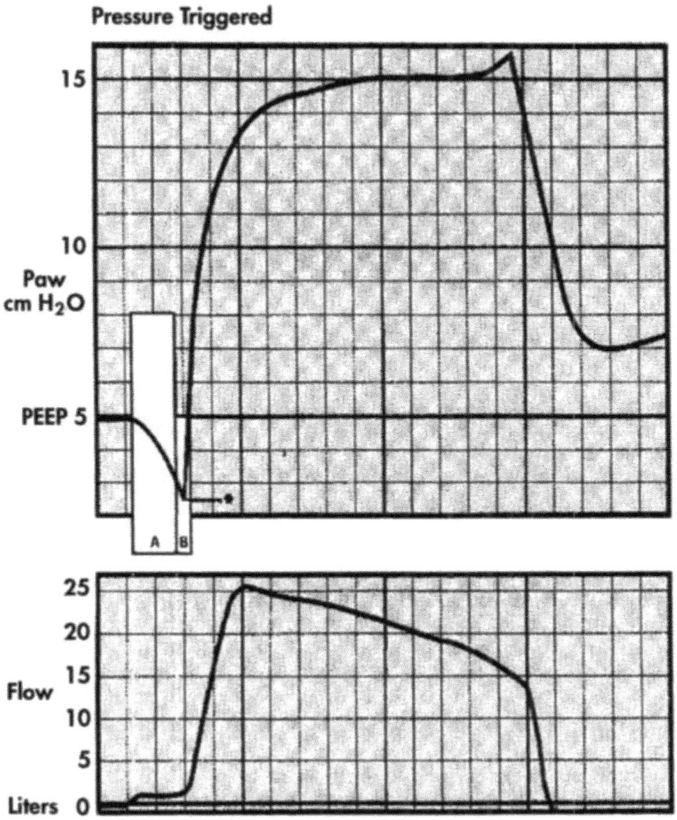

Fig. 1. Illustrative breath during pressure triggered mechanical ventilation

for flow to traverse the circuit's inspiratory limb. The continued pressure decline in P_{ao} in the post-trigger phase (Part B) is explained by insufficient initial flow delivery and is a function of the ventilator flow-pressure control algorithm. Based on these considerations she concluded that differences between pressure and flow triggering should be evaluated on the basis of events occurring during the triggering itself and after its completion [3].

We recently studied the patient-ventilator interaction during the triggering phase in SIMV [11] and during spontaneous ventilation [12] comparing pressure-triggering (set in both studies at a mean sensitivity value of 0.83 ± 0.08 cm H_2O) and flow-triggering (set at mean sensibility value of 1.5 ± 0.2 l/min with a base flow value of 10 ± 0.1 l/min). For this purpose, twenty to thirty consecutive breaths were collected in both studies after 30 to 35 min of stable breathing pattern and then averaged to provide the flow, P_{ao} and P_{es} signals of the "mean representative breath". Illustrative "mean breaths" during volume and pressure assisted breaths with both kinds of triggering systems are depicted in Fig. 2. Following

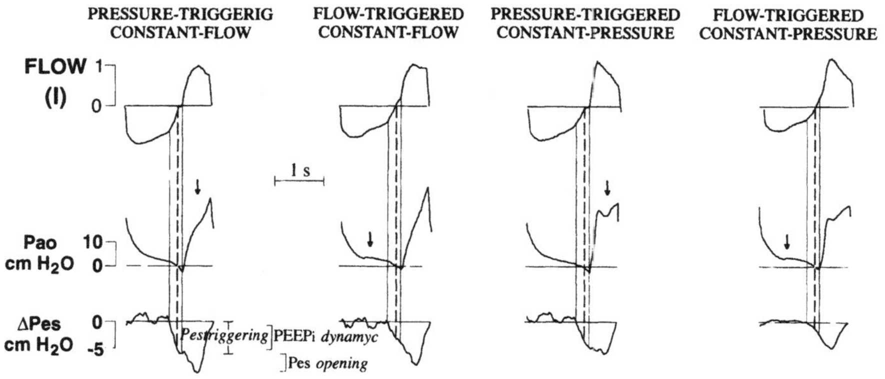

Fig. 2. Representative averaged SIMV mandatory breaths obtained under the four experimental conditions. From top to bottom, flow, airway opening pressure (P_{ao}) and esophageal pressure(ΔPes) signals are shown. Horizontal solid lines present the zero reference for the flow, P_{ao} and P_{es} signals. Vertical solid lines identify on the P_{es} signal the inspiratory effort produced during the triggering phase (P_{es} triggering). The zero reference line for P_{es} was identified as the end-expiratory position of the P_{es} signal during a short trial of controlled mechanical ventilation and inspiratory muscle inactivity previous to the experimental procedure. The dotted vertical line divides the P_{es} triggering into ($PEEP_i$) and inspiratory effort to initiate flow from the ventilator (P_{es} opening). The arrows on P_{ao} tracings during pressure-triggered constant-flow and constant-pressure mandatory breaths indicate a convexity towards the time axis. The slight PEEP level present during flow triggering is indicated by arrows on the P_{ao} tracings during constant-flow and constant-pressure mandatory breaths. SIMV: synchronized intermittent mandatory ventilation. (From [11])

Sassoon's analysis [3] we calculated the pressure-Time product (PTP) of the triggering phase (PTP *triggering*) as the area under the P_{es} signal from the onset of its negative deflection to the point on P_{es} corresponding to the onset of inspiratory flow, referred to as chest wall static recoil pressure-time curve. PTP post-triggering was therefore calculated as follows: PTP post-triggering = PTB/b - PTP triggering [3]. A close inspection of Fig. 2 reveals that the portion of P_{es} signal delimiting PTP triggering is the result of two consecutive components. First, the inspiratory muscle effort begun while expiratory flow was present and P_{ao} was progressively decreasing, these signals reaching zero-flow and atmospheric pressure, respectively. This initial portion of P_{es}, encompassed between the onset of its negative deflection and the point on P_{es} corresponding to the first zero-flow and negative P_{ao} values, represents the dynamic intrinsic positive end-expiratory pressure ($PEEP_i$) [13-14]. PTP-$PEEP_i$ was defined as the corresponding subtended area referenced to the CW static recoil pressure-time curve. Second, the P_{es} portion between the points corresponding to the first zero-flow (just prior to negative P_{ao}) value and to the last zero-flow (and maximum negative P_{ao}) values, represented the amount of inspiratory muscle effort that had to be produced to open the inspiratory valve to initiate inspiration (P_{es} opening). The corresponding time is the delay due to the pressure decline to the trigger threshold and to the response time of the pneumatic system once this threshold is reached (*time delay*) [3]. PTP-opening was defined as the area subtended to P_{es} opening referenced to the CW static recoil pressure-time curve. Tables 1 and 2 respectively show results obtained in nine patients during SIMV 50 % [11] and in six COPD patients during spontaneous ventilation through the ventilator (CPAP 0) [12]. Application of flow-triggering significantly decreased PTP-opening during SIMV (Table 1) and during CPAP (Table 2).

Differences between pressure and flow-triggering can be examined in the trigger and post-trigger phases. Differences in the trigger phase are primarily related to the time delay in opening the pneumatic system. Using a respiratory simulator Sassoon elegantly analysed the relationship between PTP-opening and the time delay for both pressure and flow-triggering [3]. She found that, for a given time delay, initial inspiratory effort during pressure and flow-triggering was similar. However, because the total time delay with flow-triggering was relatively shorter then with pressure-triggering (75 ms *vs* 115 ms during flow and pressure triggering set respectively at a flow sensitivity of 2 l/min and 1 cm H_2O), PTP-opening would be less with flow than with pressure-triggering [3]. Our data confirm Sassoon's observation in the sense that time delay during pressure-triggered SIMV was significantly ($p < 0.01$) longer than during flow-trigging for mandatory and spontaneous SIMV breaths (Table 1) and for CPAP breaths (Table 2). Furthermore, in our patients we found that P_{es} opening was significantly smaller with flow than with pressure-triggering during both mandatory SIMV breaths (12.08 ± 2.42 *vs* 7.44 ± 2.08 cm H_2O), SIMV breaths (11.90 ± 1.92 *vs* 6.04 ± 1.44 cm H_2O) and during CPAP breaths (P_{es} opening amounting to 4.08 ± 0.41 and 4.31 ± 1.01 cm H_2O during pressure and flow triggering respectively). The reduction in PTP-opening with flow-triggering observed in our patients may indeed be attributed to a shorter time delay and to a smaller negative deflection in P_{es} during the triggering phase.

It is interesting to outline that in COPD patients during CPAP 0, higher values of ΔP_{es} opening (16.08 ± 1.58 and 10.11 ± 1.63 cm H_2O during pressure and flow triggering respectively) corresponded to lower time delay (80 ± 20 and 40 ± 10 ms respectively). In contrast, in non COPD patients during spontaneous SIMV breaths, lower values of ΔP_{es} opening (11.90 ± 1.92 *vs* 6.04 ± 1.44 cm H_2O during pressure and flow triggering respectively) corresponded to longer time delay (130 ± 30 *vs* 100 ± 10 ms). This may suggest that the triggering algorithm reacts with shorter time response with higher inspiratory drive, inspiratory muscle strength and ventilatory requirements.

During pressure-triggered SIMV, $PEEP_i$ amounted to 2.81 ± 0.15 and 2.01 ± 0.11 cm H_2O during pressure-triggered assisted and spontaneous SIMV breaths respectively, while in the COPD patients during pressure triggered CPAP $PEEP_i$ amounted to 5.18 ± 1.66 cm H_2O. Application of flow-triggered SIMV significantly decreased $PEEP_i$ and consequently PTP-$PEEP_i$ in both groups of patients (Table 1) during both kinds of mandatory and during spontaneous breaths. $PEEP_i$ is a common finding in mechanically ventilated patients but different patho-physiological mechanisms may be responsible [15]. In fact, in patients with chronic obstructive lung disease (COPD) $PEEP_i$ may be caused by expirato-

Table 1. Effects of flow triggering on pressure time product at different phases of inspiratory effort in nine patients during weaning from mechanical ventilation during SIMV 50 %

	PTP *triggering* (cm H_2O•sec)			PTP *post-triggering* (cm H_2O•sec)
	PEEPi	*Opening*	*Time delay (sec)*	
Mandatory breathes				
pressure triggered	1.11 ± 0.09	1.55 ± 0.11	0.19 ± 0.01	8.38 ± 1.03
flow triggered	0.55 ± 0.08†	0.93 ± 0.09†	0.16 ± 0.01†	4.16 ± 1.01†
Spontaneous breaths				
pressure triggered	1.09 ± 0.02	1.59 ± 0.02	0.13 ± 0.02	11.50 ± 1.04
flow-triggered	0.53 ± 0.01†	0.51 ± 0.01†	0.10 ± 0.01†	7.83 ± 1.05†

Abbreviations. SIMV: synchronized intermittent mandatory ventilation; PTP: pressure time product; $PEEP_i$: intrinsic positive end-expiratory pressure

Data are mean ± SEM (Modified from [11])

† $p < 0.001$ paired t test pressure vs flow triggering

Table 2. Effects of triggering systems on pressure time product at different phases of inspiratory effort in six copd patients during cpap 0

	PTP *triggering* (cm H_2O•sec)			**PTP *post-triggering***
	PEEPi	*Opening*	*Time delay (sec)*	
Pressure triggering	2.32 ± 0.10	2.52 ± 0.10	0.08 ± 0.02	10.07 ± 3.13
flow triggerin	0.47 ± 0.32†	0.90 ± 0.16†	0.04 ± 0.01†	6.18 ± 2.33†

Abbreviations. COPD: chronic obstructive pulmonary disease; CPAP: continous positive end-expiratory pressure; PTP: pressure time product *per* breath; P_{es}: esophageal pressure; $PEEP_i$: dynamic intrinsic positive end-expiratory pressure
Data are mean ± standard error (Modified from [12])
† $p < 0.001$ paired t test pressure vs flow triggering

ry flow limitation [15]. Alternatively, increased expiratory resistance (including endotracheal tube and exhalation valve) may cause $PEEP_i$ because the lungs do not have time to reach their equilibrium volume [15]. Besides, when expiratory muscle recruitment occurs at end exhalation flow will persist to the end of the expiratory cycle and an end-expiratory gradient of alveolar to central airway pressure (i.e. a $PEEP_i$ effect) without increase in lung volume will be present [15].

Patients included in the SIMV study [11] did not have a previous history of COPD. Therefore, the observed reduction in $PEEP_i$ with flow-triggering could be attributed to its ability to decrease expiratory resistance and/or reduce abdominal muscle recruitment. A reduction in expiratory resistance with PEEP has recently been shown in mechanically ventilated patients [13]. During flow-triggered SIMV a slight PEEP was present (Fig. 5) due to the set base flow of 10 l/min. Therefore, the reduction in $PEEP_i$ could be explained by a reduction in expiratory resistance caused by the increase in lung volume due to this "PEEP effect" which occurred during flow-triggered SIMV. Besides, a careful inspection of Fig. 2 reveals that during pressure-triggered SIMV more expiratory effort was present as both P_{es} and P_{ao} were increased during expiration. This could be explained by an increase in abdominal pressure transmitted to the thorax through the diaphragm, caused by recruitment of the expiratory muscle. When flow-triggered SIMV was applied the positive swings in the end-expiratory P_{es} signals were reduced during both constant-flow and constant-pressure SIMV delivered breaths (Fig. 2). The same was true during spontaneous SIMV breaths. This may suggest that with flow-triggered SIMV the abdominal muscles were relaxed during expiration because of a better patient-ventilator interaction [16]. However, to confirm these speculations direct measurements of expiratory resistance and gastric pressure should be performed. In COPD patients during flow triggered CPAP 0 [12] a small positive end-expiratory pressure on the P_{aw} signal was evident [7]. This is due to the pressure generated by the base flow passing through the ventilator tubing system at the end of the patient's expiration when the flow triggering is made active [7]. On average this end-expiratory positive pressure amounted to 2.16 ± 0.12 cm H_2O. Recent studies have suggested that in COPD patients with expiratory flow limitation the use of continuous positive airway pressure (CPAP) in spontaneously breathing patients [14, 15-17] can counterbalance and reduce the inspiratory threshold load imposed by $PEEP_i$ without causing further hyperinflation. It is therefore not surprising that the end-expiratory positive pressure present during flow triggered CPAP 0 was able to partially unload the respiratory muscles and the diaphragm from the additional work imposed by $PEEP_i$. In fact, $PEEP_{i,dyn}$ measured during flow triggered CPAP 0 corresponded to the difference between $PEEP_{i,dyn}$ measured during pressure triggered CPAP 0 minus the end-expiratory positive pressure present during flow triggered CPAP 0.

Application of flow-triggering significantly reduced PTP post-triggering during assisted and spontaneous SIMV breaths (Table 1) and during CPAP breaths (Table 2). During spontaneous ventilation Sassoon and co-workers [7, 9] showed that the most relevant differences in pressure and flow-triggered CPAP on work of breathing and PTP are primarily related to events occurring after triggering has been completed [3]. This is a result of insufficient flow delivery in pressure-triggered CPAP. In contrast, flow-triggered CPAP is more responsive to patient ventilatory demand during the post-triggering phase. In fact, with flow-triggering P_{ao} increases immediately after trigger sensitivity is attained and is maintained above atmospheric pressure throughout inspiration, acting as a small inspiratory pressure assistance [3]. This mechanism explains the reduction in PTP post-triggering observed during flow-triggered spontaneous SIMV breaths. In contrast, the triggering methods should not affect PTP-post triggering of mandatory SIMV breaths provided that the peak inspiratory flow rate is set sufficiently high [3]. Nevertheless, our data show that the difference between pressure and flow-triggered SIMV mandatory breaths reside in both the triggering (including events during late expiration) and post-triggering events. During flow-triggered constant-flow mandatory breaths a convexity towards the time axis is evident on the P_{ao} curve during inspiration (Fig. 5). This should reflect an inadequate flow delivery in early inspiration after triggering was completed [18-20]. In fact, during constant-flow mandatory breaths, peak flow amounted to 0.66 ± 0.03 l/sec (25-27 % above the spontaneous breathing peak flow) (Table 2). However, application of flow-triggering during constant-flow mandatory SIMV breaths minimised the inspiratory sag on the P_{ao} wave form (Fig. 5) without affecting peak inspiratory flow. Our data therefore show that also flow-triggering reduces PTP post-triggering also during mandatory breaths, regardless of the peak inspiratory flow value. This effect could be related to the extra inspiratory flow provided by the flow triggering system before the beginning of the mandatory flow, while the threshold flow value is reached.

Flow triggering without flow by

Proportional assist ventilation (PAV) is a form of synchronized partial ventilatory support in which the ventilator generates pressure in proportion to patient effort; the more the patient pulls the more pressure the machine generates. The ventilator simply amplifies patient effort without imposing any ventilatory or pressure targets (Fig. 3). The objective of PAV is to allow the patient to attain whatever ventilation and breathing pattern his or her control system sees fit. The responsibility for determining level and pattern of breathing is shifted entirely from the physician to the patient. In this respect PAV differs fundamentally from all other methods of ventilatory support, where ventilator variables are, by and large, determined by machine settings [21-22]. In the case of assisted modes of mechanical ventilation breathing is accomplished by the action of both respiratory muscle pressure (P_{mus}) and the mechanical ventilator (ΔP_{ao}). Both pressures are dissipated against two forces, the elastic recoil of the respiratory system [equal to static elastance (E) time changes in lung volume (ΔV)] and the resistance to gas flow offered by the airways and tissue [equal to the resistance of the

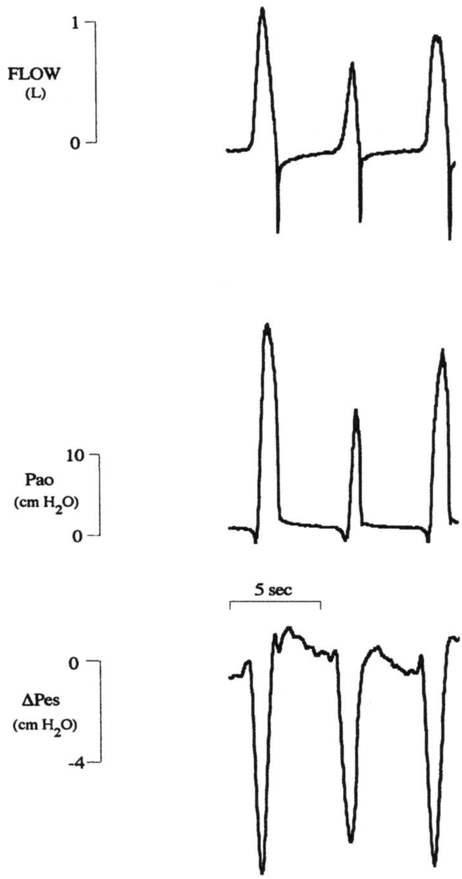

Fig. 3. Experimental record illustrating a patient during PAV. From top to bottom flow, airway opening pressure (P_{ao}) and esophageal pressure (ΔP_{es}) are shown. Note that corresponding to different inspiratory efforts, the ventilator delivers different levels of peak inspiratory flow and applied pressure

respiratory system time inspiratory flow ($\dot{V}$)]. Thus at any instant the total pressure developed during the assisted breathing is given by:

$$P_{mus} + \Delta P_{ao} = E \cdot \Delta V + R \cdot \dot{V}$$

With PAV, airway pressure is linked with, and is proportional to, P_{mus}. Any change in total pressure produced by changes in effort is amplified, resulting in greater ventilatory consequences. Thus where the proportionality ($P_{mus} / \Delta P_{ao}$) is in 2:1, a change of 1.0 cm H_2O results in a 3.0 cm H_2O change in total applied pressure [21-22].

The objective of PAV is therefore to deliver pressure in proportion to the patient's instantaneous effort. To do so the ventilator must be able to sense or estimate patient effort on an ongoing basis. Figure 4 illustrates how this is obtained. The patient is connected to a freely moving piston which is coupled to motor that generates force (pressure) in proportion to the current applied to it. The gas flow from piston to patient is monitored and the signal is integrated to provide instantaneous volume. Each signal is subjected to amplification through gain controls. The two signals are then summed and determine the current flowing to the motor. The gain of the volume signal (same units of elastance) will determine how much P_{ao} will result per unit of inspiratory volume, while the gain of the flow signal (same units of resistance) will determine how much P_{ao} will result per unit of inspiratory flow.

The critical requirement for PAV is a fast response system such that ΔP_{ao} follows P_{mus}. To do this system actually available in our lab (Winnipeg ventilator, University of Manitoba, Manitoba, Canada) consists of a freely moving piston inside a cylinder. As the patient pulls the piston moves freely into the cylinder providing an initial flow and volume (Fig. 4), when the velocity of the piston movement (i.e. inspiratory flow) reaches a pre-set threshold value the motor will start to assist the movement of the piston according to the pre-set values of volume and flow assistance. The physiological impact of this triggering mechanism (Fig. 5) is presented in Table 3 [23]. As can be seen, the triggering mechanism during PAV set with an elastic and resistive support equal to 85 % of the total elastic and resistive work, requires less effort than the classic flow triggering mechanism during mandatory and spontaneous SIMV breaths (Table 1) and during CPAP 0 breaths (Table 2). This is due to a smaller negative deflection in P_{es} during the triggering phase of PAV (ΔP_{es} opening equal to 5.45 ± 0.20 cm H_2O) [5], while the time delay of the PAV triggering mechanism is shorter than the flow by during SIMV (Table 1).

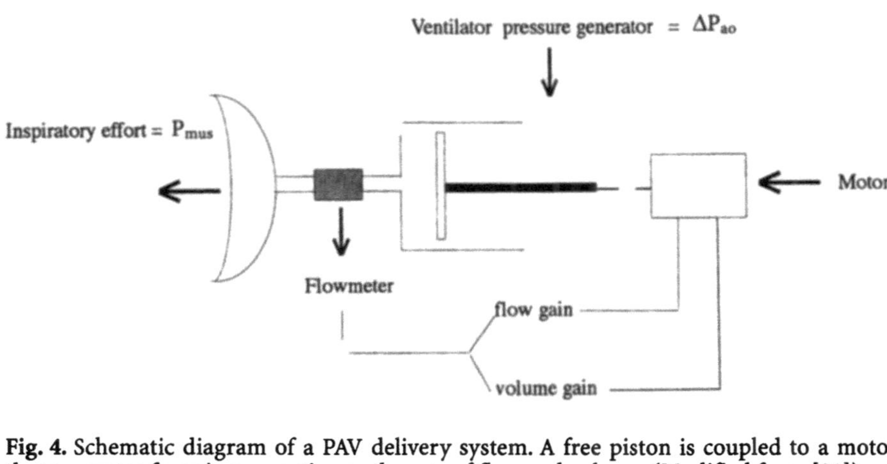

Fig. 4. Schematic diagram of a PAV delivery system. A free piston is coupled to a motor that generates force in proportion to the rate of flow and volume. (Modified from [21])

Table 3. Pressure time product at different phases of inspiratory effort in nine patients during PAV

	PTP *triggering* (cm H_2O • sec)			PTP *post-triggering*
	PEEPi	*opening*	*Time delay (sec)*	
Flow triggening	0.40 ± 0.06	0.59 ± 0.14	0.14 ± 0.02	6.28 ± 0.63

Abbreviations. PAV: proportional assist ventilation; PTP: pressure time product per breath; P_{es}: esophageal pressure; $PEEP_i$: dynamic intrinsic positive end-expiratory pressure
Data are mean ± standard error
† $p < 0.001$ paired t test pressure vs flow triggering

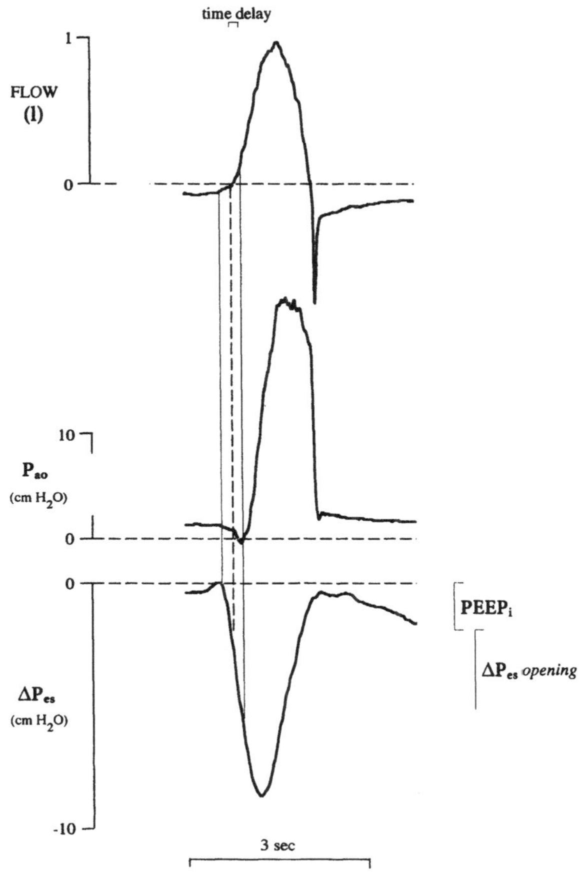

Fig. 5. The triggering mechanism during PAV

Conclusion

Our data shown that in patients connected to a mechanical ventilator the inspiratory effort necessary to initiate a breaths is a significant part of the total inspiratory effort. A correct triggering mechanism may definitely improve the patient-ventilator interaction. For reasons of space we discussed only the physiologic impact of the triggering mechanisms, without considering the other aspects (the limit variable *vs* patient's inspiratory flow and the cycle variable *vs* patient's T_i/T_{tot}) of the physiologic approach to the patient-ventilator interaction problems. We have therefore kept in mind that only the integrated analysis of all these three components will lead to the clinical optimization of the patient-ventilator interaction.

References

1. Hubmayer RD, Abel MD, Rehder K (1990) Physiologic approach to mechanical ventilation. Crit Care Med 18:103-113
2. American Association for Respiratory Care (1992) Consensus statement on the essentials of a mechanical ventilator. Respir Care 37:1000-1008
3. Sassoon CSH (1992) Mechanical ventilator design and function: the trigger variable. Respir Care 37:1056-1068
4. Chatburn RL (1991) A new system for understanding mechanical ventilators. Respir Care 36:1123-1155
5. Viale JP, Annat G, Bertrand O, et al (1985) Additional inspiratory work in intubated patients breathing with continous positive pressure systems. Anesthesiology 63:536-539
6. Beyond L, Chasse M, Harf A et al (1988) Inspiratory work of breathing during spontaneous ventilation using demand valves and continous flow system. Am Rev Respir Dis 138:300-304
7. Sassoon CSH, Giron AE, Ely EA et al (1989) Inspiratory work of breathing on flow by and demand flow continuous positive airway pressure. Crit Care Med 17:1108-1114
8. Sassoon CSH, Light RW, Lodia R et al (1991) Pressure-time product during continous positive airway pressure, pressure support ventilation and T-piece during weaning from mechanical ventilation. Am Rev Respir Dis 143:469-475
9. Sassoon CSH, Lodia R, Rheeman CH et al (1992) Inspiratory muscle work of breathing during flow by, demand flow, and continous flow sysuems in patients with chronic obstructive pulmonary disease. Am Rev Respir Dis 145:1219-1222
10. Henry WC, West GA, Wilson RS (1983) A comparison of the cost of breathing between a continous flow CPAP system and a demand flow CPAP system. Respir Care 28:1273-1281
11. Giuliani R, Mascia L, Recchia F et al (1995) Patient-ventilator interaction during SIMV: effects of flow triggering. Am J Respir and Crit Care Med 151:1-9
12. Ranieri VM, Mascia L, Giuliani R (1995) Inspiratory effort and measurement of dynamic intrinsic PEEP in COPD patients: effects of ventilator triggering systems Inten Care Med 21:896-903
13. Smith TC, Marini JJ (1988) Impact of PEEP on lung mechanics and work of breathing in severe airway obstruction. J Appl Physiol 65:1488-1499
14. Petrof BJ, Legaré M, Goldberg P et al (1990) Continous positive airway pressure reduces work of breathing and dyspnea during weaning from mechanical ventilation in severe chronic obstructive pulmonary disease. Am Rev Respir Dis 141:281-289
15. Marini JJ (1989) Should PEEP be used in airflow obstruction? Am Rev Respir Dis 140:1-3
16. Tobin MJ, Perez W, Guenther SM et al (1986) The pattern of breathing during successful and unsuccessful trials of weaning from mechanical ventilation. Am Rev Respir Dis 134:1111-1118
17. Appendini L, Patessio L, Zanaboni et al (1994) Physiologic effects of positive end-expiratory pressure and mask pressure support during exacerbations of chronic obstructive pulmonary disease. Am J Respir Crit Care Med 149:1069-1076
18. Marini JJ, Rodriguez RM, Lamb V (1986) The inspiratory workload of patient-initiated mechanical ventilation. Am Rev Respir Dis 134:902-909
19. Marini JJ, Capps JS, Culver BH (1985) The inspiratory work of breathing during assisted mechanical ventilation. Chest 87:612-618
20. Ward ME, Corbeil C, Gibbson W et al (1988) Optimization of respiratory muscle relaxation during mechanical ventilation. Anesthesiology 69:29-35

21. Younes M (1992) Proportional assist ventilation, a new aproach to ventilator support: Part I. Theory Am Rev Respir Dis 145:114-120
22. Younes M, Puddy A, Roberts D et al (1992) Proportional assit ventilation: results of an initial clinical trial. Am Rev Respir Dis 145:121-129
23. Mascia L, Caracciolo A, Ranieri M (1994) Pressure support ventilation (PSV) vs proportional assist ventilation (PAV): effects of changes in respiratory drive. Int Care Med 20:S51

Chapter 12

Volutrauma and barotrauma

D. Dreyfussl, G. Saumon

Introduction

Mechanical ventilation is a technique which, although frequently life-saving, carries nevertheless the potential risk of severe complications [1]. Of these adverse effects, some are the direct consequence of pulmonary pressure and/or volume changes induced by mechanical insufflation of diseased lungs. Barotrauma is the usual term for such complications and refers to the presence of extra-alveolar air (manifesting as interstitial emphysema, pneumomediastinum or pneumoperitoneum, pneumothorax, etc.). In addition to these "macroscopic" alterations, it has been experimentally demonstrated that lung distension during mechanical ventilation may induce alterations of lung fluid balance, increases in endothelial and epithelial permeability and severe ultrastructural damage. These abnormalities may culminate in the production of a pulmonary permeability-type edema accompanied by diffuse alveolar damage.

Pulmonary edema during high pressure/high volume ventilation

Webb and Tierney [2] have shown that rats mechanically ventilated with intermittent positive pressure ventilation with a peak airway pressure of 30 cmH_2O developed pulmonary edema very rapidly. Hence, after only one hour of such ventilation there was an increase in the extravascular lung water content, as assessed by post-mortem weighing. When the lung of these animals were examined by light microscopy, only interstitial edema was present. In contrast to such mild alterations induced by moderate increases in airway pressure, ventilating the animals with 45 cmH_2O peak pressure resulted very rapidly (less than 40 minutes) in a very severe pulmonary edema responsible for massive tracheal flooding and hypoxemia leading to the death of most animals. Extravascular lung water was considerably increased (nearly 3-fold normal values). Histological examination confirmed this severity by disclosing widespread alveolar edema.

Closely related observations were made by Kolobow et al. on a sheep model of acute respiratory failure [3]. They ventilated the animals with intermittent positive pressure ventilation and a peak inspiratory pressure of 50 cmH_2O for two days. This resulted in important alterations of lung compliance and gas exchange, leading to the death of some animals. At gross examination the lungs appeared severely damaged. The same team has also confirmed on larger animals the observations by Webb and Tierney that peak inspiratory pressure of moderate range, but applied for longer periods could also be deleterious to the lungs [4]. Indeed, sheep ventilated with a peak inspiratory pressure of only 30 cmH_2O for 48 hours had a progressive deterioration in total static lung compliance, functional residual capacity and arterial blood gases. Post-mortem examination disclosed severe pulmonary atelectasis, increased wet lung weight and an increase in the surface tension of saline lung lavage fluid (reflecting altered surfactant function).

Several studies aimed at assessing the nature (hydrostatic or of permeability origin) of ventilation-induced edema. An increased microvascular permeability has been demonstrated in isolated lung lobes after ventilation with high peak airway pressure [5]. Alveolar epithelial permeability may increase as the result of lung distension and may even allow free diffusion of albumin when high levels of distension are reached [6]. These permeability alterations at the endothelial and epithelial levels might reflect a "stretched pore" phenomenon resulting from important tensions on cells connections.

In order to assess whether pulmonary edema is of the hydrostatic or of the permeability type, we conducted experiments on intact rats ventilated for various durations (5, 10 and 20 minutes) with intermittent positive pressure ventilation with a peak inspiratory pressure of 45 cmH_2O [7]. In addition to measuring indexes of pulmonary edema such as extravascular lung water content and the distribution space of ^{22}Na in lungs, we also estimated microvascular permeability by measuring the post-mortem extravascular dry lung weight (whose increase reflects the amount of extravasated proteins) and the albumin uptake by lungs of intravenously injected radiolabelled albumin. Permeability edema was present as soon as after 5 minutes of challenge, as attested by significant increases of all edema and permeability indices. The severity of these alterations increased with the duration of the experiment. Hence, after 20 minutes of such ventilation, a significant increase in edema was observed. The animals had copious amounts of tracheal fluid, with an albumin concentration close to that of plasma. Electron microscopic examination of lungs of rats having received 20 minutes of intermittent positive pressure ventilation with 45 cmH_2O peak airway pressure disclosed a pattern of diffuse alveolar damage with Type I cell destructions and hyaline membranes.

Other authors using different approaches have confirmed the presence of altered microvascular permeability during mechanical ventilation-induced pulmonary edema [8, 9]. In addition to permeability alterations, hydrostatic force changes may also contribute to edema formation. Parker et al. [8] have shown in open-chest dogs that ventilation with very high (64 cmH_2O) peak inspiratory pressure resulted in the compound of the two effects (i.e. hydrostatic and permeability changes) on lung microcirculation. Indeed, they observed first an increase in the estimated mean microvascular pressure of 12.5 cmH_2O (derived from Swan-Ganz measurements) and second an increase in microvascular permeability. Increases in vascular pressure of the same magnitude have been reported by others during ventilation with high peak airway pressure in closed chest lambs

[9]. This mild to moderate increase in vascular pressure seems unable to produce a permeability-type edema, especially of the severity of that observed after high volume ventilation, but can enhance the extravasation of fluid and proteins through an altered microvasculature.

Respective responsibilities of high airway pressure and high lung volume

In lungs with a normal compliance high peak airway pressure such as that used in our study results in a high tidal volume. It seemed therefore important to determine the respective roles of pressure and volume in the genesis of high permeability edema. We addressed this point in experiments where airway pressure and lung volume were made to vary independently [10]. We compared the effects of high pressure-high volume ventilation, as previously described, to those of high airway pressure alone (ventilating the animals with intermittent positive pressure ventilation with 45 cmH_2O peak pressure, but with a normal tidal volume obtained by thoracoabdominal strapping) and to those of high volume ventilation with low (negative) airway pressure (ventilating the animals by means of an iron lung).

Permeability edema occured in both groups submitted to high volume ventilation whether airway pressure was high or low. At the ultrastructural level severe alterations of the alveolar-capillary barrier were present. In contrast, after high pressure-low tidal volume ventilation both extravascular lung water and indices of microvascular permeability remained within normal range and no ultrastructural damage was observed. The observation that volume changes are responsible for both edema and permeability changes and that high airway pressure has no deleterious effect per se has been confirmed in larger animals by other teams [9, 11].

Effects of the different components of lung volume

The issue on the effects of PEEP during acute lung injury is sill debated. Indeed, during mechanical ventilation-induced pulmonary edema, for a same teleinspiratory pressure, less edema was present in animals ventilated with PEEP than in those ventilated with ZEEP [2, 10]. Does this mean that PEEP has some "protective" effect against volutrauma (in contrast with no reduction or even the increase in edema observed with PEEP during most types of experimental edema), or is it simply the result of hemodynamic alterations due to the higher mean intrathoracic pressure during ventilation with PEEP? This question pertains to the problem of the respective responsibility of large pressure-volume excursions and of the absolute level of lung distension in the genesis of ventilator-induced lung injury. To assess this point rats were ventilated with increasing tidal volumes starting from different levels of positive end-expiratory pressure [12]. Pulmonary edema with permeability alterations occurred regardless of the level of PEEP, provided that the increase in tidal volume was large enough. Similarly, edema occurred even during normal tidal volume ventilation provided the increase in PEEP was large enough. It is worth noting that moderate increases in tidal volume or PEEP that were innocuous when applied alone, produced edema when combined. Similar observations were made in animals ventilated with negative inspiratory pressure indicating that the effect of PEEP was not the consequence of raised airway pressure but of the increase in functional residual capacity. Thus, it appears that end-inspiratory volume is probably the main determinant of ventilation-induced edema, rather than level of functional residual capacity or tidal volume. However, although permeability alterations were similar edema was less marked in animals ventilated with PEEP than in those ventilated with ZEEP with the same end-inspiratory pressure. This "beneficial" effect of PEEP was probably the consequence of hemodynamic alterations. Indeed, infusion of dopamine to correct the drop in systemic arterial pressure that occurred during PEEP ventilation resulted in a significant increase in pulmonary edema.

Effects of mechanical ventilation on previously injured lungs

Most previously mentioned studies were conducted on animals with healthy lungs. It is conceivable that diseased lungs are more susceptible than healthy ones to the deleterious effects of mechanical ventilation. Bowton and Kong [13] studied the effects of varying tidal volume during mechanical ventilation of oleic acid-injured, isolated perfused rabbit lungs. Lungs ventilated with a high tidal volume of 18 ml/kg had a significantly greater weight gain than those ventilated with a small tidal volume of 6 ml/kg. Hernandez and colleagues studied the effects of oleic acid alone, mechanical ventilation alone and the conjunction of both interventions on the capillary filtration coefficient of isolated perfused young rabbit lungs [14]. Low doses of oleic acid or mild overinflation during mechanical ventilation did not significantly affect the filtration coefficient when studied separately. In contrast, when oleic acid administration was followed by mechanical ventilation a significant increase in this coefficient was observed. The effects of superimposing high peak inspiratory pressure (45cmH_2O) ventilation on lungs mildly injured by hydrochloric acid, oleic acid or alpha-naphtylthiourea were investigated in intact rats [15]. Pulmonary edema and permeability alterations were more important in animals submitted to combined aggression (ventilation plus toxic injury) than in those submitted to a single aggression.

Mechanisms of pulmonary edema during high pressure/high volume ventilation

As explained above changes in hydrostatic forces are minorly involved (on a quantitative basis) in the genesis of this edema. Two mechanisms can lead to increased vascular pressure during lung distension. First, surfactant abnormalities which have been evidenced after high volume ventilation [16, 17] can promote an increase in alveolar surface tension. This leads in turn to a decrease in the pressure surrounding alveolar microvessels and, therefore, to an increased transmural pressure of these vessels. Second, lung distension results in an augmentation of the transmural pressure of extraalveolar vessels [18] which in turn enhances fluid filtration at this level.

A possible explanation for the severe permeability alterations observed during mechanical ventilation-induced edma may be the occurrence of mechanical failure of both alveolar epithelium and microvascular endothelium due to the very high alveolar distending pressures. Indeed, the similarities in the ultrastructural aspect of the lungs observed during mechanical ventilation-induced lung injury and during the capillary stress failure that occurs after very important increases in capillary transmural pressure (40 mmHg or more) [19] are quite remarkable and may indicate that both are manifestations of the same spectrum of mechanical lung failure. Thus, pulmonary edema after high pressure-high volume ventilation is likely to be the result of the synergistic effects of a very severe microvascular permeability alteration and of increased filtration pressure. This would explain the fulminating course of such edema which may be produced by very short periods of overinflation in small animals [20].

In conclusion, cyclic lung overinflation results in pulmonary edema. This edema is of the permeability type and associated with diffuse alveolar damage. It is worth noting that such injury is not the consequence of "barotrauma" but rather of "volutrauma". These observations might be clinically relevant. Indeed, it has been shown that during ARDS the distribution of lung lesions is not homogeneous [21]. Therefore, owing to uneven distribution of pulmonary compliance, some overdistension of the less damaged zones may occur during mechanical ventilation of such patients, especially when high peak airway pressures are required. The possibility that protracted regional overinflation may worsen preexisting lesions is worth consideration.

References

1. Pingleton SK (1988) Complications of acute respiratory failure. Am Rev Respir Dis 137:1463-1493
2. Webb HH, Tierney DF (1974) Experimental pulmonary edema due to intermittent positive pressure ventilation. Protection by positive end-expiratory pressure. Am Rev Respir Dis 110:556-565
3. Kolobow T, Moretti MP, Fumagalli R, Mascheroni D, Prato P, Chen V, Joris M (1987) Severe impairment in lung function induced by high peak airway pressure during mechanical ventilation. An experimental study. Am Rev Respir Dis 135:312-315
4. Tsuno K, Prato P, Kolobow T (1990) Acute lung injury from mechanical ventilation at moderately high airway pressures. J Appl Physiol 69:956-961
5. Parker JC, Townsley MI, Rippe B, Taylor AE, Thigpen J (1984) Increased microvascular permeability in dog lungs due to high peak airway pressures. J Appl Physiol 57:1809-1816
6. Egan EA, Nelson RM, Olver RE (1976) Lung inflation and alveolar permeability to non-electrolytes in the adult sheep in vivo. J Physiol 260:409-424

7. Dreyfussl D, Basset G, Soler P, Saumon G (1985) Intermittent positive-pressure hyperventilation with high inflation pressures produces pulmonary microvascular injury in rats. Am Rev Respir Dis 132:880-884
8. Parker JC, Hernandez LA, Longenecker GL, Peevy K, Johnson W (1990) Lung edema caused by high peak inspiratory pressures in dogs. Role of increased microvascular filtration pressure and permeability. Am Rev Respir Dis 142:321-328
9. Carlton D, Cummings JJ, Scheerer RG, Poulain FR, Bland RD (1990) Lung overexpansion increases pulmonary microvascular protein permeability in young lambs. J Appl Physiol 69:577-583
10. Dreyfussl D, Soler P, Basset G, Saumon G (1988) High inflation pressure pulmonary edema. Respective effects of high airway pressure, high tidal volume and positive end-expiratory pressure. Am Rev Respir Dis 137:1159-1164
11. Hernandez LA, Peevy KJ, Moise AA, Parker JC (1989) Chest wall restriction limits high airway pressure-induced lung injury in young rabbits. J Appl Physiol 66:2364-2368
12. Dreyfussl D, Saumon G (1993) Role of tidal volume, FRC and end-inspiratory volume in the development of pulmonary edema following mechanical ventilation. Am Rev Respir Dis 148:1194-1203
13. Bowton DL, Kong D L (1989) High tidal volume ventilation produces increased lung water in oleic acid-injured rabbit lungs. Crit Care Med 17:908-911
14. Hernandez LA, Coker PJ, May S, Thompson AL, Parker JC (1990) Mechanical ventilation increases microvascular permeability in oleic-acid injured lungs. J. Appl Physiol 69:2057-2061
15. Dreyfussl D, Soler P, Saumon G (1991) High volume ventilation produces more severe damage in previously injured lungs. Am Rev Respir Dis 143 [Suppl.]:A251 (Abstract)
16. Forrest JB (1972) The effect of hyperventilation on pulmonary surface activity. Brit J Anaesth 44:313-319
17. Wyszogrodski I, Kyei Aboagye K, Taeusch HW Jr, Avery ME (1975) Surfactant inactivation by hyperventilation: conservation by end-expiratory pressure. J Appl Physiol 38:461-466
18. Permutt S (1979) Mechanical influences on water accumulation in the lungs. In: Fishman AP, Renkin EM (eds) Pulmonary edema. Clinical Physiology Series. American Physiological Society, Bethesda, pp 175-193
19. West JB, Tsukimoto K, Mathieu-Costello O, Prediletto R (1991) Stress failure in pulmonary capillaries. J Appl Physiol 70:1731-1742
20. Dreyfussl D, Soler P, Saumon G (1992) Spontaneous resolution of the pulmonary edema caused by short periods of cyclic overinflation. J Appl Physiol 72:2081-2089
21. Maunder RJ, Shuman WP, Mc Hugh JW, Marglin SI, Butler J (1986) Preservation of normal lung regions in the adult respiratory distress syndrome. Analysis by computed tomography. JAMA 255:2463-2465

Chapter 13

Pulmonary and system factors of gas exchanges

J. Roca

Introduction

The chief function of the lung is pulmonary gas exchange, which requires adequate levels of ventilation and perfusion of the alveoli. The lung must match pulmonary O_2 uptake (VO_2) and elimination of CO_2 (VCO_2) to the whole body metabolic O_2 consumption and CO_2 production, whatever the O_2 and CO_2 partial pressures in the arterial blood

In order to best manage patients with respiratory failure in both the intensive and the medical care setting, proper assessment of pulmonary gas exchange is crucial. Arterial blood respiratory gases (O_2 and CO_2) and acid-base status are the directly measurable variables used by most clinicians for this purpose. However, while respiratory gases have become increasingly easy to obtain in recent years, their interpretation has become progressively more difficult, especially in the intensive care setting. This is because of deepening awareness that factors other than intrapulmonary abnormalities can alter arterial PO_2 and PCO_2. Ideally, it would be of great practical interest to clinicians to handle respiratory blood gas measurements as an index on the state of the lungs, such that improved or impaired results could be equated to improvement or impairment lung function, respectively. The situation is that arterial PO_2 and PCO_2 reflect not only the state of the lung, at least as a gas exchanger, and thereby intrapulmonary determinants (i.e. ventilation-perfusion (V_A/Q) mismatch, intrapulmonary shunt and alveolar-end-capillary diffusion limitation for oxygen) but also the conditions under which the lung is operating, namely the composition of inspired gas and mixed venous blood, i.e. the extrapulmonary factors.

We will focus essentially on the pathophysiologic determinants of arterial PO_2 and PCO_2 in the light of the results obtained with the multiple inert gas elimination technique, in order to provide a solid framework for the proper interpretation of the interplay of the extra- and intrapulmonary factors determining respiratory gases. This analysis is exclusively addressed to conditions characterized by hypercapnic respiratory failure, henceforth called ventilatory failure, more specifically caused by chronic obstructive pulmonary disease (COPD).

Physiological background

Table 1 shows the intrapulmonary factors that may contribute individually or combinedly to hypoxemia and hypercapnia as well as the extrapulmonary factors that, either directly or indirectly (through their effect on mixed venous oxygen tension, PvO_2), can also influence arterial PO_2 and PCO_2. It is important here to emphasize the key role of PvO_2 and how extrapulmonary factors (other than inspired PO_2 and total ventilation) may contribute to reduce PaO_2 through their effects on PvO_2. In this regard, a diminished PvO_2 may result from a low cardiac output, an increased oxygen uptake, and/or a decreased blood oxygen content due to several alterations in the principal factors modulating the oxyhemoglobin dissociation curve [1].

Table 1. Factors determining arterial hypoxemia

Intrapulmonary		Extrapulmonary
- *V_A/Q mismatching* *	**Main factors:**	↓ *Minute ventilation*
- *Shunt*		↓ *Cardiac output*
- Alveolar-end O_2 diffusion limitation		↓ *capillaryInspired PO_2*
		↑ *O_2 uptake*
	Secondary factors:	↓ P_{50} ↓ Hb concentration ↑ pH ↓ Temperature ↑ VCO_2

*V_A/Q: ventilation-perfusion; Hb: haemoglobin; P_{50}: PO_2 that corresponds to 50% oxyhaemoglobin saturation. *In italics*: the most relevant

Factors determining PO_2

The most prominent clinical intrapulmonary factor determining the pathophysiology of hypoxemia in ventilatory failure caused by COPD is undoubtedly abnormal V_A/Q relationships [2, 3]. Although shunt may also have some relevance in modulating hypoxemia, particularly when COPD patients suffer from acute respiratory failure and have retained secretions and abundant mucus plugging [4] or when there is a reopening of foramen ovale, its amount is by and large small [2, 3]. By contrast, the role played by diffusion limitation for oxygen in COPD is almost negligible [5].

The PO_2 and PCO_2 values in any alveolar unit, and hence the end-capillary PO_2 and PCO_2 of each lung, are basically determined by the composition of the inspired gas, the composition of mixed venous blood and, even more importantly, by the ratio of gas flow (ventilation) to blood flow (perfusion) -V_A/Q- of the unit. The V_A/Q ratio may vary from completely unventilated but perfused units (0=shunt) to completely unperfused but ventilated units (dead space). While breathing room air lung units with very low V_A/Q ratios (not completely unventilated) have alveolar gas tensions very close to mixed venous blood values such that they behave very similarly to shunt from a gas exchange standpoint. As the V_A/Q ratio increases above 0.1, while end-capillary PO_2 increases rapidly, $PaCO_2$ also falls rapidly. Arterial blood saturates fully approaching the V_A/Q ratio of 1.0, but it is of note that once the V_A/Q ratio is above 1.0, the end-capillary PO_2 increases progressively as long as the V_A/Q ratios increase until reaching inspired gas levels. However, this has little effect on the transfer of O_2 due to the alinear (sigmoid) shape of the oxyhemoglobin dissociation curve. Likewise, the $PaCO_2$ will approach the inspired gas composition as long as the V_A/Q ratios continue to increase. Because of the more linear characteristics of the CO_2 hemoglobin dissociation curve,the lung units with high V_A/Q ratios will continue to be progressively useful for CO_2 output. The distributions of V_A/Q ratios are crucial in determining the levels of PO_2 and PCO_2. Thus, in the presence of acute or chronic pulmonary disease, V_A/Q distributions become markedly abnormal such that it is common to see areas of low and/or high V_A/Q ratios and different patterns of V_A/Q distributions (bimodal bloodflow and/or ventilation distributions) [1].

During acute exacerbation of COPD several abnormal V_A/Q distributions have been documented [3]. These are, however, qualitatively similar to what is seen in less severe clinical forms of COPD [2]. Not uncommonly, a combined bimodal pattern including the bloodflow distribution and also the ventilation distribution may be one of the most representative V_A/Q abnormalities. This means that a large proportion of bloodflow is perfusing lung units with low or very low V_A/Q ratios; likewise, a large proportion of ventilation is diverted to lung units with high or very high V_A/Q ratios. In other occasions, however, COPD patients show a bimodal blood flow distribution together with a broadly unimodal ventilation curve; and vice versa, the bimodal pattern is disclosed sometimes at the level of the alveolar ventilation distribution alone, whereas the bloodflow pattern is abnormally broader only. Units with low V_A/Q ratios are likely to represent regions subtended by airways partially blocked by mucus secretions, smooth muscle hypertrophy, bronchospasm, distortion or some combination of these abnormalities. By contrast, lung units with high VA/Q ratios are likely produced by continued ventilation of regions of alveolar destruction, which presumably greatly reduce blood flow in these areas, hence leading to units with high V_A/Q ratios. Conceivably, they represent emphysematous regions where destruction of the alveolar walls results in the loss of the vascular cross-sectional areas [2]. Alternatively, it is considered that the relative small amounts of shunt are due to the efficiency of collateral ventilation in maintaining alveolar ventilation beyond obstructed airways.

Among the extrapulmonary factors determining arterial PO_2, the most relevant from the clinical standpoint (in italics in Table 1) are inspired PO_2 total (overall) ventilation, cardiac output (CO) and oxygen uptake. Total (overall) ventilation is considered an extrapulmonary factor because it is primarily the result of tidal volume (less series dead space common to more than one V_A/Q unit) times frequency, which are set by extrapulmonary breathing control mechanisms [1]. Although important from a physiological viewpoint, hemoglobin concentration, body temperature, acid-base status and position of the oxyhemoglobin dissociation curve (e.g. characterized by P_{50}) do less influence PaO_2.

Regarding the effects of inspired O_2 fraction in the presence of V_A/Q mismatching, arterial PO_2 is very sensitive to this extrapulmonary factor as opposed to when shunt is the predominant mechanism of hypoxemia [6]. In fact, inspired PO_2 has little effect in increasing the alveolar PO_2 of lung units with very low V_A/Q ratios (although not completely unventilated) such that substantial levels of inspired oxygen fraction are needed to improve PaO_2. Thus, it has been shown that fully saturating PaO_2 in the presence of moderate to severe V_A/Q abnormalities is required to increase FiO_2.

By using a multicompartments lung model, West [7] was able to show that increases in overall ventilation have a powerful effect on gas exchange when V_A/Q distributions are normal, PaO_2 increasing and $PaCO_2$ decreasing. However, when V_A/Q distributions are abnormal, this is usually accompanied by an increase in $PaCO_2$ (other factors being equal) which is rapidly brought down to normal values by an increase in ventilation.

Interestingly, PaO_2 also increases with further increases in ventilation, although when V_A/Q distributions are impaired normal values cannot be regained easily. Yet, with further increases in ventilation there is little effect on the PO_2. Since increasing V_A/Q mismatch reduces the transfer of O_2 and CO_2, it might be expected that this situation will lead always to both hypoxemia and hypercapnia. However, small increases in $PaCO_2$ may activate chemoreceptors, thus causing hyperventilation as long as the ventilatory system works appropriately and the patient is able to respond. This increased ventilation distributed to well ventilated areas will increase their V_A/Q ratios causing a raise in end-capillary PO_2 and a fall in PCO_2. When the ability to increase ventilation is exceeded by the degree of V_A/Q mismatching there is an increase in $PaCO_2$. Maintaining a relatively increased minute ventilation effectively prevents simultaneous increases in the levels of $PaCO_2$ provided that there is no parallel increase in the work of breathing [8]. In patients who cannot maintain a high rate of ventilation due to the increased work of breathing and in those whose respiratory drive increases slightly when $PaCO_2$ is high, hypercapnia can ensue.

There are three potential ways in which CO may influence pulmonary gas exchange [9]. The most influential one is through the effect on the O_2 content of the mixed venous blood. This may occur directly through changes in CO and its effect on arterial-venous O_2 difference, by failure of the cardiovascular system (cardiac output) to respond to changes in O_2 delivery (CO • arterial O_2 content) with reduction in the extraction fraction of oxygen (O_2 consumption/O_2 delivery). A second way in which CO may alter pulmonary gas exchange is by modifying the transit time of the red blood cell spent in the pulmonary capillary. If CO increases then the transit time decreases such that abnormal gas exchange due to incomplete alveolar end-capillary equilibration may, at least in theory, occur. However, this is only possible when there is combined diffusion limitation for oxygen, as happens in idiopathic pulmonary fibrosis not only during exercise but also under resting conditions [10]. A third way by which CO may alter pulmonary gas exchange is by redistributing pulmonary blood flow within the lungs. Alterations in blood flow may be achieved in different ways. One way is through the well-known, although poorly understood, positive association between intrapulmonary shunt and CO, such that shunt fraction increases when CO rises, and vice versa [11, 12].

Another way may also be achieved by modification of the pulmonary vascular tone, which is basically sensed by the levels of alveolar oxygen tension, the major determinant of pulmonary vascular resistance. However, PvO_2 may also play a key role in influencing pulmonary vascular tone through an as yet undetermined pathway [13, 14]. Finally, increases and decreases in intracardiac and intrapulmonary artery pressures may also lead to redistribution of pulmonary blood flow [9].

Changes in oxygen consumption may represent another way of modulating the levels of PaO_2. Using a lung model essentially characterized by V_A/Q mismatching Wagner [15] has shown that changes in oxygen utilization have marked effects on PaO_2. Thus, a 10 % change in O_2 uptake can alter PaO_2 by 10 mmHg in either direction. This is in contrast with what happens when the major mechanism of hypoxemia is intrapulmonary shunt, where arterial PO_2 is less sensitive to a change in oxygen uptake. This is explained by the shape of the oxyhemoglobin dissociation curve. Thus, when PaO_2 lies on the flat (top) part of the oxyhemoglobin curve, as happens under the conditions of V_A/Q inequality, changes in PaO_2 are much larger than when it falls in the steep part of the curve, where the effects on PaO_2 are reduced.

Factors modulating PCO_2

From a clinical standpoint, three major factors can modulate the levels of $PaCO_2$ (Table 1). One corresponds to an intrapulmonary factor, i.e. V_A/Q inequality, already alluded to above, and the other three are extrapulmonary factors, namely overall ventilation, changes in acid-base status and carbon dioxide production [16].

Among alterations in overall ventilation, abnormalities in respiratory mechanics, namely respiratory muscle fatigue, abnormal neuromuscular function and/or structural changes in the chest wall, and changes in the control of ventilation, emerge as the major extrapulmonary factors. Changes in overall ventilation may be produced by quantitative or qualitative abnormalities in the breathing pattern, increases in dead space, or both. A decrease in alveolar ventilation is always associated with an increase in $PaCO_2$. Hypercapnia due to metabolic alkalosis can be also contemplated, to some extent, as a condition which is accompanied by a depression in the ventilatory control system with normal lungs. Finally, changes in the metabolic rate (CO output) due to alterations in the level of activity, fever, disease or carbohydrate metabolism (for instance, high glucose loads during parenteral nutrition) may be major causes of hypercapnia. Usually, if the lungs are normal, ventilation increases simultaneously and, therefore, the retention of carbon dioxide is prevented. Patients with lung disorders, unable to increase appropriately their degree of ventilation, may show hypercapnia.

Clinical implications

Influence of cardiac output and ventilation

Torres et al. [17] studied V_A/Q inequalities in 8 patients with COPD during mechanical ventilation and also during weaning (spontaneous breathing) from mechanical ventilation required for acute respiratory failure. While there were no differences in most of the pulmonary and systemic hemodynamic parameters between the two conditions CO increases significantly when patients were removed from the ventilator. Interestingly, while neither PaO_2 no $AaPO_2$ and venous admixture showed significant changes between the two conditions, both PvO_2 and O_2 delivery increased significantly when patients were removed from mechanical ventilation. Oxygen uptake (calculated by the Fick principle) did not change. Another important finding at spontaneous breathing was that, while minute ventilation remained essentially unchanged, respiratory frequency increased and tidal volume fell significantly. In other words, the efficiency of breathing fell such that $PaCO_2$ increased and pH decreased also significantly. Substantial alterations in low V_A/Q areas (i.e. increase in the percentage of bloodflow to these regions) were shown during spontaneous ventilation. Moreover, both the dispersion of ventilation and one of the overall indices of V_A/Q heterogeneity (so called, DISP R-E*) increased (worsened) significantly. The variable DISP R-E* is an overall index of heterogeneity of lung function and represents the combined dispersion of both bloodflow and ventilation distributions [18]. It corresponds to the root mean square difference between retentions (R) and excretions (E) after correcting for series dead space (using acetone data). By contrast, shunt, the dispersion of bloodflow and inert dead space remained essentially unchanged.

These results show that patients with COPD, during spontaneous ventilation after removal from mechanical ventilation, further worsened the V_A/Q mismatch. This worsening can be explained by alterations in breathing pattern and also by changes in CO. It is of note that dispersion of pulmonary bloodflow did not increase despite the increase in perfusion observed in low V_A/Q areas during spontaneous ventilation, since the V_A/Q distributions shifted to the left because of a reduction in overall V_A/Q ratio. Yet, neither the PaO_2 nor the $AaPO_2$ underwent major changes, indicating that respiratory blood gas measurements may not sufficiently reflect changes in V_A/Q relationships because other factors such as minute ventilation and CO were influencing pulmonary gas exchange in this clinical setting. Indeed, CO increased substantially after cessation of mechanical ventilation because of a concomitant increase in venous return. The importance of the latter and other hemodynamic changes has been stressed by Lemaire et al. [19] during unsuccessful weaning in patients with COPD. Additional factors contributing to respiratory weaning failure could be myocardial infarction and left ventricular failure due to abrupt alterations in venous return. According to Permutt [20] an increase of gastric pressure during spontaneous ventilation with subsequent increased splanchnic flow could also be an additional pathogenic mechanism. Simultaneously, there were increases in PvO_2 and O_2 delivery due to an increase in CO (extrapulmonary factor). The resulting beneficial effect of the latter on PaO_2 was thus offset by the impairment in PaO_2 due to further worsening of V_A/Q relationships (increased dispersion of ventilation, intrapulmonary factor), enhanced (decreased overall V_A/Q ratio) in turn by a concomitant less efficient breathing pattern (increased respiratory frequency and decreased tidal volume, extrapulmonary factors). Interestingly, in this particular setting, the qualitative alterations in minute ventilation had a powerful effect on pulmonary gas exchange. The finding that the dispersion of ventilation was one of the most significantly altered V_A/Q variables, together with the overall index of V_A/Q heterogeneity, suggests that maldistribution of ventilation may play a key role in the worsening of V_A/Q mismatch during weaning. By contrast, inert dead space did not play any role.

More recently, in order to investigate the time-course and pattern of V_A/Q relationships Ferrer et al. [21] have studied sequentially 10 patients with acute hypercapnic respiratory failure not receiving mechanical ventilation. It is of note that most of the respiratory and inert gas data improved one month following the initial episode. More specifically, PaO_2 increased and $PaCO_2$ decreased and both the dispersion of alveolar ventilation and one of the overall indices of V_A/Q heterogeneity decreased (improved) significantly. Furthermore, there was a significant relationship between the improvement in the dispersion of ventilation distribution and that of FEV_1, one of the best functional descriptions of the degree of airway obstruction. This suggests, therefore, that some of the V_A/Q abnormalities observed in patients with COPD with ventilatory failure may be related to reversible functional abnormalities related, in part, to maldistribution of ventilation (namely, bronchoconstriction, edema, mucus plugging, air trapping and also intrinsic or auto-PEEP) in addition to other irreversible structural lesions, such as airways (inflammation, fibrosis and smooth muscle hypertrophy, among other major lesions) and emphysema abnormalities [22].

Barberà et al. [22] in our laboratory have shown, by using the multiple inert gas elimination technique in patients with mild COPD before lung resection due to a small localized neoplasm and subsequently determining the degree of small airways abnormalities and of pathologic emphysema, the significant correlations between these structural changes and the dispersion of blood flow and ventilation. Accordingly, it has been hypothesized that a non-homogeneous distribution of inspired air, as a result of the airway narrowing, would be at the origin of the increased dispersion of ventilation distribution. Alternatively, the loss of alveolar attachments of bronchiolar walls observed in pulmonary emphysema may result in both distortion and narrowing of the lumen of bronchioles. The latter may cause reduced alveolar ventilation in the dependent alveolar units, which will produce lung units with continued bloodflow and thus low V_A/Q ratios. This abnormality in V_A/Q relationship would become evident in the bloodflow curve as an increased dispersion of perfusion. In addition, emphysema was related to abnormalities of ventilation distribution. The latter may be related, at least in part, to the loss of pulmonary capillary network associated to alveolar destruction of emphysematous spaces (namely, wasted ventilation). This would lead in turn to the development of lung units with high V_A/Q ratios and hence to increased dispersion of ventilation. Accordingly, the bimodal ventilation distribution alluded to before earlier [2, 3] would be an extension of this phenomenon likely reflecting large areas of destroyed parenchyma.

Influence of oxygen uptake and ventilation

Lemaire et al. [19] studied carefully the hemodynamic effects of rapid weaning from mechanical ventilation in 15 patients with severe advanced COPD and preexisting cardiovascular disease. Although inert gas exchange data were not measured, it is of interest to note that there was a significant impairment in both PaO_2 and $PaCO_2$ together with an increase in CO and the presence of significant deleterious hemodynamic events. Interestingly, oxygen uptake increased significantly; unfortunately, measurements of breathing pattern were not documented. The important conclusion that can be drawn from this study, however, is that the increased metabolic (extrapulmonary factor) demands of these patients could have influenced negatively the final PaO_2, thus overwhelming the beneficial effects on the latter variable produced by the accompanying increase in CO (extrapulmonary factor). According to our experience, underlying V_A/Q relationships (intrapulmonary factor, not measured) should have worsened. The latter variable, possibly with an expected less efficient breathing pattern could have contributed to further worsen respiratory blood gases (decreased PaO_2 and increased $PaCO_2$), just as they did in our patients [17]. Interestingly, Annat et al. [23] also showed in eight COPD patients during weaning from mechanical ventilation to both continuous positive pressure ventilation and inspiratory pressure support ventilation, increases in both oxygen consumption and decreases in minute ventilation. In addition, there was a marked increment in $PaCO_2$ without changes in PaO_2. Conceivably, the concomitant increase in CO (not measured) would be at the origin of the results of arterial blood gases. An increased CO_2 would have raised mixed venous PO_2, thus counterbalancing the combined deleterious effects on PaO_2 of both the reduced ventilation and the increased oxygen uptake. Just as with the study of Lemaire et al. [19], the increase in oxygen uptake was one of the most outstanding findings compared to the work of Torres et al. [17]. The absence of an increased oxygen consumption in the latter study may be, however, perfectly explained by the large variability of CO measurements with the thermodilution technique in the clinical setting, used to calculate oxygen uptake through the Fick principle. Furthermore, in the experimental setting the Fick method can underestimate oxygen consumption measured at the mouth because bronchial and thebesian veins empty into the systemic circulation such that the oxygen consumed by parts of the lung and the heart may not be reflected necessarily in the Fick measurement [24, 25]. In brief, it is considered that oxygen consumption measured from the mixed expired samples at the mouth is more accurate than that calculated from the CO and the arterial-mixed venous oxygen contents. Although the differences between each measurement are not statistically significant, it has been shown that their correlation is relatively weak [26]. Alternatively, in Annat et al. [23] the outstanding influence of a decreased overall ventilation in worsening pulmonary gas exchange needs also to be emphasized.

Conclusion

In summary, taken together these findings highlight the key role of the interplay of extrapulmonary and intrapulmonary factors governing pulmonary gas exchange in COPD patients with ventilatory failure under different clinical conditions. According to their respective role, respiratory blood gases may be influenced in either direction, or remain unaltered in different clinical settings. In these patients V_A/Q mismatching emerges undoubtedly as the principal intrapulmonary determinant of pulmonary gas exchange, the role of shunt being almost negligible. In addition, the contribution of CO and overall ventilation among other predominantly extrapulmonary factors may play a key role in modulating the observed arterial respiratory gases. The influence of CO and total ventilation need to be particularly highlighted since each of them is able to offset the effects of changes on PaO_2 and $PaCO_2$ produced by further worsening in V_A/Q mismatch per se. The important message for the clinician though is that arterial blood gas measurements may be totally insensitive to properly reflect the alterations operating at the level of the extrapulmonary and intrapulmonary determinants of pulmonary gas exchange.

References

1. Rodriguez-Roisin R, Wagner PD (1989) Clinical relevance of ventilation-perfusion inequality determined by inert gas elimination. Eur Respir J 3:469-482
2. Wagner PD, Dantzker DR, Dueck R, Clausen JL, West JB (1977) Ventilation-perfusion inequality in chronic obstructive pulmonary disease. J Clin Invest 59:203-216
3. Dantzker DR (1984) Gas exchange. In: Montenegro HD (ed) Chronic obstructive pulmonary disease. Churchil Livingstone, Edinburg, pp 141-160
4. Glauser FL, Pollaty RC, Sessler CN (1988) Worsening oxygenation in the mechanically ventilated patient. Causes, mechanisms and detection. Am Rev Respir Dis 138:458-4565
5. Agustí AGN, Barberà JA, Roca J, Wagner PD, Guitart R, Rodriguez-Roisin R (1990) Hypoxic pulmonary vasoconstriction and gas exchange in chronic obstructive pulmonary disease. Chest 97:268-275
6. Dantzker DR (1987) Ventilation-perfusion inequality in lung disease. Chest 91:749-754

7. West JB (1969) Causes of carbon dioxide retention in lung disease. N Engl J Med 284:1232-1236
8. West JB (1971) Causes of carbon dioxide retention in lung disease. N Engl J Med 284:1232-1236
9. Dantzker DR (1983) The influence of cardiovascular function on gas exchange. Clin Chest Med 4:149-159
10. Agusti AGN, Roca J, Gea J, Wagner PD, Xaubet A, Rodriguez-Roisin R (1991) Mechanisms of gas exchange impairment in idiopathic pulmonary fibrosis. Am Rev Respir Dis 143:219-225
11. Lynch JP, Mhyre JG, Dantzker DR (1979) Influence of cardiac output on intrapulmonary shunt. J Appl Physiol 46:315-321
12. Breen PH, Schumacker PT, Hedenstierna G, Ali J, Wagner PD, Wood LDH (1982) How does increased cardiac output increase shunt in pulmonary edema? J Appl Physiol 53:1487-1495
13. Hyman Al, Higashida RT, Spannhake EW, Kadowitz PJ (1981) Pulmonary vasoconstrictor responses to graded decreases in precapillary blood PO_2 in intact-chest cat. J Appl Physiol 51:1009-1016
14. Benumof Jl, Pirio AF, Johanson I, Trousdale FR (1981) Interaction of PvO_2 on hypoxic pulmonary vasoconstrictor. J Appl Physiol 51:871-874
15. Wagner PD (1982) Ventilation-perfusion inequality in catastrophic lung disease. In: Prakash O (ed) Applied physiology in clinical respiratory care. Martinus Nijhoff, The Hague, pp 363-379
16. Weinberger SE, Schwartzstein RM, Weiss JW (1989) Hypercapnia. N Engl J Med 321:1223-1231
17. Torres A, Reyes A, Roca J, Wagner PD, Rodriguez-Roisin R (1989) Ventilation-perfusion mismatching in chronic obstructive pulmonary disease ventilator weaning. Am Rev Respir Dis 14:1246-1250
18. Gale GE, Torre-Bueno JR, Moon RE, Saltzman HA, Wagner PD (1985) Ventilation-perfusion inequalities in normal humans during exercise at sea level and simulated altitude. J Appl Physiol 58:978-988
19. Lemaire F, Teboul JL, Cinotti L, et al (1988) Acute left ventricular dysfunction during unsuccessful weaning from mechanical ventilation. Anesthesiology 69:171-179
20. Permut S (1988) Circulatory effects of weaning from mechanical ventilation: the importance of transdiaphragmatic pressure. Anesthesiology 69:157-160
21. Ferrer A, Roca J, Barberà JA, Agusti AGN, Wagner PD, Rodriguez-Roisin R (1990) Evolution of ventilation perfusion mismatch during exercebations of chronic obstructive pulmonary disease. Eur Respir J 3 [suppl 10]:101S (abstract)
22. Barberà JA, Ramirez J, Roca J, Wagner PD, Sanchez-Lloret J, Rodriguez-Roisin R (1990) Lung structure and gas exchange in mild chronic obstructive pulmonary disease. Am Rev Respir Dis 141:895-901
23. Annat G, Viale JP, Dereymez CP, Bouffard YM, Delafosse BX, Motin JP (1990) Oxygen cost of breathing and diaphragmatic pressure-time index. Measurement in patients with COPD during weaning with pressure support ventilation. Chest 98:411-414
24. Caldwekk PRB, Echeverri U, Kilcoyne MM, Fritts HW Jr (1979) Observations on a model of proliferative lung and disease: II. Description of pulmonary gas exchange and comparison of Fick and dye cardiac outputs. J Clin Inves 49:1311-1315
25. Light RB (1988) Intrapulmonary oxygen consumption in experimental pneumococcal pneumonia. J Appl Physiol 64:2490-2495
26. Hubmayr RD, Loosbrock LM, Gillespie DJ, Rodarte JR (1988) Oxygen uptake during weaning from mechanical ventilation. Chest 94:1149-1155

Chapter 14

Mechanical ventilation and lung perfusion

A. VERSPRILLE

Introduction

All mechanisms causing a decrease in cardiac output will decrease lung perfusion. During mechanical ventilation a decrease occurs by inflation and by superimposing a positive end-expiratory pressure (PEEP) on a ventilatory pattern. Both conditions cause an increase in central venous pressure, which causes the decrease in cardiac output by virtue of its back pressure on venous return. If a change in PEEP is established for a period longer than a minute, the time is long enough for the circulatory control mechanisms to counteract the negative effects. During a ventilatory cycle central venous pressure rises and then decreases again in only a few seconds. The time period of a ventilatory cycle is too short to modulate circulatory control activity synchronously with the changes in central venous pressure, cardiac output and arterial pressure, even at a low ventilatory rate of 10 per minute. During inflation the primary response to the rise in central venous pressure is a decrease in venous return, causing a decrease in right ventricular (RV) output. After a delay of 2-5 heart beats also LV output decreases. This delay is an important phenomenon in relation to the tidal changes in pulmonary perfusion and blood volume and the decrease in mean flow by inflation relative to end-expiratory flow. To analyse these events, firstly, the cyclic changes in haemodynamic variables occurring during a ventilatory cycle will be described. Thereafter, we will consider the mechanisms of tidal changes in lung perfusion and pulmonary blood volume.

Cyclic events

Since 1966 cylic events during mechanical ventilation have been reported by many authors [1] but only during the last decade has quantitative analyses been done thanks to the possibilities of extensive computer analyses. Detailed information on the experimental conditions to sample heart beat-to- beat data of haemodynamic changes during the ventilatory cycles has been published elswhere [1, 2], here I will summarize the results. Numerical data of the beat-to-beat analyses during a ventilatory cycle during normovolaemic conditions are shown in Fig. 1. Intrathoracic (P_{it}), central venous (P_{cv}) and transmural central venous pressure ($P_{cv,tm}$), the latter as a substitute of right ventricular (RV) filling pressure, are

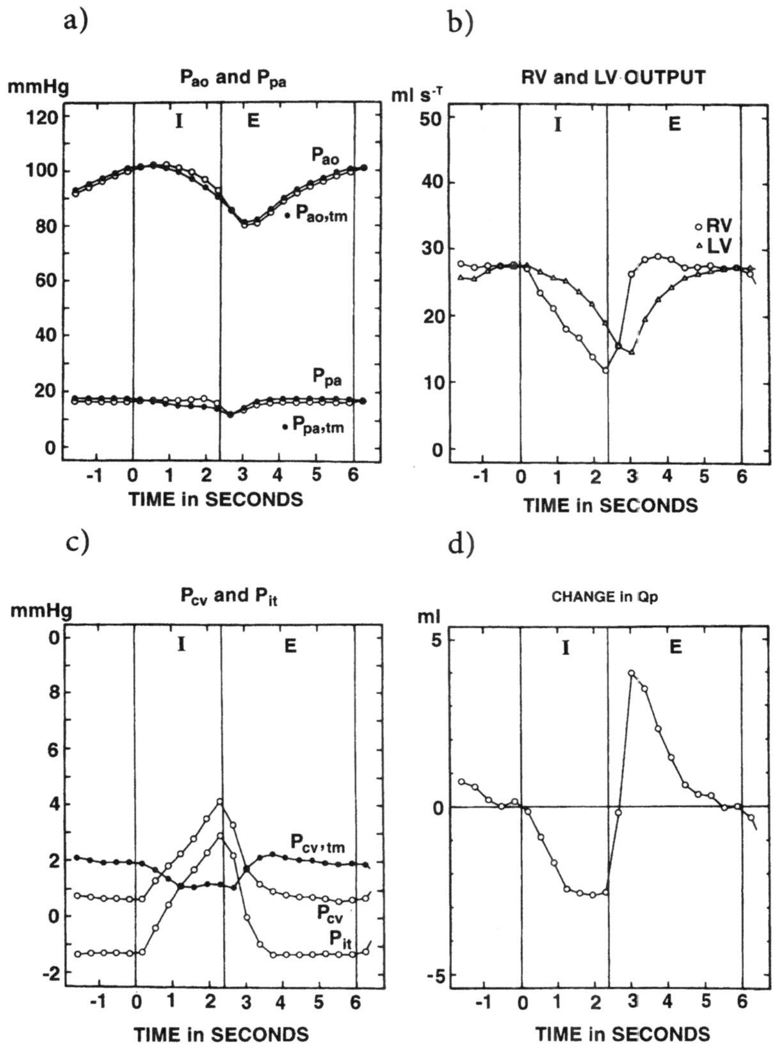

Fig. 1. Haemodynamic changes during a ventilatory cycle under conditions of normovolaemia, all plotted against time. Inflation starts at time zero; negative time is the time of the preceeding cycle. A ventilatory cycle lasted 6 s and this ventilatory rate was 10 per minute. Inflation (I) was 2.4 s and spontaneous expiration (E) 3.6 s

a. Open circles: aortic (P_{ao}) and pulmonary arterial pressure (P_{pa}) relative to ambient air pressure. Closed circles: the transmural values relative to intrathoracic pressure
b. Right (RV) and left ventricular (LV) output in ml per s
c. Open circles: central venous (P_{cv}) and intrathoracic (actually pericardial) pressure (P_{it}). Closed circles: transmural P_{cv}; $P_{cv,tm} = P_{cv} - P_{it}$.
d. The difference between stroke volume of the RV and that of the LV, representing the change in pulmonary blood volume (Q_p) per heart beat. The sum of negative values represents total blood shift from the pulmonary to the systemic circulation during inflation; the positive values represent the increase in Q_p per heart beat during expiration

plotted in Fig.1, c. During inflation the increase in P_{cv} is smaller than that in P_{it}, implying a fall in filling pressure, $P_{cv,tm}$. We also demonstrated such changes in RV end-diastolic transmural pressure, $P_{rved,tm}$ [1]. The fall in filling pressure at the right side of the heart is obviously due to a fall in preload, i.e. a decrease in venous return. The decrease in venous return is represented by the fall in RV output (Fig.1b). Heart rate did not change more than 3 % during a ventilatory cycle. The lowest value of RV-output occurred at maximal inflation, its fast recovery during early expiration coinciding with a recovery of $P_{cv,tm}$. The recovery in RV output to its end-expiratory value occurred via an overshoot of a few beats, with a delay of 3 beats the fall in LV-output followed the fall in RV-output. The delay is about 2-3 beats in hypo-and normovolaemia and larger in hypervolaemia [2]. Parallel to the fall in LV-output a decrease in left ventricular filling pressure ($P_{lv,ed,tm}$) occurred [1], the nadir of the fall in LV stroke volume being always found a few beats after the start of expiration when the intrapulmonary pressure fell to its end-expiratory level. Thereafter, a gradual recovery of stroke volume and filling pressure to the end-expiratory plateau occurred.

In spite of a large decrease in RV output, only a slight decrease in transmural pulmonary arterial pressure ($P_{pa,tm}$) occurred during inflation, which recovered during expiration. If the input into a vessel or system of vessels is decreased, the filling pressure, and therefore the volume of the vessel, will only remain constant if also the output is concomitantly and equally decreased. Therefore, we explained the almost constant transmural pulmonary arterial pressure during inflation by an increasing obstruction of outflow from the pulmonary arterial system due to an increasing alveolar pressure, aortic pressure (P_{ao}) falling approximately in parallel with LV output (Fig. 1a).

During early inflation an increase rather than a decrease can be seen, the reason is certainly not an increased LV output. During normovolaemic conditions we did not find a significant change in LV output during the first few beats of the inflation phase; the value was similar to the end-expiratory output. Only during hypervolaemia did we observe a significant increase in LV output during the first four strokes in the inflation period [2].

Tidal change in lung perfusion

The decrease in RV output during inflation is not fully compensated for by the increase in flow during expiration to obtain a mean flow equal to end-expiratory flow; only a small overshoot in early expiration compensates for the loss in flow during inflation. During conditions of normovolaemia a loss in flow of about 10 % on average is caused by inflation if ventilatory rate is 10 per minute [1, 2], in simple terms this means that mean cardiac output is about 10 % lower than end-expiratory flow.

During inflation the rise in central venous pressure causes an accumulation of blood in the venous capacities. Thus, a relevant question to consider is why the decrease in flow during inflation is not fully compensated for by an increased flow during expiration, when all accumulated blood will be released from the venous capacities. A first answer is that during a ventilatory cycle central venous pressure is higher on average than at end-expiration due to the increase and fall as observed in Fig.1c. The overall higher P_{cv} will decrease venous return, but this rise in central venous pressure of a few mm Hg represents only a very small part (a few percent) of the total arterial-to-venous pressure gradient. A more detailed answer can be derived from Fig.1. Due to the accumulation of blood in the venous system RV output is decreased much more than the rise in P_{cv} predicts from the arterial-to-venous pressure gradient, this decrease in RV output is followed by a similar decrease in LV-output with its lowest value during the first beats in early expiration. Concomitantly, a decreased aortic pressure occurs and, therefore, decreases the driving force of blood into the venous system. The decreased input into the venous system and the blood released from the venous capacities make up the venous return, which by itself is larger than the end-expiratory flow, but far too little to compensate for the loss in flow during inflation. The coincidence of a release of the accumulated venous blood and the low basic venous input flow is due to the capacity function of the pulmonary vascular system and the alveolar pressure acting upon it, causing a delay between the output decrease of the right and left ventricle.

Comparing volaemic conditions our results revealed (Table 1) that during hypervolaemia the tidal loss in flow in ml • s^{-1} • kg^{-1} is lower than during normovolaemia [2]. As a percentage the loss in flow relative to end-expiratory flow is even more reduced compared to that during normovolaemia, because the loss is related to the higher end-expiratory flow during hypervolaemia.

In Table 1 the changes in central venous pressure are also presented. During hypervolaemia the rise in central venous pressure by inflation was significantly smaller than that during normo- and hypovolaemia. As inflation volume was the same in all volaemic conditions the rise in intrathoracic pressure was also the same, implying that the fall in transmural central venous pressure was largest during hypervolaemic conditions. We attributed this larger fall in filling pressure for a smaller decrease in flow during hypervolaemia, compared to normo- and hypovolaemia, to the typical character of a ventricular function curve [2]. During hypervolaemia cardiac function was related to the less steep part at higher load and filling pressure compared to the other two volaemic conditions. A smaller increase in P_{cv} during inflation will certainly contribute to a smaller tidal decrease in venous return. However, the smaller increase in P_{cv} cannot fully explain the difference in tidal flow loss between hypervolaemia and normo- and hypovolaemia.

An additional explanation for the smaller decrease in flow during inflation under conditions of hypervolaemia could be a higher filling state of the venous capacities. During hypervolaemia central venous pressure is substantially increased compared to normovolaemia, and upstream the venous pressure will be relatively even higher, in accordance with the higher flow. If a vessel is filled upto the level of a steep rise in pressure for a given volume increase, a smaller volume will be accumulated for a similar or even higher rise in intravascular

Table 1. Tidal loss in right ventricular flow and tidal rise in central venous pressure during inflation

	RV FLOW LOSS % of end-exp flow mean, sd, p	ml • s^{-1} • kg^{-1} mean, sd, p	RISE IN P_{cv} mm Hg mean, sd, p
Normovolaemia-1	9.0 3.0 0.15	0.20 0.084 0.05	2.6 0.39 0.9
Hypervolaemia	2.2 2.0 0.002	0.06 0.065 0.005	1.7 0.66 0.0
Normovolaemia-2	10.7 3.7	0.26 0.1	2.6 0.66
Hypovolaemia	15.6 3.8 0.008	0.25 0.07 0.88	2.7 0.67 0.64

n is 48 in all volaemic series
p: p-values from paired t-test versus normovolaemia-2. The volaemic conditions were created in the order given top-down in the table
Normovolaemia-1: the blood volume after surgery with normal composition
Hypervolaemia: + 15 ml per kg dextran solution
Normovolaemia-2: - 15 ml per kg bleeding
Hypovolaemia: - 15 ml per kg bleeding
(The table is taken from [2], by courtesy of Pflügers Archiv)

pressure. During inflation the rise in central venous pressure is about the same for normo- and hypervolaemia, which together with a higher filling state might explain the smaller accumulation of blood under hypervolaemic conditions.

During hypovolaemia the tidal loss in flow in $ml.s_{-1}.kg_{-1}$ was the same as during normovolaemia, but it was higher in percentage due to the lower end-expiratory flow. Apparently, during hypovolaemia as well as during normovolaemia the filling state of the venous capacity is in the linear part of its pressure-volume relationship, implying a similar accumulation of blood for a similar rise in venous pressure.

Tidal changes in pulmonary blood volume

If we regard RV and LV output as input and output of the pulmonary circulation respectively, we can calculate from the heart beat-to-beat differences in ventricular output the changes in pulmonary blood volume. The differences between the stroke volumes of both ventricles are presented in Fig.1d as can be seen, because the input of blood into the pulmonary circulation fell immediately after the start of inflation, while output from it remained constant for several beats (Fig. 1b), a loss of blood from the pulmonary circulation occurred during inflation. During expiration this loss was recovered due to a larger input into than output from the pulmonary circulation. The tidal change in blood volume was larger if inflation volume was larger, which we determined during inspiratory pause procedures after inflation of various volumes. The accumulated differences between the input and output of the pulmonary circulation yielded an S-shape relationship between the change in blood volume and inflation volume [1]. At an inflation volume of approximately 25 ml/kg body weight (bw) the maximal tidal change in blood volume was found at about 1.5 ml/kg bw. We calculated that approximately 7 % of this value came from the decrease in LV volume due to the decrease in preload (filling pressure). If we extrapolate these data to human beings, a shift of 15-20 % of the total pulmonary blood volume to the systemic circulation during inflation could occur during mechanical ventilation at 10 strokes per minute.

Quantitative data regarding the contribution to this shift by either the arteries, the capillaries or the veins is unknown but we have some evidence to conclude that the contribution of the pulmonary arterial system is relatively small, because we observed only a small decrease in transmural pulmonary arterial pressure during inflation (Fig. 1a). If the blood volume in the arteries does not change much during inflation, the tidal shift of blood from the pulmonary circulation will be mainly delivered by the capillaries and veins, which implies a relatively larger loss of capillary and venous blood volume during inflation than 15 - 20 %, calculated for the tidal shift of blood related to the total pulmonary blood volume.

Two mechanisms causing the shift of blood from the pulmonary circulation into the systemic circulation might be involved:

1. the normal function of the pulmonary vascular volume capacity, implying an emptying if input is decreased;
2. an effect of squeezing of these capacities due to the rise in alveolar and intrathoracic pressure [1].

During expiration the squeezing effect is omitted and the increased input into the pulmonary circulation will fill the vascular capacities again. We also compared the tidal shifts in blood volume during mechanical ventilation under conditions of hypo-, normo- and hypervolaemia during ventilation at a rate of 10 per minute [2]. Hypovolaemia was 15 ml blood per kg body weight below normovolaemia and hypervolaemia 15 ml/kg bw above it. The tidal change in pulmonary blood volume was about 1 ml per kg during normo- and hypovolaemia (Table 2). During hypervolaemia the tidal shift was 40 % lower.

We considered two hypotheses to explain these data:

1. a similar tidal shift in blood volume during normo- and hypovolaemia for a similar rise in extravascular pressures (intrathoracic and intrapulmonary pressure) indicates that the pressure-volume relationship of the pulmonary circulation is in its linear part. This view fits with the linear model of the pulmonary vascular bed [3]. The smaller blood shift from the pulmonary circulation during hypervolaemia could be due to a higher filling state of the pulmonary vasculature system, up to the non-linear part of the P-V relationship, where a pressure change coincides with a smaller volume change;
2. another explanation could be the smaller decrease in RV output by inflation during hypervolaemia compared to the fall during normo- and hypovolaemia [2]. A small decrease in input into a capacity will only cause a slight decrease in volume and output.

Table 2. Tidal shift in pulmonary blood volume during inflation

	mean ml kg^{-1}	sd ml kg^{-1}	p ml kg^{-1}
Normovolaemia-1	10.96	0.17	0.34
Hypervolaemia	0.61	0.27	0.000
Normovolaemia-2	0.99	0.24	
Hypovolaemia	1.04	0.17	0.18

p: p-values from paired t-test versus normovolaemia-2
The volaemic conditions are defined in the legends of Table 1
(This table is taken from [2], by courtesy of Pflügers Archiv)

An objection against the first explanation is that arterial pulmonary pressure was only increased a few mm Hg relative to the value during the other volaemic conditions. Therefore, it seems unlikely that the filling state of the arterial system was at the higher non-linear part of the P-V relationship. We regard the slightly increased pulmonary arterial pressure during hypervolaemia too small to accept a filling state at the non-linear level of the P-V relationship. On the other hand we have to be careful to make a definite choice. Firstly, we concluded above that the arterial system will contribute only slightly to the tidal shift of blood. Secondly, we have no information about the filling state of the pulmonary system downstream of the arterial system. The pulmonary arterial pressure depends on either the vascular flow resistance or the level of alveolar pressure causing the Starling resistors (which is the analogy of the height of the rim of a waterfall) or a combination of the two. Because the mode of ventilation was the same during all volemic conditions, the alveolar pressure will have caused a similar threshold pressure at capillary level to the arterial flow (height of the rim). [In such a situation the slightly increased pulmonary arterial pressure during hypervolaemia can be explained by the higher flow over the upstream arterial and arteriolar flow resistance]. The consequence of a rim of a waterfall is the functional separation of the upstream part of a flow from its downstream part. A downstream pulmonary venous pressure rise will not influence the upstream pulmonary arterial pressure if the venous pressure is below the pressure of the rim. Therefore, we cannot definitely exclude a higher filling state of the venous part of the pulmonary vascular system during hypervolaemia, but, if the lung veins are filled up more during hypervolaemia, would they not cause a larger shift of blood rather than a smaller one during compression by inflation if the rise in intrathoracic pressure is about the same? It will be obvious that we are at a level of speculation and that we have no definite answer.

In contrast to the first hypothesis the second has no controversial considerations in itself, though this is not the only reason that I have a preference for the second explanation. The data verifying this mechanism were experimentally observed (Table 2), whereas the first explanation is wholly unsupported by experimental evidence.

Consequences during disease

During inflation the increase in alveolar volume will increase the area of the diffusion membrane between alveolar air and lung capillary blood, which favours gas exchange. The corresponding decrease in capillary blood volume and blood flow will cause a negative effect on total gas transfer. Thus, besides its positive effect on gas exchange by unfolding of alveolar membranes and recruitment of alveoli, inflation has a negative effect by decreasing capillary blood volume. In acute respiratory distress the compliant parts of the lung, i.e. the more healthy parts which are essential for keeping the patient alive, will receive a larger part of tidal volume than the parts with low compliance. As a consequence, during inflation blood volume will decrease more in the compliant parts than in the less compliant parts, the consequence of which if true, is a disadvantage for gas exchange.

Overall, mechanical ventilation has a positive effect, otherwise it would not be a therapy in the treatment of patients suffering from acute respiratory distress. Undoubtedly, the positive effect of unfolding and recruitment of membrane for gas transfer, implying a recruitment of shunt blood for oxygen uptake, exceeds the negative effect on oxygen uptake in the less diseased areas attributed to a decrease in capillary blood volume. Our results indicated that this negative effect can be diminished by blood transfusion because the tidal shift in pulmonary blood volume is decreased if total blood volume is increased.

References

1. Versprille A, Jansen JRC, Frietman RC, Hulsmann AR, Klauw MM (1990) Negative effect of insufflation on cardiac output and pulmonary blood volume. Acta Anaesthesiol Scand 34:607-615
2. Versprille A, Jansen JRC (1993) Tidal variation of pulmonary blood flow and blood volume in piglets during mechanical ventilation during hyper-, normo- and hypovolaemia. Pflgers Arch Eur J Physiol 424:255-265
3. Shoukas AA (1975) Pressure-flow and pressure-volume relations in the entire pulmonary vascular bed of the dog determined by two port analysis. Circ Res 37:809-818

Chapter 15

Monitoring respiratory mechanics during controlled mechanical ventilation

G. MUSCH, M.E. SPARACINO, A. PESENTI

Introduction

Monitoring the mechanics of the respiratory system in the critical care setting has become increasingly popular and feasible since modern ventilators and other respiratory monitoring equipment allow easy measurement of airway and esophageal pressure, airflow and volumes during mechanical ventilation. It is thus possible to assess the basic physiologic properties of the respiratory system - compliance and resistance - which are important to the physician since they bear diagnostic, prognostic and therapeutic relevance to the patient.

This discussion will be limited to the assessment of respiratory mechanics during controlled mechanical ventilation in muscle relaxed patients. Before getting into the practical and computational details of the problem though, a brief overview of some of the mathematical models currently employed to explain the behaviour of the respiratory system is needed in order to gain a deeper understanding of what will follow.

Modelling of respiratory system mechanics

A wide variety of respiratory system models have been used by physiologists so far [1-8]; these can be characterized by the number of compartments they assume, where a compartment is meant as any physiological entity whose dynamics are described by a linear first order differential equation [2]. We will not deal with the mathematical aspects of such models, which are fully treated elsewhwere [1, 9, 7], but we will try to give a qualitative explanation of the behaviour of those models that might be helpful in interpreting respiratory mechanics data during controlled meehanical ventilation.

We will make two simplifying assumptions:

1. that the models are linear i.e. their mechanical characteristics are indeed parameters independent of flow, volume and pressure;
2. that inertial components of the models are negligible. This assumption seems valid for the respiratory system in the range of normal breathing frequencies up to 2 Hz [10].

Linear one-compartment model

A graphical representation of a one compartment-model is depicted in Fig. 1a; such a system consists of an elastance E ("balloon") served by a resistance R ("pipe").

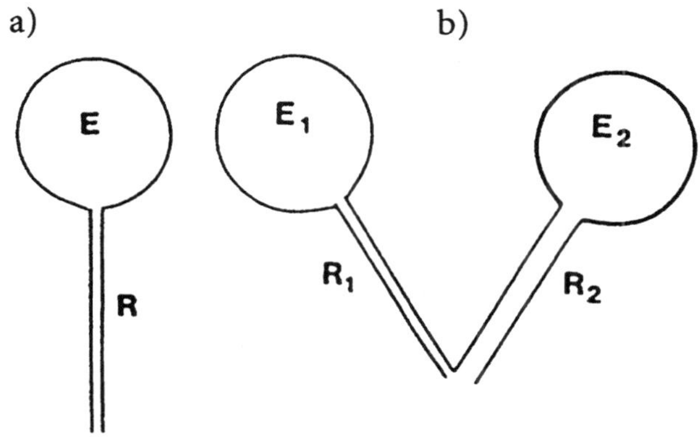

Fig. 1. a. One-compartment model of the respiratory system, featuring single constant elastance (E) and resistance (R). b. Two-compartment model of the respiratory system consisting of two single-compartment models joined in parallel. (From [9], with permission)

Its equation of motion is [1, 9]

$$P(t) = R \cdot \dot{V}(t) + E \cdot V(t) \tag{1}$$

where P(t) is the pressure applied to the system at time t, measured at the proximal, "open", end of the pipe, V(t) is flow through R at time t and V(t) is volume above resting volume at time t. Equation (1) is a linear first-order differential equation; it shows that the applied pressure P(t) has to counterbalance the elastic recoil of the balloon and to drive airflow through the resistance R. Figure 2 shows the time course of P(t), flow and volume when the balloon is inflated at constant flow over a certain time, followed by rapid occlusion of the pipe for a given time interval and then allowed to deflate passively. The instantaneous pressure rise at inspiratory flow onset equals the rapid pressure drop that is observed when constant inspiratory flow stops and is given by [9]: R • V(t). Dividing this pressure change by flow yields an estimate of R. Furthermore, dividing the pressure value recorded after occlusion by the volume inflated allows computation of the elastance E [9].

When deflation begins, P(t) drops to zero and volume decreases exponentially with a time constant = R • C (where C=1/E denotes compliance); if deflation was abruptly interrupted, P(t) would rise instantaneously to a plateau value representing the elastic recoil of the balloon at the time of interruption [2, 9].

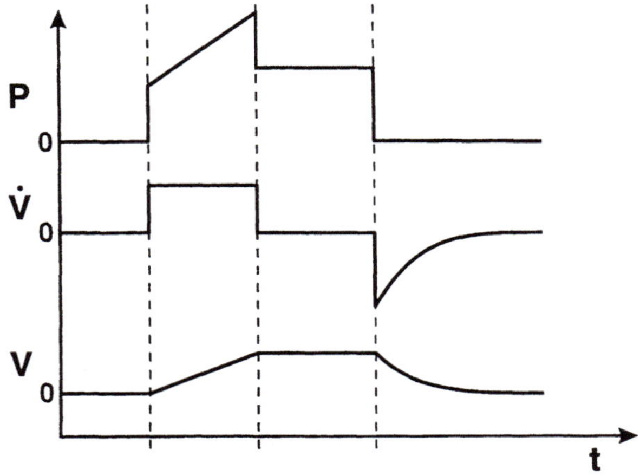

Fig. 2. Time course of pressure P (recorded at the open end of the resistance R), flow $\dot{V}$ inflated volume V, during constant flow inflation and successive deflation of the one-compartment model in Fig. 1a

Linear parallel two-compartment model

A second compartment may be added in parallel to the previous model either by including another "pipe with balloon" structure with a different time constant (Fig. 1b), or by adding a viscoelastic component that behaves as a slow compartment [3]. These two different kinds of two-compartment models have been referred to as "gas redistributive" and "rheologic" respectively [2].

Figure 3 shows the pressure, volume and flow time course of the two-compartment model during flow conditions equal to those mentioned above for the one- compartment model. Two points here need to be stressed.

First, there is no way of differentiating between the rheologic and the gas redistribution model from the pressure and volume recordings; it can be shown

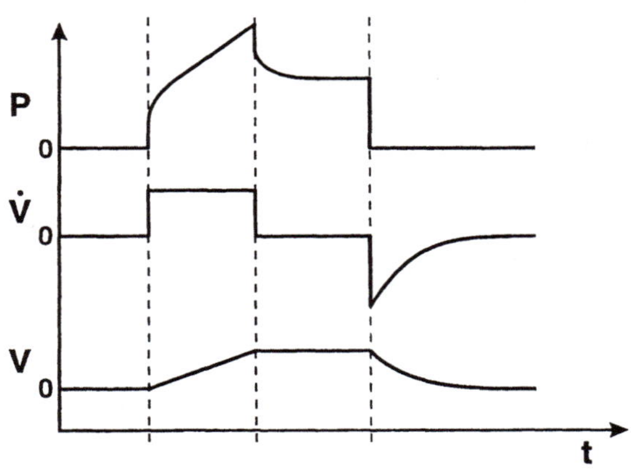

Fig. 3. Time course of pressure P (recorded at the open, common, end of the resistances R_1 and R_2), flow $\dot{V}$ and inflated volume V, during constant flow inflation and successive deflation of the two-compartment model in Fig. 1b

mathematically that the equations describing the parallel gas redistribution model (1) and viscoelastic rheologic model [7] have exactly the same form.

Second, there are important differences in pressure and volume tracings as compared with the one-compartment model: after constant flow interruption there is a rapid decrease in pressure that reflects either the pipe's resistance [1], equal to $R_1 \cdot R_2/(R_1+R_2)$ (parallel resistors), or the resistance of the fast compartment [3], depending on the kind of model we adopt. This ideally instantaneous drop is then followed by a slower pressure transient, which can be shown to follow exponential kinetics [9, 7], and that is due to either gas redistribution between the two units with different time constants ("pendelluft") or to stress relaxation of the viscoelastic component.

Similar slow pressure transients might be observed if passive deflation were suddenly interrupted: an immediate rise in pressure would be followed by an asymptotic exponential rise to a plateau value [1]. Furthermore, the volume-time profile during deflation would follow a double rather than a single exponential function. Two-compartment models have been shown to describe respiratory mechanics data better than one-compartment ones [3, 5, 6, 11-13]; the second compartment has been interpreted as representing either stress relaxation of lung and chest wall tissues [7, 14,-16], as seems to be the case for healthy lungs, at least in animals, and/or gas redistribution between alveolar units with different time constants [17, 18]. It seems likely that in diseased lungs both processes may contribute to the pressure transients that follow constant flow interruption.

We will now go through the most important respiratory mechanics variables and some of the methods available for their assessment during controlled mechanical ventilation.

Respiratory resistance

Illustrate are some of the methods available for the assessment of inspiratory and expiratory resistance during controlled mechanical ventilation.

Inspiratory resistance

A technique that has gained popularity in recent years is the flow interruption technique during constant flow inflation [1, 9]; it is basically a combination of the interrupter [19] and elastic subtraction [20] methods proposed by Von Neergaard and Wirtz. Experimental tracings in Fig. 4 show the time course of airway and esophageal pressure during an end inspiratory occlusion after constant flow inflation: airway pressure shows a rapid drop followed by a slower decay. Three values may thus be identified on this tracing: peak airway pressure ($P_{eak,aw}$) i.e. airway pressure immediately preceding occlusion, "zero flow" airway pressure ($P_{1,aw}$) i.e. airway pressure immediately following occlusion, that can be determined either inspectively or by back extrapolation of the slow pressure decay to the time of occlusion [21], and plateau pressure ($P_{2,aw}$) i.e. airway pressure at the

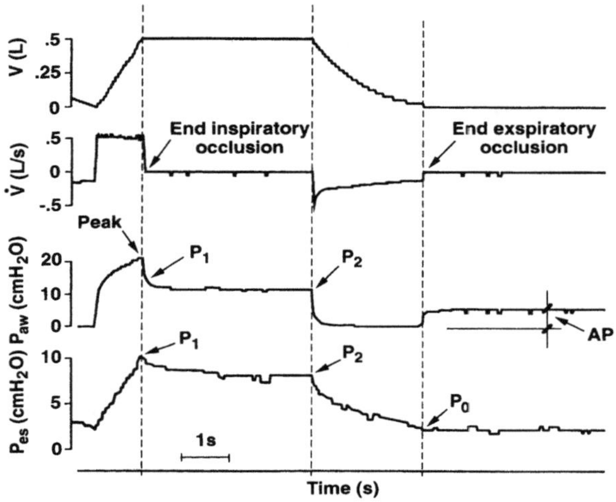

Fig. 4. End inspiratory occlusion followed by an end expiratory port occlusion. Experimental tracing. AP: Auto-PEEP; P_{aw}: airway pressure; P_{es}: esophageal pressure; $\dot{V}$: airflow; V: volume

end of the inspiratory hold; this last value depends on the duration of occlusion but 3 s are commonly recognized as sufficient to reach a value that well approximates static recoil pressure of the respiratory system [3, 22].

In the esophageal pressure tracing shown, only a peak ($P_{1,es}$) and a plateau ($P_{2,es}$) value may be identified. There is contrasting evidence concerning the existance of a rapid drop in esophageal pressure following airway occlusion and hence an esophageal contribution to R_{min} (see below): studies on animals have been able to identify such rapid decay in esophageal pressure [11, 12] although other Authors did not find a rapid initial drop in esophageal pressure after end inspiratory occlusion in human subjects [22, 13]. The pressure drops that follow flow interruption represent the gradients required to drive end inspiratory airflow into the respiratory system and to maintain motion of lung and chest wall tissues; they are therefore used to calculate inspiratory resistance.

By dividing these pressure changes by the preceding constant flow, several components of inspiratory resistance may be computed and they may be partitioned into lung and chest wall resistance [3, 22, 23, 13]:

1. "Ohmic" resistance (denoted as R_{init}, R_{int}, R_{min}) is computed as $R_{min} = (P_{eak,aw} - P_{1,aw})/\dot{V}$. In intubated patients it mainly represents airway resistance [1, 14] and it has been shown to vary with inspiratory flow, at a given lung volume, according to the Rohrer equation (3)

$$R_{min} = a + b \cdot \dot{V}$$

where a and b are two coefficients reflecting laminar and turbulent flow components respectively. Rmin has been shown to decrease with increasing lung volume at a given flow rate [3].

2. "Additional" resistance (that we will denote as ΔR) reflects the pressure drop due to tissue viscoelasticity (stress relaxation) and/or time-constant inhomogeneities (pendelluft). It is not a "pure" resistance since flow has already stopped during the slow pressure decay of either airway or esophageal pressure; therefore, the term "additional pulmonary impedance" has been suggested [24]. Additional resistance may be calculated for the lung and the chest wall separately if esophageal pressure is available:

$$\Delta R_L = [(P_{1,aw}-P_{1,es})-(P_{2,aw}-P_{2,es})]/V$$
$$\Delta R_{cw} = [P_{eak,es}-P_{2,es}]/V$$

R_{min}, ΔR_L and ΔR_{cw} are all that is needed to compute respiratory system additional resistance ($\Delta R_{rs} = \Delta R_L+\Delta R_{cw}$), respiratory system total resistance ($R_{max,rs} = \Delta R_{,rs}+R_{min}$) and lung total resistance ($R_{max,L} = \Delta R_L+R_{min}$).

As we have previously stated, experimental evidence at present suggests an esophageal contribution to R_{min} in humans to be negligeable, if any; therefore $R_{min,rs}$ equals $R_{min,L}$.

We still have two important points left.

First, a correction for the values of R_{min} is needed due to the fact that the closing time of the ventilator valve is finite and hence some inspiratory flow continues between the onset of valve closure and full valve closure [11, 25].

Second, if airway pressure is not measured at the tip of the endotracheal tube but at its proximal end, the resistive pressure drop due to the artificial airway needs to be subtracted from peak airway pressure before calculating inspiratory resistances. Several Authors have dealt with the problem of estimating flow resistance of the artificial airway in mechanically ventilated patients. Behrakis et al. [26] determined the pressure flow relationship of various endotracheal tubes in vitro, using the same gas mixture as in the in vivo study; by fitting Rohrer's equation to such a relationship they calculated the resistance of the tubes. Since, in their in vivo experiment, they measured airway pressure at the proximal end of the tube, they subtracted its calculated flow resistance from total measured respiratory resistance to obtain intrinsic respiratory flow resistance. Later, though, Wright et al. [27], questioned the validity of this method: they found the in vivo resistance of the endotracheal tubes, measured through an intratracheal catheter, to exceed their in vitro resistance and attributed this finding to deformations, kinking and secretions that may narrow the lumen of the endotracheal tube in intubated patients. Very recently Navalesi et al. [28] have substantially confirmed these results. Furthermore, they studied the effect of the site of tracheal pressure measurement on tube resistance and concluded that there were no relevant differences in inspiratory tube resistance when the tip of the tracheal catheter was placed either 2 cm inside, at the tip of, or 2 cm outside the endotracheal tube. In contrast, expiratory tube resistance appeared to be much affected by the position of the intratracheal catheter, decreasing progressively as the tip of the catheter was moved from outside to inside the tube. They explained this finding as due to the airflow velocity increase that results from the reduction in cross sectional area from the trachea to the tube during expiration.

Endotracheal tubes with intramural catheter channels that open at the tip of the tube might provide a valuable alternative to intraluminal catheters; since they do not reduce the tube's cross sectional area, they do not increase tube resistance. Furthermore, the fixed position and orientation of their opening may contribute to obtaining more reliable tracheal pressure measurements than with intraluminal catheters [28].

Increased respiratory resistance is a hallmark of obstructive pulmonary disease and several Authors have shown an increase of both ohmic and additional resistances in COPD patients [29, 22]. Recently, however, evidence of an abnormally increased resistance in ARDS patients has gathered also [29-31], present data suggesting an increase of both additional and ohmic resistances, the latter being, at least partially, reversed by bronchodilators [30].

Expiratory resistance

We will illustrate three methods for the assessment of expiratory resistance (R_{ex}) in muscle relaxed mechanically ventilated patients.

Flow interruption technique

If expiratory flow is interrupted, airway pressure rises to a plateau value that corresponds to a weighted average of alveolar pressures at the time of occlusion. Subtracting airway pressure just before the interruption from the post occlusion plateau value and dividing by the expiratory flow that was present just prior to interruption yields an estimate of expiratory resistance at that given lung volume [1, 7]. Here also, if airway pressure is not measured at the tip of the endotracheal tube, the resistive pressure losses due to the artificial airway and, possibly, to the ventilator circuit have to be subtracted from the post occlusion plateau in airway pressure [26].

Passive exhalation time constant method

If the respiratory system is assumed to behave as a single compartment, the exhalation time course of lung volume above resting volume is fitted by a single exponential equation [33]. Its time constant τ, i.e. the product of resistance (R_{ex}) and compliance (C_{rs}), represents the time needed to exhale 63 % of lung volume above resting volume [34]. Tau may be calculated from the expiratory volume-time curve and expiratory resistance computed as $R_{ex} = \tau/C_{rs}$. This value of expiratory resistance, however, includes also the resistance of the expiratory pathway from the endotracheal tube to the expiratory port. Furthermore, one-compartment modelling of the respiratory system does not seem adequate in most instances, as we have previously recalled.

Alveolar pressure estimation method

Noninvasive measurement of alveolar pressure without flow interruption is not possible; however, alveolar pressure may be estimated during exhalation if respiratory system compliance (C_{rs}) and exhaled volume are known:

$$P_{alv}(t) = P_{2,aw} - V(t)/Crs$$

where $P_{alv}(t)$ is the estimated alveolar pressure at the time a volume equal to V(t) has been exhaled. Expiratory flow resistance may thus be estimated as [26]:

$$R_{ex} = [P_{alv}(t) - P_{aw}(t)]/[\dot{V}(t)]$$

where $P_{aw}(t)$ and $\dot{V}(t)$ are airway pressure and flow,respectively, at the time V(t) was exhaled.

Here also correction is due if P_{aw} is not measured at the distal end of the endotracheal tube.

Auto-PEEP

The difference between alveolar and airway opening pressures at end expiration is defined as auto-PEEP [35]. In muscle relaxed mechanically ventilated patients Auto-PEEP is always associated with dynamic hyperinflation, i.e. an increase of end expiratory lung volume above resting volume [36]. Two distinct forms of Auto-PEEP may occur in relaxed mechanically ventilated patients, depending on the presence or absence of flow limitation [36].

Dynamic hyperinflation without flow limitation occurs when the lungs do not have enough time to reach their resting volume during passive deflation because of high ventilatory requirements coupled with brief expiratory time and/or high resistance. This may be the case in ARDS patients in whom very high minute volumes are necessary to compensate for the reduced efficiency of ventilation in order to maintain reasonable arterial carbon dioxide levels despite a high shunt fraction and dead space. Furthermore, prolonged inspiratory time, commonly regarded as beneficial for arterial oxygenation, is used in the ventilatory management of ARDS patients; this implies a brief expiratory time that fosters the development of Auto-PEEP. Findings of Auto-PEEP in mechanically ventilated ARDS patients have actually been reported [29, 37].

Even in normal anesthetized subjects the added resistance of the endotracheal tube, the expiratory circuit and the exhalation valve may substantially increase total expiratory resistance (from less than 4 cm H_2O/l/s to greater than 10 cm H_2O/l/s) thus delaying lung emptying and fostering the development of Auto-PEEP if minute ventilation is high (usually greater than 20 l/s).

Dynamic hyperinflation with flow limitation is seen in patients with very severe airflow obstruction, usually with asthma or acute exacerbation of COPD.

Flow limitation was originally described in spontaneously breathing emphysematous subjects by Fry [38] and later in ventilated patients (see for instance ref. 39). It is defined as the independence of expiratory flow on transpulmonary pressure as observed from isovolume pressure-flow curves. This means that either increasing transpulmonary pressure, as may occur in spontaneously breathing subjects performing greater expiratory effort, or decreasing transpulmonary pressure, as may be the case in mechanically ventilated subjects to whom PEEP is applied, does not change the rate of lung emptying. A decreased lung recoil coupled with high expiratory resistance and, eventually, flow limitation, are the factors that foster the development of Auto-PEEP in patients with COPD.

Several theories have been put forward to explain flow limitation and have been reviewed by Hyatt [40]. One of these, the "equal pressure point theory", assumes that intrathoracic airway collapse occurs where intrabronchial and extrabronchial pressures are equal, this choke point being named the equal pressure point (EPP). In this situation any pressure change downstream of the EPP would not affect expiratory flow rate and pressure upstream of the EPP, unless it reversed the dynamic airway collapse. This is of particular importance in understanding the interactions between Auto-PEEP and any externally applied PEEP: if flow limitation is present, PEEP at least when lower than a critical value estimated to be about 85 % of Auto-PEEP [41], does not cause further hyperinflation and may actually be advantageous during assisted mechanical ventilation by reducing work of breathing and effective triggering sensitivity [36, 33]. Conversely, if Auto-PEEP without flow limitation occurs, any externally applied PEEP represents a back pressure to expiratory flow that further reduces lung emptying and increases lung hyperinflation [36], with increased risk of barotrauma and hemodynamic deterioration. This might explain apparent inconsistencies in the findings of different Authors [41, 33, 42].

Recognition of flow limitation is therefore fundamental for proper ventilatory management. Valuable information may be provided by the expiratory flow-time tracing: high flow transients following occlusion release, a linear and/or biphasic flow profile and failure of added resistance to influence expiratory flow rate indicate flow limitation and dynamic airway collapse [35]. A PEEP test may be performed to evaluate whether Auto-PEEP remains constant or decreases at increasing PEEP levels.

Auto-PEEP can be measured by several methods during passive ventilation. The most popular one is the end expiratory port occlusion method [43], when the expiratory port of the ventilator is occluded at end exhalation and airflow is thus interrupted, airway pressure rises to a plateau value that represents a compliance weighted average of end expiratory alveolar pressures of different lung units (Fig. 4). Notice from Fig. 4 that the time course of the pressure rise after the end expiratory occlusion is smooth, consistent with a multi-compartment model interpretation of the respiratory system [1].

An alternative method to evaluate Auto-PEEP [44] is based on the consideration that inspiratory flow will not start until airway pressure overcomes alveolar pressure; the airway pressure change that is necessary to initiate inflation yields an estimate of Auto-PEEP that is usually referred to as "dynamic" Auto-PEEP as opposed to "static" Auto-PEEP measured by the end expiratory port occlusion method.

Other methods to assess Auto-PEEP during controlled mechanical ventilation are based upon so called "external PEEP counterbalancing" where Auto-PEEP is estimated as the lowest level of PEEP that causes an increase in lung volume, measured by impedance plethysmography [45]. This technique, though, may yield reliable results only if flow limitation is the pathophysiologic condition underlying airflow obstruction [36].

The main pathophysiologic consequences of dynamic hyperinflation are related to a potential risk for barotrauma and hemodynamic compromise, with decreased cardiac output and blood pressure and misleadingly high values of heart filling pressures [41-43].

Compliance

The change in volume per unit change in applied static pressure is defined as compliance.

In muscle relaxed patients total respiratory system compliance may be determined by inflating the lungs with a given volume of gas and recording the associated airway pressure rise under static (i.e. no flow) conditions when airway pressure (P_{aw}) equals the elastic recoil pressure of the respiratory system ($P_{el,rs}$) [46]. If esophageal pressure, which estimates pleural or intrathoracic pressure, is available, total respiratory system compliance (C_{rs}) may be partitioned into its lung (C_L) and chest wall (C_{cw}) components with formulas

$$C_{rs} = TV/\Delta P_{el,rs} \qquad C_L = V_t/\Delta P_L \qquad C_{cw} = V_t/\Delta P_{es}$$

where V_T is the inflated volume and $\Delta P_{el,rs}$, $\Delta P_{,es}$ and ΔP_L the changes in static airway pressure, static esophageal pressure and static transpulmonary pressure ($P,_L = P_{el,rs}\text{-}P_{es}$) associated with TV inflation.

Simple algebric calculations from the above formulas show that:

$$1/C_{rs} = 1/C_L + 1/C_{cw} \quad \text{or}$$
$$E_{rs} = E_L + E_{cw}$$

where E = 1/C denotes elastance, the inverse of compliance. The two equations above show that the lung and chest wall are modelled as being in series.

Another important equation derived from easy arithmetical workup of the above formulas is:

$$\Delta P_{es} = P_{el,rs} \bullet (C_L\,(C_L + C_{cw}))$$

this implies that the fraction of an alveolar pressure change which is transmitted to the pleural space depends on the relative stiffness of the lung and chest wall. This is important because the hemodynamic consequences of positive pressure breathing depend upon the increase in intrathoracic pressure that, for a given alveolar pressure, will be higher with compliant lungs and/or stiff chest wall than with stiff lungs [47]. Chest wall volume and compliance determine the value of intrathoracic pressure.

Respiratory compliance may be evaluated in several ways in the critical care setting during controlled mechanical ventilation.

A supersyringe may be used to draw the pressure volume curve of the respiratory system in paralyzed patients [48, 49]. The patient is first administered several large breaths from the ventilator possibly to standardize for previous volume history, and is then connected to the supersyringe which has been previously filled with approximately 20 ml/Kg of pure oxygen. A manometer needs to be placed on the syringe so that if an Auto-PEEP is present it can either be accounted for in the drawing of the P-V curve or the patient be disconnected and allowed an apnea sufficient to reach resting volume. Fernandez et al. [50] have shown that an isovolumetric pressure increment (IPI) that corresponds to Auto-PEEP can be detected when the supersyringe is connected to patients with dynamic hyperinflation at the end of the expiratory time set in the ventilator; failure to take IPI into account may lead to erroneous parameters derived from the P-V curve. Once the supersyringe has been connected to the patient, the respiratory system is inflated in 50-200 ml steps allowing a 2-3 s pause between successive inflations to reach an airway pressure plateau which is recorded together with the corresponding volume change. When either an airway pressure of about 50 cm H_2O or a total inflated volume of 20 ml/Kg, which should approximately correspond to total lung capacity, has been reached inflation should stop and the thorax be deflated in the same stepwise fashion so that both the inflation and deflation limbs of the P-V curve may be drawn.

In ARDS patients, at least at some point in ARDS natural history, marked alterations of the P-V curve profile ensue [51] and this has allowed the definition of some indexes that bear important consequences for the ventilatory management of the patient [48, 52]. Different values of compliance may be estimated from the P-V curve as shown in Fig. 5. C_{start} has been defined as the compliance pertaining to the first 100 ml inflation, C_{inf} and C_{def} as the respective slopes of the inflation and deflation limb of the P-V curve in their most linear segments. The ratio of C_{inf} to C_{start} has been shown to correlate with alveolar recruitment and the lowest pressure value at which the slope of the P-V curve corresponds to C_{inf} has been claimed as a rational value at which to set PEEP, and thus named Best-PEEP. Other indexes derived from the P-V curve include the unrecovered volume (UV), i.e. the volume not recovered from the lung into the syringe at the end of deflation and the hysteresis area (HA), i.e. the area within the inflation and deflation limbs of the P-V curve. When the P-V curve is drawn with the supersyringe method a number of factors, including continuing gas exchange with a time dependent discrepancy between oxygen subtracted from and carbon dioxide added to the system, temperature and humidity changes in the inhaled gas, may

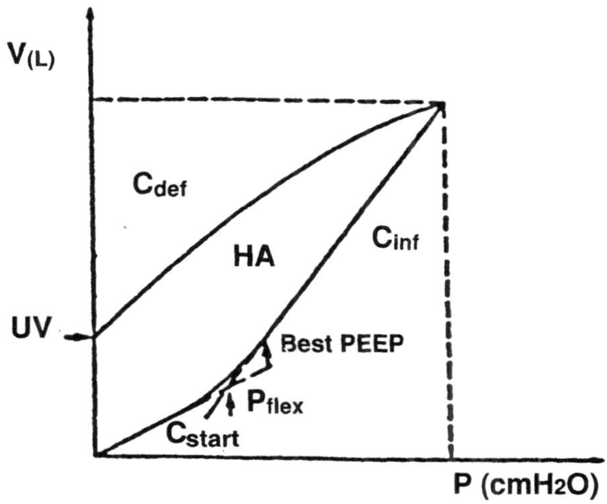

Fig. 5. P-V curve of total respiratory system obtained with the supersyringe method. See text for further explanation. (From [48])

misleadingly affect the shape of the curve. The derived parameters should thus be properly corrected for the above factors [53]. This is particularly true for those indexes calculated on the deflation limb of the P-V curve, and especially for UV and HA.

During routine mechanical ventilation in muscle relaxed patients static compliance may be calculated through an end inspiratory hold manouver, as shown in Fig.4 [3, 32, 22, 44, 23, 43], which allows the determination of lung, chest wall and total respiratory system static compliance according to the following standard formulas:

$$C_L = V_t/[(P_{2,aw}\text{-}P_{2,es})\text{-}[(PEEP+Auto\text{-}PEEP)\text{-}(P_{0,es})]$$
$$C_{cw} = V_t/[P_{2,es}\text{-}P_{0,es}]$$
$$C_{rs} = V_t/[P_{2,aw}\text{-}(PEEP+Auto\text{-}PEEP)]$$

where V_T is tidal volume, $P_{0,es}$ is end expiratory esophageal pressure, $P_{2,es}$ and $P_{2,aw}$ are end inspiratory occlusion esophageal and airway pressures respectively.

As discussed above, when an end inspiratory hold manouver follows constant flow inflation, a "zero flow" airway pressure ($P_{1,aw}$) may be identified before $P_{2,aw}$ is reached; this allows the computation of the dynamic respiratory system compliance ($C_{dyn,rs}$) [3]:

$$C_{dyn,rs} = V_t/[P_{1,aw}\text{-}(PEEP+Auto\text{-}PEEP)]$$

$C_{dyn,rs}$ may then be partitioned into lung ($C_{dyn,L}$) and chest wall ($C_{dyn,cw}$) dynamic compliance [13].

References

1. Bates JHT, Baconnier P, Milic-Emili J (1988) Theoretical analysis of interrupter technique for measuring respiratory mechanics. J Appl Physiol 64:2204-2214
2. Similowski T, Bates JHT (1991) Two-compartment modelling of respiratory system mechanics at low frequencies: gas redistribution or tissue rheology? Eur Resp J 4:353-358
3. D'Angelo E, Calderini E, Torri G, Robatto FM, Bono D, Milic-Emili J (1989) Respiratory mechanics in anesthetized paralyzed humans: effects of flow, volume, and time. J Appl Physiol 67:2556-2564
4. Bates JHT, Brown K, Kochi T (1987) Identifying a model of respiratory mechanics using the interrupter technique. Proc Ninth Am Conf IEEE Eng Med Biol Soc 1802-1803
5. Mead J (1969) Contribution of compliance of airways to frequency dependent behaviour of lungs. J Appl Physiol 26:670-673
6. Otis AB, McKerrow CB, Bartlett RA, Mead J, McIlroy MB, Selverstone NJ, Radford EP (1956) Mechanical factors in distribution of pulmonary ventilation. J Appl Physiol 8:427-443
7. Bates JHT, Brown KA, Kochi T (1989) Respiratory mechanics in the normal dog determined by expiratory flow interruption. J Appl Physiol 67:2276-2285
8. Zin WA, Rossi A, Milic-Emili J (1983) Model analysis of respiratory responses to inspiratory resistive loads. J Appl Physiol 55:1565-1573
9. Bates JHT, Rossi A, Milic-Emili J (1985) Analysis of the behaviour of the respiratory system with constant inspiratory flow. J Appl Physiol 58:1840-1848
10. Sharp JT, Henry JP, Sweany SK, Meadows WR, Pietras RJ (1964) Total respiratory inertance and its gas and tissue components in normal and obese men. J Clin Invest 43:503-509
11. Kochi T, Okubo S, Zin WA, Milic-Emili J (1988) Chest wall and respiratory system mechanics in cats: effects of flow and volume. J Appl Physiol 64:2636-2646
12. Bates JHT, Decramer M, Chartrand D, Zin WA, Boddener A, Milic-Emili J (1985) The volume-time profile during relaxed expiration in the normal dog. J Appl Physiol 59:732-737
13. D'Angelo E, Robatto FM, Calderini E, Tavola M, Bono D, Torri G, Milic-Emili J (1991) Pulmonary and chest wall mechanics in anesthetized paralyzed humans. J Appl Physiol 70(6):2602-2610
14. Bates JHT, Ludwig MS, Sly PD, Brown K, Martin JG, Fredberg JJ (1988) Interrupter resistance elucidated by alveolar pressure measurement in open-chested normal dogs. J Appl Physiol 65:408-414
15. Stamenovic D, Glass GM, Barnas GM, Fredberg JJ (1988) A model of imperfect elasticity of the human chest wall. The Physiologist 31:A220
16. Similowski T, Levy P, Corbeil C, Albala M, Pariente R, Derenne JP, Bates JHT, Milic-Emili J (1989) Viscoelastic behaviour of the lung and chest wall in dogs determined by flow interruption. J Appl Physiol 67:2219-2229
17. Fredberg JJ, Ingram RH, Castile FG, Glass GM, Drazen JM (1985) Nonhomogeneity of lung response to inhaled histamine assessed with alveolar capsules. J Appl Physiol 58:1914-1922
18. Bates JHT, Decramer M, Zin WA, Harf A, Milic-Emili J, Chang HK (1986) Respiratory resistance with histamine challenge by single breath and forced oscillation methods. J Appl Physiol 61:873-880

19. von Neergaard K and Wirtz K (1927) Die Messung der Stromungswiederstände in der Atemwege des Menschen, insbesondere bei Asthma und Emphysem. Z Klin Med 105:51-82
20. von Neergaard Kand Wirtz K (1927) Über eine Methode zur Messung der Lungenelastizitat am lebenden Menschen, insbesondere beim Emphysem. Z Klin Med 105:35-50
21. Bates JHT, Hunter I, Sly PD, Okubo S, Filiatrault S and Milic-Emili J (1987) The effect of valve closure time on the determination of the respiratory resistance by flow interruption. Med Biol Eng Comput 25:136-140
22. Polese G, Rossi A, Appendini L, Brandi G, Bates JHT, Brandolese R (1991) Partitioning of respiratory mechanics in mechanically ventilated patients. J Appl Physiol 71:2425-2433
23. Rossi A, Gottfried SB, Higgs BD, Zocchi L, Grassino A, Milic-Emili J (1985) Respiratory mechanics in mechanically ventilated patients with respiratory failure. J Appl Physiol 58(6):1849-1858
24. Milic-Emili J (1989) Pulmonary flow resistance. Lung 167:141-148
25. Kochi T, Okubo S, Zin WA, Milic-Emili J (1988) Flow and volume dependence of pulmonary mechanics in anesthetized cats. J Appl Physiol 64:441-450
26. Behrakis PK, Higgs BD, Baydur A, Zin WA, Milic- Emili J (1983) Respiratory mechanics during halothane anesthesia and anesthesia-paralysis in humans. J Appl Physiol 55:1085-1092
27. Wright PE, Marini JJ, Bernard GR (1989) In vitro versus in vivo comparison of endotracheal tube airflow resistance. Am Rev Resp Dis 140:10-16
28. Navalesi P, Hernandez P, Laporta D, Landry J, Maltais F, Navajas D, Gottfried SB (1994) Influence of site of tracheal pressure measurement on in situ estimation of endotracheal tube resistance. J Appl Physiol 77(6):2899-2906
29. Broseghini C, Brandolese R, Poggi R, Polese G, Manzin E, Milic-Emili J, Rossi A (1988) Respiratory mechanics during the first day of mechanical ventilation in patients with pulmonary edema and chronic airways obstruction. Am Rev Resp Dis 138:355-361
30. Pesenti A, Pelosi P, Rossi N, Aprigliano M, Brazzi L, Fumagalli R (1993) Respiratory mechanics and bronchodilator responsiveness in patients with the adult respiratory distress syndrome. Crit Care Med 21(1):78-83
31. Pesenti A, Pelosi P, Rossi N, Virtuani A, Brazzi L, Rossi A (1991) The effects of PEEP on respiratory resistance in patients with ARDS and in normal anesthetized subjects. Am Rev Resp Dis 144:101-107
32. Gottfried SB, Rossi A, Higgs BD, Calvery PMA, Zocchi L, Bozic C, Milic-Emili J (1985) Noninvasive determination of respiratory system mechanics during mechanical ventilation for acute respiratory failure. Am Rev Resp Dis 131:414-420
33. Smith T, Marini J (1988) Impact of PEEP on lung mechanics and work of breathing in severe airflow obstruction. J Appl Physiol 65:1488-1499
34. Nunn JF (1977) Applied respiratory physiology. 2nd ed., Butterworths, Boston
35. Marini J (1991) Monitoring the mechanics of the respiratory system. In: Contemporary management in critical care. Churchill Livingstone, M Tobin (ed), London
36. Marini JJ (1989) Should PEEP be used in airflow obstruction? Am Rev Resp Dis 140:1-3
37. Tantucci C, Corbeil C, Chasse M, Robatto FM, Nava S, Braidy J, Matar N, Milic-Emili J (1992) Flow and volume dependence of respiratory system flow resistance in patients with ARDS. Am Rev Resp Dis 145:355-360
38. Fry DL, Ebert RV, Stead WW, Brown CC (1954) The mechanics of pulmonary ventilation in normal subjects and in patients with emphysema. Am J Med 16:80-97

39. Kimball WR, Leith DE, Robins AG (1982) Dynamic hyperinflation and ventilator dependence in COPD. Am Rev Resp Dis 126:991-995
40. Hyatt R (1983) Expiratory flow limitation. J Appl Physiol 55(1):1-8
41. Ranieri VM, Giuliani R, Cinella G, Pesce C, Brienza N, Ippolito E, Pomo V, Fiore T, Gottfried SB, Brienza A (1993) Physiologic effects of PEEP in patients with COPD during acute ventilatory failure and controlled mechanical ventilation. Am Rev Resp Dis 147:5-13
42. Tuxen D (1989) Detrimental effects of PEEP during controlled mechanical ventilation of patients with severe airflow obstruction. Am Rev Resp Dis 140:5-9
43. Pepe P, Marini J (1982) Occult PEEP in mechanically ventilated patients with airflow obstruction. Am Rev Resp Dis 126:166-170
44. Rossi A, Gottfried SB, Zocchi L, Higgs BD, Lennox S, Calvery PMA, Begin P, Grassino A, Milic-Emili J (1985) Measurement of static compliance of the total respiratory system in patients with acute respiratory failure during mechanical ventilation. Am Rev Resp Dis 131:672-677
45. Hoffman RA, Ershowsky P, Krieger BP (1989) Determination of auto-PEEP during spontaneous and controlled ventilation by monitoring dogs in end expiratory thoracic gas volume. Chest 96(3):613
46. Rahn H, Otis AB (1946) The pressure-volume diagram of the thorax and lung. Am J Physiol 146:161-178
47. O'Quinn R, Marini JJ, Culver BH, Butler J (1985) Transmission of airway pressure to the pleural space during lung edema and chest wall restriction. J Appl Physiol 59(4):1171
48. Gattinoni L, Pesenti A, Avalli L, Rossi F, Bombino M (1987) Pressure volume curve of total respiratory system in acute respiratory failure: computed tomographic scan study. Am Rev Resp Dis 136:730-736
49. Beydon L, Lemaire F, Jonson B (1991) Lung mechanics in ARDS: compliance and pressure volume curves. In: Zapol WM, Lemaire F (eds) Adult Respiratory Distress Syndrome. Marcel Dekker, New York
50. Fernandez R, Mancebo J, Blanch L, Benito S, Calaf N, Net A (1990) Intrinsic PEEP on static pressure-volume curves. Int Care Med 16:233-236
51. Matamis D, Lemaire F, Brun-Bruisson C, Ansquer JC, Atlan G (1984) Total respiratory pressure-volume curves in the Adult Respiratory Distress Syndrome. Chest 86:58-66
52. Gattinoni L, Pesenti A, Caspani ML et al (1984) The role of total static lung compliance in the management of severe ARDS unresponsive to conventional treatment. Int Care Med 10:121-126
53. Gattinoni L, Mascheroni D, Basilico E, Foti G, Pesenti A, Avalli L (1987) Volume-pressure curve of total respiratory system in paralyzed patients: artifacts and correction factors. Int Care Med 13:19-25

Chapter 16

Aspects of monitoring during ventilatory support ($P_{0.1}$)

R. Brandolese, U. Andreose

Introduction

Gas exchange (O_2 and CO_2) in the lungs is dependent on the respiratory pump to inflate the lungs and on the functioning of the lungs themselves. When the respiratory system is unable to mantain normal work, respiratory failure can develop. The respiratory pump includes the neurological respiratory control mechanism, peripheral nerves, respiratory muscles and chest wall structures. The act of breathing depends entirely on the stimulation of respiratory muscles by the action of the respiratory center, which is composed of several widely scattered neurons located bilaterally in the medulla oblungata and pons. Information from the chemoreceptors sensitive to respiratory gases and from the mechanoreceptors are integrated in the brain stem and spinal cord. It is useful to divide the respiratory control system into a voluntary and automatic. The voluntary system adapts respiration to rapidly changing environmental factors.

The automatic system coordinates the chemoreceptors and the mechanoreceptors inputs and adjusts ventilation according to metabolic requirements and the mechanical properties of the respiratory system (lungs, chest wall and respiratory muscles). The blood gases are maintained constant and the work of breathing is minimised [1].

The time courses of inspiratory and expiratory phases are entirely controlled by the respiratory centre: inspiration starts and is then terminated, in some circumstances, by afferent impulses from the stretch receptors of the lungs [2], but the mechanoreceptors of the chest wall and the chemoreceptors of course also play a role. The expiration is affected by less certain factors than inspiration, but may be influenced by carotid bodies [3, 4].

If minute ventilation increases, the tidal volume (V_t) also initially increases too, followed by a rise in respiratory rate according to the formula of work of breathing (WOB) [5]:

$$WOB = 1/2\ V_t^2/C_{dyn} + 1/4\ \pi^2 \cdot V_t^2\ Rf$$

where C_{dyn} is dynamic compliance of total respiratory system, V_T is tidal volume and f is respiratory rate.

The expiratory time (T_e) shortens more than the inspiratory time (T_i) [6]. The rise in V_T despite a fall in T_i implies that the velocity of shortening of the muscle fibers increases, in other words, the mean inspiratory flow (V_t/T_i) becomes more rapid when V_t increases. The mean inspiratory flow rate is influenced by the mechanical properties of the lungs and the chest wall, the intensity of stimulation of the inspiratory muscles and their strength [7, 8]. Control of T_i, T_e and V_t/T_i enables any combination of V_t and respiratory rate to be achieved. The metabolic demand of the tissues governs minute ventilation, the chemoreceptors ensure an alveolar ventilation adequate to maintain normal blood gases and a breathing pattern adjusted to minimize the work of breathing [1].

Mechanical properties of chest wall

The contraction of the inspiratory muscles inflates the lungs, overcoming the elastic properties of the lung and chest wall, the air flow resistances and the small viscosity and inertia of the tissue. This may be expressed by the following formula:

$$P_{mus,i} = P_{el,rs} + P_{res,rs} \quad (1)$$

Moreover $P_{mus,i}$ must counterbalance the intrinsic positive end expiratory pressure if any. The formula (1) has to be corrected into:

$$P_{mus,i} = P_{el,rs} + P_{res,rs} + P_{eepi}$$

$P_{mus,i}$ representing the mechanical workload for the inspiratory muscles.

The elastic recoil of the chest wall is closely related to its volume and the relationship is approximately linear in the range of tidal volume during quiet breathing. The compliance of the chest wall falls at both high and low lung volume so that more energy is required to inflate and deflate the lungs [9, 10].

If the chest wall is separated from the lungs, the volume that it reaches owing to its elastic recoil is considerably greater than the volume assumed by the lungs.The volume at which these two opposite forces are balanced is the Functional Residual Capacity (FRC). This is the end expiratory rest volume if there is no expiratory muscle activity and no available elastic recoil pressure to further expiratory flow. The force of the inspiratory muscles decreases when pulmonary volume increases because inspiratory muscle becomes shorter and are in a disavantaged position in their force-length relationship [11].

Contractile properties of respiratory muscles

The force developed by a muscle is dependent on its mass or cross-sectional area and the number of activated fibers, the mass being influenced by nutritional state, age and pathological disorders of the muscles. The mass of contracting muscle employed to cope with any applied respiratory load, can be increased by recruiting other types of muscles [11]. Failure to recruit muscles may be due to a lack of motivation or to an impairment of the central respiratory control.

The tension developed during a single muscle twitch is less than that which occurs with repeated stimulation. In general, the force developed is about 25 % of maximum at 10 Hz, 70 % of maximum at 20 Hz and finally 100 % at 100 Hz [11].

The muscle length is an important determinant of the force generated by the respiratory muscles. The inspiratory muscle are more powerful near RV (residual volume) where they are longest and the expiratory muscles at TLC where they are stretched. The volume of the lung is a rough guide to establish the length of the respiratory muscles, but the length of the respiratory muscle may vary from breath to breath even at the same lung volume.

The more rapidly a muscle shortens the less is the tension that is developed [11]. More muscle energy is necessary if the muscle shortens rapidly and it has been seen that respiratory muscle fatigue is more likely if the mean inspiratory flow increases [12].

The contractility of the respiratory muscles is decreased by hypoxia [13], hypercapnia [14], alteration of acid-basic balance. It is aiso decreased by fatigue [11].

Weakness of a muscle is an inability to generate an expected force, while fatigue is the inability to sustain an established force. It is very important to differentiate the fatigue arising in the muscle or at neuromuscular junction from the fatigue determined because of an insufficient drive from the central nervous system, or because of mechanical insufficiency of the muscle [11].When muscle fatigue is developing, there is normally a compensatory increase in the firing frequency and in the number of active motoneurons. The adequacy of the respiratory drive has to be assessed in order to establish the presence or absence of fatigue. Two types of muscle fatigue have been recognized:

- high frequency fatigue;
- low frequency fatigue.

High frequency fatigue is characteristic of myastenia gravis, and the force generated by the muscles is reduced at stimulation frequency of 100 Hz. Recovery from this type of fatigue is rapid, approximately ten minutes [15].

Low frequency fatigue is seen in primary muscle disorders such as the myopathies. Low frequency fatigue is characteristic of COPD decompensated patients and takes days for recovering [15, 11].

Airway occlusion pressure

In 1973 Milic-Emili et al. first performed the airway occlusion manouvre occluding the trachea of anesthetized cats at FRC [16]. In this way it was possible to measure the pressure generated during occluded inspiratory efforts. At elastic equilibrium volume of total respiratory system (FRC) the elastic recoil is nil and therefore the pressure measured is the net pressure developed by the inspiratory muscles [17, 18]. During inspiratory efforts at occluded airways there is no flow of gas and the intrathoracic gas volume does not change, so that the measurement performed is not influenced by the elastic and resistive properties of the respiratory system. The airway occlusion pressure may be a useful index of neuromuscular inspiratory drive [19] (Fig. 1). The occlusion manouvre is performed allowing the subject, if not intubated, to breath through a mouthpiece with a valve that allows inspiration and expiration to be performed in separate modes. The operator, while the subject is breathing out, closes the inspiratory line of the respiratory circuit so that the next inspiration is performed at occluded airways generating a negative inspiratory pressure at the mouthpiece. After a short time the subject perceives that the tube is blocked and continues to make some abnormal inspiratory efforts [20, 21]. However, the pressure generated during the first 100-300 msec represents the force generated by the inspiratory muscles in isometric conditions under the same respiratory neural stimulus as an unobstructed breath. This technique requires, unlike inspiratory work, no esophageal balloon and a minimum of electronic devices. When the airways of a subject are occluded, he struggles against the occluded device so that the inspiratory peak pressure may be quite different breath by breath and the measure is not correlated to an unobstructed respiratory drive. However, it has been demonstrated that there is a delay of no less than 150 msec between the application of the occlusion and the subject's recognition and reaction. Hence the pressure measured at 100 msec after having occluded the airways is independent from the attitude (cortical responses) [21] of the subject and has been considered as an index of respiratory central drive. This index has the additional advantage of being independent from lung volume vagally mediated reflexes. If a subject breaths mixtures with different concentration of CO_2, the occlusion mouth pressure wave increases its amplitude without changing its shape [21]. We can say in other words that the occlusion pressure is proportional to the output of the respiratory centers. It is important

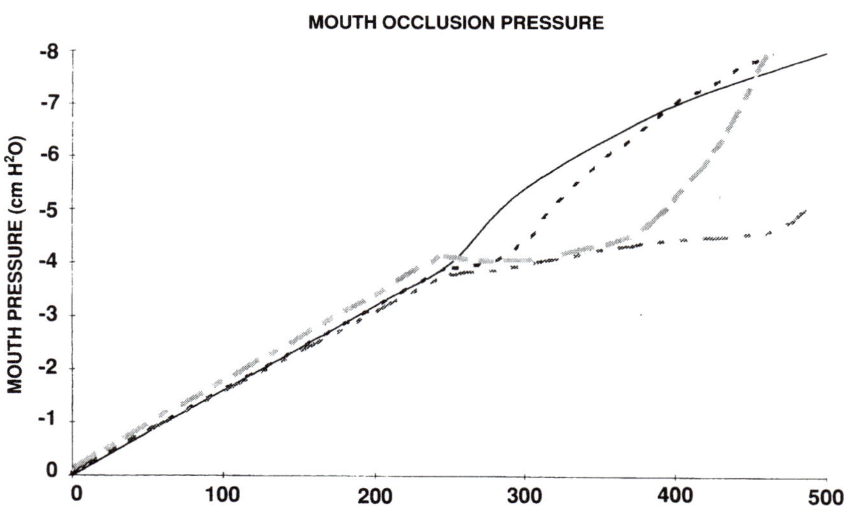

Fig. 1. Consecutive series of occlusion pressure waves from a representative subject breathing air. These waves are very similar in the first section, up to 250 msec from the start of inspiration

that measurements of mouth occlusion pressure ($P_{0.1}$) be made at constant lung volume, since the relationship between the stimulus leaving the respiratory centers and the pressure developed by the respiratory muscles changes with volume variation because of altered geometry of the respiratory system and force-length properties of the inspiratory muscles [22, 23]. In the assessment of $P_{0.1}$ the supine position is suitable, because in this posture the ratio of functional residual capacity to total lung capacity changes less than in the upright position. Moreover, in the supine position the contraction of the respiratory muscles is more uniform from subject to subject [24]. Other factors may affect the measurement of $P_{0.1}$, such as neuromuscular diseases, drugs and reflexes that arise from the intercostal muscles during airway occlusion [21]. Interestingly, it has been demonstrated that for the same chemical respiratory drive conscious men are able to respond to application of respiratory load by increasing the airway occlusion pressure measured after 100 msec of occlusion. There is a sensitivity of central neural drive to chemical stimuli but also to mechanical loading. $P_{0.1}$ is a good index of neurorespiratory drive output and is dependent only on the neuronal discharge and on the effectiveness of the inspiratory muscles [21]. The measurement of $P_{0.1}$ may be obtained using a pressure transducer connected to a mouthpiece, to the proximal portion of an endotracheal tube if the patient is intubated, or to an air-tight face mask. The pressure occlusion signal is transmitted to a previously calibrated recording system. If an esophageal balloon is positioned in the third portion of the oesophagus, we can record $P_{0.1}$ esphageal using the same apparatus.

Which $P_{0.1}$ must we utilize in clinical settings: mouth, tracheal or esophageal? Marazzini at al. [25] compared the pressure generated at mouth and at esophagus during the first 100 msec after occlusive manouvre in normal subjects and in COPD patients during CO_2 rebreathing. They found that normal subjects had similar responses to CO_2 in terms of mouth and esophageal pressure, whereas COPD patients had a greater response to CO_2 in $P_{0.1}$ measured in the esophagus than at the mouth. This phenomenon may be explained on the basis of the different magnitude of the time constant of the upper airways in the normal subject in comparison to COPD patients. But if the upper airways are by-passed via a tracheal or tracheostomy tube one would expect that the time constant should be drastically reduced. To verify this hypothesis Murciano at al. [26] compared esophageal and tracheal pressure in patients mechanically ventilated due to acute exacerbation of their chronic airway obstruction. Their results agreed whith the hypothesis and no difference was found between the esophageal and tracheal occlusion pressure in COPD mechanically ventilated patients. In normal adult subjects mouth occlusion pressure is as high as 1 cm H_2O during quiet breathing and is not related to age and sex [24, 27]. Minute ventilation is a direct consequence of the central respiratory drive and in each subject there is a linear relation between minute ventilation and $P_{0.1}$ [21, 28]. If $P_{0.1}$ increases, minute ventilation also increases; approaching a $P_{0.1}$ of 10-12 cm H_2O there is a drastic enhancement in minute ventilation up to 70 l/min. In contrast, the resting $P_{0.1}$ value is quite different in patients with lung diseases, both restrictive or obstructive [27]. At equal minute ventilation the driving neuromuscular pressure is greater in COPD patients than in normal subjects, so that the $V_e/P_{0.1}$ ratio is less in the first group [27]. These patients spend much more to produce much less.

In stable COPD patients the value of mouth occlusion pressure varies in the range of 3-5 cm H_2O becoming as high as 10-15 cm H_2O in decompensated COPD patients [29], with a minute ventilation only feebly increased and an alveolar ventilation decreased because of breathing pattern [30] (rapid shallow breathing, which determines a greater ventilation of dead space) (Fig. 2). All COPD patients were found to have an abnormal value of $P_{0.1}$ and the hypercapnic blue bloaters are not distinguishable from the normocapnic pink puffers by measuring mouth occlusion pressure. In COPD patients the measurements of ventilation are not indicative for assessment of central neural drive because minute ventilation is low and this is due to high value of respiratory resistance. At this point the introduction of mouth occlusion pressure in clinical practice has offered a solution to this problem because the measure is independent of flow resistance and elastance [21]. We mentioned above that mouth occlusion pressure is related to mechanical workload: in other words patients whose respiratory impedence is high (increased

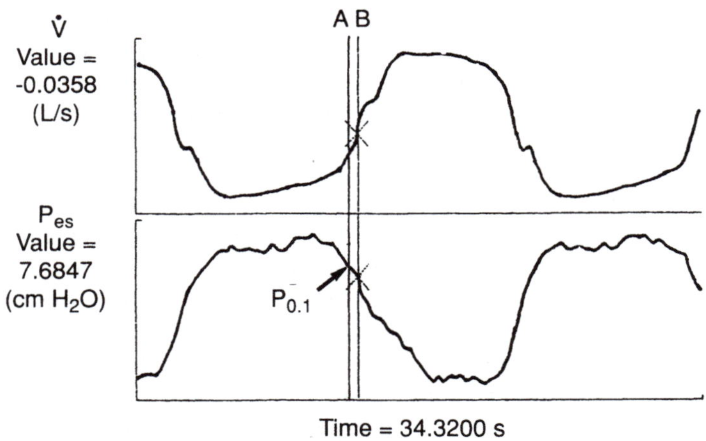

Fig. 2. Up and down tracings of respiratory flow and esophageal pressure in a patient with acute exacerbaton of chronic airways obstruction during spontaneus breathing in CPAP mode. This figure displays a complete respiratory cycle. The deflection in esophgeal pressure before start of inspiratory flow defines the presence of $PEEP_{i,dyn}$ (intercept of vertical line B with esophageal pressure tracing at the point of zero flow). The "occlusion pressure" is also shown ($P_{0.1es}$) measured at the point were vertical line A intersects the esophageal pressure tracing after a time interval of 100 msec from the beginning in the drop of the esophageal pressure. The values of $P_{0.1es}$ and $PEEP_{i,dyn}$ are 5.7 and 7.6 cm H_2O respectively. In this case, because of the presence of $PEEP_i$, the occlusion of the airways at the end of expiration has not been performed, because pleonastic. In fact, until the whole $PEEP_i$ is counterbalanced by an isometric contraction of the inspiratory mucles, the end expiratory lung volume remains unchanged and consequently there is no dissipation in the pressure generated. In other words, the airways become reopened when $PEEP_i$ has been overcome

respiratory resistances, elastance and hyperinflation, $PEEP_i$) were shown to have an increased respiratory central drive. If these patients have to be mechanically ventilated the measurements of $P_{0.1}$ can be an optimal guide to application of an adequate pressure at airway opening by the ventilator. The value of preset pressure during pressure support ventilation will be varied in relation to the $P_{0.1}$ trend. This modulation in preset pressure will determine the use of high ventilatory pressure in presence of a high $P_{0.1}$ and, conversely, the application of low pressure if respiratory drive is small. The monitoring of mouth occlusion pressure in the clinical setting is important to differentiate patients who cannot be weaned from the respirator (high $P_{0.1}$) from those who are able to resume spontaneous breathing (low $P_{0.1}$) [31, 32]. It should be noted that we do not know if this elevated drive means a bigger workload, whether they have higher inspiratory output or elevated resistance and consequently a change in $P_{0.1}$ without a parallel change in output.

Moreover we must keep in mind that in myotonic dystrophya authors have observed a normal $P_{0.1}$ in presence of low ventilation and this may be explained on the basis of an unexpected upper airway resistance which determines a phase-lag in the transmission of occlusion pressure [33]. But we must consider that $P_{0.1}$ measurement is only one of the many parameters used during a weaning trial and it has been widely discussed elsewhere [34-36]. In the clinical setting the ratio $P_{0.1}/P_{imax}$ is also used as an index that links ventilatory drive and the ability of the respiratory muscles to generate pressure [37, 38].

Briefly, maximum inspiratory pressure (P_{imax}) is the force that respiratory muscles are able to generate during an occlusive manouvre at prefixed volume, usually at FRC. But though the measurement of P_{imax} is feasible in cooperating subjects, it is not always reliable in critically ill mechanically ventilated patients. P_{imax} alone is not a sensitive predictive index for a successfull weaning from the ventilator, but the ratio $P_{0.1}/P_{imax}$ seems to be a better index than P.01 alone, in a correct evaluation of low values of $P_{0.1}$ determined by a relative ineffectiveness of the respiratory muscles and not by a low respiratory central drive [38]. Hence P_{imax} makes possible the identification of patients who fail to exhibit a high P0.1 value due to muscles weakness and/or muscle fatigue. Montgomery et al. [39] demonstrated that $P_{0.1}$ alone was not significantly different between patients that had been weaned and those whose weaning trial was unsuccessful. But if $P_{0.1}$ was measured after CO_2 stimulation it was able to separate the two groups of patients. The ratio $P_{0.1}/P_{0.1}$ (CO_2) appears to be an index of the respiratory reserve based on the real clinical status of every patient rather than on theoric standard predictive parameters. Marini [40] has demonstrated that during assisted mechanical ventilation the work of breathing done by the ventilated patient may be a consistent part of the total work performed by the machine. The same author has found a close correlation between the work of the patient during mechanical ventilation and the magnitude of the discharge rate of the inspiratory central drive [40].

Relation between positive end expiratory pressure (PEEP) and $P_{0.1}$

The simplified equation of motion of the air into the respiratory system is defined by the following equation:

$$P = Vt/C_{dyn} + R_{rs}(V_t/T_i) + P_{eepi}$$

This equation establishes the magnitude of the inspiratory muscle load which has been overcome to generate flow across the airways [41]. It is clear that the determinants of inspiratory workload are the elastic and resistive components of total respiratory system. But in the equation we can see an adjunctive elastic component $PEEP_i$ i.e. elastic recoil pressure at end expiration. $PEEP_i$ is a corollary of dynamic pulmonary hyperinflation which is a constant feature of decompensated COPD patients during mechanical ventilation [41-43]. $PEEP_i$ can be defined as the inspiratory threshold load that inspiratory muscles have to counterbalance before starting inspiration. Hence PEEPi represents an adjunctive extra burden for the respiratory muscles and so the mechanical workload is further enhanced. Smith and Marini [44] have studied the interrelations between Peepi and central neural drive measured on the negative deflection of esophageal pressure tracing. These authors applied a positive expiratory pressure (PEEP) in COPD patients affected by a severe airway obstruction and mechanically ventilated; many respiratory mechanics variables were measured and among these they related $P_{0.1}$ to PEEPi. The addition of external PEEP influenced the $P_{0.1es}$. Whereas the application of 5 cm H_2O PEEP determined a feable decrease in $P_{0.1es}$ (15 %), 10 cm H_2O PEEP caused a relevant and significant reduction in the central inspiratory drive (47 %).The decrease in $P_{0.1es}$ is attributed to a lesser degree of inspiratory treshold load because PEEPe replaced PEEPi (Table 1).

$P_{0.1}$ has been related to other parameters of respiratory and pulmonary func-

Table 1. Individual values of $P_{0.1es}$ and ΔP_{es} in a representative COPD patient during different degrees of pressure support and during spontaneus breathing. Note that inspiratory center drive output expressed as $P_{0.1es}$ varies in relation to different mechanical loads sustained by the respiratory muscles (ΔP_{es}). $P_{0.1es}$ is airway occlusion pressure measured at 100 msec on the esophageal pressure tracing. ΔPes is the gratest difference in esophageal pressure generated by the inspiratory muscle during tidal breathing

	Spontaneus breathing			**Pressure support**			
	T Tube	*CPAP 0*	*CPAP 5*	*10/5**	*15/5**	*15/0**	*10/0**
$P_{0.1es}$ (cm H_2O)	4.00	5.60	2.90	1.36	1.40	2.60	3.40
ΔP_{es} (cm H_2O)	19.63	16.00	12.79	4.00	5.00	13.00	13.48

* PEEP value set by the ventilator

tion. The ratio of $P_{0.1}$ and mean inspiratory flow define a parameter called "effective inspiratory impedence" which relates the central neural drive to effectiveness of airflow [45]. In other words this parameter illustrates the effective tranformation of neural drive discharge into flow. Finally, $P_{0.1}$ has been related to tidal volume (Vt), obtaining the effective elastance, which indicates the degree of neural drive required to achieve effective ventilation [46].

Summarizing, $P_{0.1}$ is the only noninvasive measure of output that leaves the central nervous system reaching the appropriate effector (respiratory muscles) across conditions where respiratory mechanics is changed. Moreover $P_{0.1}$ alone or in combination with other indexes would be an important predictor of a successful weaning of mechanically ventilated patients from the ventilator. It is essential when measuring $P_{0.1}$ to close the airway exactly at the point of zero flow or at the end of a tidal expiration avoiding an uncorrected gauge.

References

1. Otis AB, Fenn WO, Rahn H (1950) The mechanics of breathing in man. J Appl Physiol 2:592-607
2. von Euler C (1983) On the central pattern generator for the basic breathing rhytmicity. J Appl Physiol 55:1647-1659
3. Bowes G, Andrey SM, Kozar LF, Philipson EA (1982) Role of the carotid chemoreceptors in regulation of inspiratory onset. J Appl Physiol 52:863-868
4. Bowes G, Andrey SM, Kozar LF, Phillipson EA (1983) Ventilatory response to conspiratory flow-resistive loads in awake and sleeping dogs. J Appl Physiol 54:1195 1201
5. Hey EN, Lloyd BB, Cunningham DJC, Jukes MGM, Bolton DP (1966) Effects of various respiratory stimuls on the depth and frequency of breathing in man. Respiratory Physiology 1:193-205
6. Newsom Davies J, Stagg DJ (1975) Inter-relationship of the volume and time components of individual breaths in resting man. J Physiol 245:481-498
7. Milic-Emili J, Grassino AE, Whitelaw WA, In.: Horbein TF (ed) (1981) Regulation of breathing. Part 2. Marcel Dekker, New York, pp 675-743
8. Milic-Emili J, Grunstein MM (1976) Drive and timing components of ventilation. Chest 70:131-133
9. Smith JC, Loring SH. Passive mechanical properties of the chest wall. In: Fishman AP, Macklem PT, Mead J, Geiger SR (eds) Handbook of Physiology. The Respiratory System. Mechanics of Breathing. Section 3, vol III, part 2, chap. 25 American Physiological Society, Bethesda, pp 429-442
10. Roussos CH, Campbell EJM. Respiratory muscles energetics. In: Fishman AP, Macklem PT, Mead J, Geiger SR (eds) Handbook of Physiology. The Respiratory System. Mechanics of breathing. Section 3, Vol. III. part 2, chap. 28 American Physiological Society, Bethesda, pp 481-509
11. Roussos CH, Macklem PT. Inspiratory muscles fatigue. In: Fishman AP, Macklem PT, Mead J, Geiger SR (eds) Handbook of Physiology. The Respiratory System. Mechanics of breathing. Section 3, Vol. III, part 2 American Physiological Society, Bethesda, pp 511-527
12. McCool FD, McCann DR, Leith DE, Hopping FG Jr (1986) Pressure-flow effects on endurance of inspiratory muscles. J Appl Physiol 60:299-303

13. Jardim J, Farkas G, Prefaut C, Thomas D, Macklem PT (1981) The failing inspiratory muscles under normoxic hypoxic carditions. Am Rev Respir Dis 124:274-279
14. Juan G, Calverley P, Talamo C, Schnader J, Roussos CH, NEJM (1984) Effect of carbon dioxide on diaphragmatic function in human beings. 310:874-879
15. Aubier M, Farkas G, de Troyer A, Mozes R, Roussos CH (1981) Detection of diaphragmatic fatigue in man by phrenic stimulation. J Appl Physiol 50:538-544
16. Grunstein M, Younes M, Milic-Emili J (1973) Control of tidal volume and respiratory frequency in anesthetized cats. J Appl Physiol 35:463-476
17. Siafakas NM, Peslin R, Bonora M, Gautier H, Duron B, Milic-Emili J (1981) Phrenic activity respiratory pressure and volume changes in cats. J Appl Physiol 51:109-121
18. Whitelaw WA, Derenne JP, Couture J, Milic-Emili J (1976) Adaptation of anesthetized men into breathing through a respiratory resistor J Appl Physiol 41:285-291
19. Milic-Emili J, Zin W. Relationship between neuromuscular respiratory drive and ventilatory output. In: Fishman AP, Macklem PT, Mead J, Geiger SR (eds) Handbook of Physiology. The Respiratory System. Mechanics of breathing. Section 3, vol. III, part 2. Chap. 35 American Physiological Society, Bethesda, pp 631-646
20. Milic-Emili J, Whitelaw WA, Derenne J (1975) Occlusion pressure, a simple measure of the respiratory center's output. NEJM November 13:1029-1030
21. Whitelaw WA, Drenne JP, Milic-Emili J (1975) Occlusion pressure as a measure of respiratory center output in conscious man. Respir Physiol 23:181-199
22. Marshall R (1962) Relationships between stimulus and work of breathing at different lung volumes. J Appl Physiol 17:917-921
23. Pengelly LD, Alderson A, Milic-Emili J (1971) Mechanics of the diaphragm. J Appl Physiol 30:796-805
24. Derenne JP, Grassino AE, Whitelaw WA et al (1975) Occlusion pressure in normal, supine men. Am Rev Respir Dis 111:907
25. Marazzini L, Cavestri R, Gori D, Gatti L, Longhini E (1978) Difference between mouth and esophageal occlusion pressure during CO_2 rebreathing in chronic obstructive pulmonary disease. Am Rev Respir Dis 118:1027-1033
26. Murciano D, Aubier M, Bussi S, Derenne JP, Pariente R, Milic-Emili J (1982) Comparison of esophageal and mouth occlusion pressure in patients with chronic obstructive pulminary disease during acute respiratory failure. Am Rev Respir Dis 126:837-841
27. Graham CS, Burki N (1990) The relationship of resting ventilation to mouth occlusion pressure - An index of resting respiratory function. Chest 900-906
28. Burki N, Mitchell LK, Chaudhary BA, Zeckman FW et al (1977) Measurements of mouth occlusion pressure as an index of respiratory center output in men. Clin Sci Mol Med 53:117-123
29. Herrera M, Blasco J, Venegas J, Berba A, Doblas A, Marquez E (1985) Mouth occlusion pressure in acute respiratory failure. Int Care Med 11:134-139
30. Sorly J, Grassino A, Lorange G, Milic-Emili (1975) Control of breathing in patients with chronic obstructive pulmonary disease. Cli Sci Mol Med 54:295-304
31. Sassoon C, Te TT, Mahutte CK, Light RW (1987) Airway occlusion pressure. An important indicator for successfull weaning in patients with chronic obstructive pulmonary disease. Am Rev Respir Dis 135:107-113
32. Soma K, Otsuka H, Tomita T (1988) Mouth Occlusion pressure as a useful indicator for weaning from mechanical ventilation. Tohuku J Exp Med 156:181-187
33. Whitelaw WA, Derenne JP (1993) Airway occlusion pressure. J Appl Physiol 1475-1483
34. Pierson DJ (1983) Weaning from mechanical ventilation in acute respiratory failure: concepts, indication, and techniques. Respir Care 28:646-660
35. Sahn SA, Lakshminarayan S (1973) Bedside criteria for discontinuation of mechani-

cal ventilation. Chest 63:1002-1005

36. Brandolese R, Andreose U (1995) The problem of weaning in COPD patients. In: Gullo A (ed) Anaesthesia, Pain, Intensive Care and Emergency Medicine, Springer-Verlag, Milano
37. Fernandez (1990) Inspiratory occlude airway pressure. In: Benito A, Net A (eds) Pulmonary Function in Mechanically Ventilated Patients. Springer-Verlag. Berlin. pp 39-49
38. Fernandez R, Cabrera J, Calaf N, Benito S (1990) P0, 1/Pimax An index for assessing respiratory capacity in acute respiratory failure. Int Care Med 16:175-179
39. Montgomery AB, Holle HO, Neagley SR, Pierson D, Schoene R (1987) Prediction of successfull ventilator weaning using airway occlusion pressure and hypercapnic challenge. Chest 91:496-499
40. Marini JJ, Rodriguez M, Lamb V (1986) The inspiratory workload in patients initiated mechanical ventilation. Am Rev Respir Dis 134:902-909
41. Poggi R, Polese G, Brandolese R, Rossi A (1992) Respiratory workload during mechanical ventilation. In: Gullo A (ed) Anaesthesia, Pain, Intensive Care and Emergency Medicine, Springer-Verlag, Milano, pp 223-229
42. Broseghini C, Brandoles R, Poggi R, Polese G, Milic-Emili J, Rossi A (1988) Respiratory mechanics during the first day of mechanical ventilation in patients with pulmonary edema and chronic airway obstruction. Am Rev Respir Dis 138:355-361
43. Pepe PE, Marini JJ (1982) Occult positive end-expiratory pressure in mechanically ventilated patients with airflow obstruction. Am Rev Respir Dis 126:166-170
44. Smith T, Marini JJ (1988) Impact of PEEP on lung mechanics and work of breathing in severe airway obstruction. J Appl Physiol 65:1488-1499
45. Hussain S, Pardy R, Dempsey J (1985) Mechanical impedance as determinant of inspiratory neural drive during exercize in humans. J Appl Physiol 59:365-375
46. Milic-Emili J, Whitelaw WA, Grassino A (1981) Measurements and testing of respiratory drive. In: Hornbein Th (ed) Regulation of breathing. Dekker, New York pp 675-743

Chapter 17

End-tidal PCO_2 monitoring during ventilatory support

L. Blanch, P. Saura, U. Lucangelo, R. Fernandez, A. Artigas

Introduction

Capnography is the technique that allows the measurement and the graphic waveform display of CO_2 at the patient's airway during the respiratory cycle. The displayed waveform is called a capnogram and many authors agree that the graphic display allows the validity of the measured PCO_2 to be assessed. Currently available systems for breath-by-breath CO_2 analysis include mass spectrometry and infra-red light absorption with infra-red CO_2 analyzers being mainly used in intensive care medicine. Major reasons are price, simplicity to calibrate and use, and each one is dedicated to a single patient. The range of response time oscillates between 100 and 200 miliseconds which is enough for breath by breath monitoring purposes. Two types of CO_2 analyzers based on the infrared radiation principle are available. Mainstream analyzers have a very rapid response time (less than 200 milliseconds) and the advantage of being a part of the ventilatory circuit. Sidestream analyzers pump the gas sample from the airway in a range between 150 to 500 ml/min through a small tube to a remote analyzer. Tubing obstruction of pulmonary secretions or water condensation and a response time longer than mainstream analyzers are their major disadvantages. The normal capnogram has a square wave pattern in which inspired PCO_2 equals zero at expiratory phase (Fig. 1). The expiratory capnogram consists of three successive phases. Phase I contains gas from the apparatus and anatomic dead space and the shape is not different from the previous inspiration. Phase II represents a rapid increase in PCO_2 resulting from progressive emptying of alveoli. Phase III represents the elimination of alveolar air and this phase is referred to as the plateau because its appearance is almost flat in patients with normal lungs and is the highest point is the end-tidal PCO_2 ($PetCO_2$). In clinical prac-

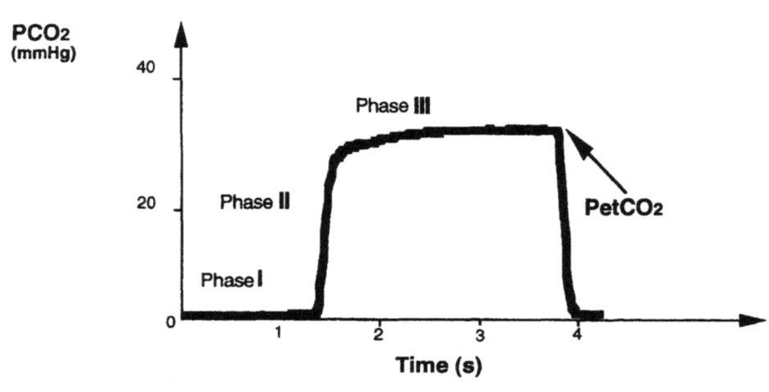

Fig. 1. Expired capnogram, $PetCO_2$ = End tidal CO_2

tice, the best measure of $PetCO_2$ will be obtained when tidal volumes are larger than dead space, by using low sample aspiration rates when using sidestream analyzers and when the waveform is displayed for plateau and $PetCO_2$ analysis [1-4].

Relationship between arterial PCO_2 and $PetCO_2$ during total ventilatory support

End-tidal PCO_2 will approximate $PaCO_2$ when CO_2 equilibrium is achieved between end-capillary blood and alveolar gas and when normal V/Q relationships are present in the lung. Both CO_2 production from tissues and mixed venous blood flow determine the amount of CO_2 released to alveoli, whereas alveolar CO_2 clearance is influenced by alveolar ventilation. As a result, in low V/Q compartments alveolar PCO_2 approximates mixed venous blood whereas in high V/Q compartments alveolar PCO_2 approximates inspired air PCO_2. Due to the fact that the capnogram is constituted by air coming from millions of alveolar units with different V/Q relationships, $PetCO_2$ is the result of the very different alveolar PCO_2. Therefore, it was established that $PetCO_2$ could be as low as PCO_2 of inspired air, or as high as mixed venous PCO_2 but not higher than mixed venous PCO_2 [5, 6].

The use of $PetCO_2$ as a reflection of $PaCO_2$ has been explored and controversy exists regarding its utility as a noninvasive method to approximate $PaCO_2$ during mechanical ventilation. Several studies analyze the relationship between $PaCO_2$ and $PetCO_2$ in critically ill patients receiving mechanical ventilation. Donati et al [7] found a $PaCO_2$-$PetCO_2$ gradient less than 4 mmHg in the recovery period after cardiac surgery. Takki et al [8] changed alveolar ventilation during anesthesia and found similar results and Perrin et al [9] showed that at different levels of alveolar ventilation, changes in alveolar PCO_2 were useful to predict variations in $PaCO_2$. On the other hand, other authors have shown the opposite. Raemer et al [10] found great variability in the gradient to accurately predict changes in $PaCO_2$. Our group have also found that the estimation of $PaCO_2$ from $PetCO_2$ in order to calculate cardiac output using the indirect Fick method did not yield enough accuracy in patients with lung disease [11]. Recently, Hoffman and associates [12] found good correlation of $PetCO_2$ and $PaCO_2$ in 20 critically ill patients; however, when ventilation was acutely altered to test the monitoring precision of $PetCO_2$, 4 of the 20 patients showed a negative correlation between $PaCO_2$ and $PetCO_2$, thus the investigators concluded that $PetCO_2$ monitoring may provide misleading trends of $PaCO_2$ when gradients change.

To examine whether additional factors, other than changes in the ventilatory pattern, could have influenced the capnogram, we reasoned that time constant inequalities within the lung may have an effect on the relationship between $PaCO_2$ and $PetCO_2$. Therefore, we analyzed the effect of autoPEEP on the relationship between $PaCO_2$ and $PetCO_2$ [13]. We studied 24 consecutive sedated and paralyzed patients under controlled mechanical ventilation for acute respiratory failure. They were grouped according to whether or not they had autoPEEP and were randomly ventilated at 3 different levels of minute ventilation. The $PaCO_2$-$PetCO_2$

gradient only remained stable in those patients without autoPEEP in whom the mean value of the $PaCO_2$-$PetCO_2$ gradient was lower than 3.6 mmHg. Despite the fact that $PaCO_2$ and $PetCO_2$ showed significant correlations in both groups, an accurate prediction of $PaCO_2$ from $PetCO_2$ could only be carried out in patients without autoPEEP. These results indicate that, in patients with acute respiratory failure under controlled mechanical ventilation, the presence of autoPEEP is associated with inaccuracy in the calculation of predicted $PaCO_2$ from $PetCO_2$.

Relationship between arterial PCO_2 and $PetCO_2$ during weaning

The decision to start a weaning trial in a critically ill patient often implies having correct arterial blood gases. The fact that capnography could provide a noninvasive tool to assess alveolar ventilation and therefore $PaCO_2$, some investigators have evaluated the utility of capnography during weaning periods. However, these studies have yielded controversial results. Niehoff et al [14] evaluated the use of capnography in 40 ICU patients under mechanical ventilation and found that $PetCO_2$ of > 40 torr predicted hypercarbia with a sensitivity of 28 %. However, the same authors found during the weaning period (IMV method) that a group of post-cardiac surgery patients randomized to a capnography/pulse oxymetry monitoring group had fewer arterial blood gas determinations than a control group weaned with periodic arterial blood sampling. Healey et al [15] compared changes in $PetCO_2$ and $PaCO_2$ before and after withdrawal of mechanical ventilation in 20 patients predisposed to hypercarbia. After switching the patients from assist/control to spontaneous breathing, changes in $PaCO_2$ were closely paralleled by changes in $PetCO_2$ ($r = 0.82$). Nine of 20 patients had an increased $PaCO_2$ of 10 torr or greater, and $PetCO_2$ rose by at least 5 torr in 7 of these patients concluding that changes in $PetCO_2$ were predictive of important $PaCO_2$ increases. Withington et al [16] evaluated the use of capnography during weaning in 40 patients following cardiac surgery reporting a 79 % sensitivity for detection of hypercarbia using $PetCO_2$. These investigators conclude that once a gradient between $PaCO_2$ and $PetCO_2$ has been calculated, capnography can be used to guide respiratory management until extubation. However, the opposite has also been found. Hess et al [17] evaluated the use of $PetCO_2$ as an indication of changes in $PaCO_2$ in 24 adult patients being weaned from mechanical ventilation. After each change in the weaning process (SIMV rate, T-piece trial) a total of 113 data sets were collected. Despite of the fact that good correlation was found between $PaCO_2$ and $PetCO_2$, in 43 % of the cases the change in $PetCO_2$ incorrectly indicated the direction of change in $PaCO_2$.

Recently, Morley et al [18] evaluated simultaneous $PaCO_2$ and $PetCO_2$ determinations during MV and again during a spontaneous breathing trial just before returning the patient to mechanical ventilation. These authors found that capnography offers a reasonable estimate of changes in $PaCO_2$ during weaning in patients without lung disease. However, for ± 5 mmHg change in $PetCO_2$, capnography had a sensitivity of 59 % and a specificity of 80 % for patients with parenchymal lung disease, particularly patients with emphysema. Interestingly and very important for clinical practice, all severe episodes of hypoventilation, defined as 10 mmHg or higher increse in $PaCO_2$, were identified by capnography. Therefore, the majority of the episodes of hypoventilation missed would be of mild to moderate severity.

We have also studied the utility of capnography in patients undergoing weaning from mechanical ventilation [19]. The objective was to analize the ability of $PetCO_2$ to identify clinically relevant episodes of hypercapnia during weaning. Our weaning protocol consisted in 2 hours breathing on 5 cm H_2O of continuous positive airway pressure (CPAP). We determined $PaCO_2$ and $PetCO_2$ in assist/control mode, after 1 hours and 2 hours (before extubation) on CPAP, or immediately before returning to assist/control mode in those patients who failed the weaning trial. We evaluated 30 patients (53 determinations) and found that changes in $PaCO_2$ and in $PetCO_2$ varied in opposite direction in only two determinations. Episodes of hypoventilation ($PaCO_2 > 42$ mmHg or and increment of 8 mmHg in $PaCO_2$ in hypercapnic patients) were detected by an increment > 3 mmHg in $PetCO_2$ with a sensitivity of 82 % and a specificity of 76 %. Like others, we can conclude that $PetCO_2$ might provide a reasonable estimate of $PaCO_2$ during weaning although false positives may occur in patients who are not hypercapnic, thus resulting in unnecessary invasive blood gas determinations.

Capnography in airway obstruction

The factors that influence the waveform of the expired capnogram are the ventilation perfusion mismatch of some lung zones, airway gas mixing and CO_2 sequential expiration [3, 5, 20]. Bronchial obstruction is associated with regional decreases in airflow, consequently reductions in alveolar ventilation and responsible for the heterogeneity of the ventilation/perfusion relationship. Therefore, the increasing expired CO_2 slope observed in some patients may be a result of the serial mixing of gas flowing from units with different time constants. Several studies conducted in asthmatic patients showed the existence of a significant correlation between indices describing the shape of the capnogram and the usual spirometric parameters. You et al [21] demonstrated the existence of a very good correlation ($p < 0.001$) between the end-tidal slope of the alveolar plateau and the forced expiratory volume in one second as a percentage of predicted. Later on the same group [22] studied different indices taken from the succesive phases of the expired capnogram and found significant correlations between spirometry and capnographic indices. In subjects receiving mechanical ventilation Watson et al [23] found very good correlation between the expired CO_2 slope and respiratory resistance in patients with normal lungs during general anesthesia.

Critically ill patients under mechanical ventilation may often exhibit high respiratory system resistance (R_{rs}) due to a variety of reasons [24, 25]. As the expiratory capnogram is correlated with spirometric indices, we investigated the relationship between R_{rs} and expired capnogram in a population of patients under mechanical ventilation admitted in a general intensive care service [26]. In addition, we assessed whether the expired CO_2 slope and $PaCO_2$-$PetCO_2$ gradient could be a sensitive parameter to predict R_{rs} during total ventilatory support. Regression analysis found a close correlation between R_{rs} and expired CO_2 slope ($r = 0.86$; $p < 0.001$) and prediction interval limits at the 95 % confidence level for R_{rs} were ± 7.39 cm H_2O/l/s from the predicted value obtained by the regression equation, where $R_{rs} = 11.42 + 2.28$. Expired CO_2 Slope. Weak correlation was found between R_{rs} and the $PaCO_2$-$PetCO_2$ gradient ($r = 0.48$; $p < 0.01$). In line with the results of Watson et al [23] in intubated subjects with normal lungs, and You et al [22] in asthmatic patients, we found a strong correlation between the expired CO_2 slope and R_{rs}. All these observations suggest that CO_2 elimination is impaired by a flow resistive mechanism and that the degree of airways obstruction modulates the PCO_2 rise rate during expiration. However, despite the strong correlation found between R_{rs} and the expired CO_2 slope, wide prediction intervals were obtained for a given value of estimated R_{rs} using the regression equation. Therefore, the expired CO_2 slope has limited clinical applicability in order to accurately predict R_{rs} at the bedside.

In contrast, we found a weak correlation between $PaCO_2$-$PetCO_2$ gradients and R_{rs} [26]. Because the $PaCO_2$-$PetCO_2$ gradient is not only influenced by structural airway abnormalities but also by high and low V/Q regions [27-29], it could explain why determinate patients may exhibit wide $PaCO_2$-$PetCO_2$ gradient together with both normal R_{rs} and expired CO_2 slope. Finally, low cardiac output states may widen the $PaCO_2$-$PetCO_2$ gradient as pulmonary perfusion decreases whereas lung mechanical properties remain unchanged [30]. These observations suggest that CO_2 elimination in critically ill patients is strongly modulated by lung, airway, endotracheal tube and ventilator equipment resistances. Although continuous capnogram waveform monitoring at the bedside might be useful to assess Rrs, very accurate predictions could only be done in determinate patients.

References

1. Hess D (1990) Capnometry and capnography: technical aspects, physiologic aspects, and clinical applications. Respir Care 35:557-576
2. Jubran A, Tobin MJ (1994) Monitoring gas exchange during mechanical ventilation. In: Tobin MJ (ed) Principles and practice of mechanical ventilation.McGraw-Hill Inc, New York, pp 919-943
3. Stock MC (1988) Non invasive carbon dioxide monitoring. Crit Care Clin 4:511-526
4. Clark JS, Votteri B, Ariagno RL et al (1992) Non invasive assessment of blood gases. Am Rev Respir Dis 145:220-232
5. Nunn JF (1987) Applied respiratory physiology. 3rd ed. Butterworths, London
6. Scheid P, Piiper J (1980) Blood/gas equilibrium of carbon dioxide in lungs. A critical review. Respir Physiol 39:1-31
7. Donati F, Maille J, Blain R et al (1985) End-tidal carbon dioxide tension and temperature changes after coronary artery bypass surgery. Can Anaesth Soc J 32:272-277
8. Takki S, Aromaa U, Kauste A (1972) The validity and usefulness of the end-tidal PCO_2 during anesthesia. Ann Clin Res 4:278-284
9. Perrin F, Perrot D, Holzapfel L et al (1983) Simultaneous variations of $PaCO_2$ and $PACO_2$ in assisted ventilation. Br J Anaesth 55:525-530

10. Raemer DB, Francis D, Phiplip JH et al (1983) Variation in PCO_2 between arterial blood and peak expired gas during anesthesia. Anesth Analg 62:1065-1069
11. Blanch Ll, Fernandez R, Benito S, Mancebo J, Calaf N, Net A (1988) Accuracy of an indirect carbon dioxide Fick method in determination of the cardiac output in critically ill mechanically ventilated patients. Int Care Med 14:131-135
12. Hoffman RA, Krieger BP, Kramer MR et al (1989) End-tidal carbon dioxide in critically ill patients during changes in mechanical ventilation. Am Rev Respir Dis 140:1265-1268
13. Blanch Ll, Fernandez R, Artigas A (1991) The effect of auto PEEP on the $PaCO_2$-$PetCO_2$ gradient and expired CO_2 slope in critically ill patients during total ventilatory support. J Crit Care 6:202-210
14. Niehoff J, DelGuercio C, LaMorte W et al (1988) Efficacy of pulse oxymetry and capnometry in postoperative ventilatory weaning. Crit Care Med 16:701-705
15. Healey CJ, Fedullo AJ, Swinburne AJ, Wahl GW (1987) Comparison of noninvasive measurements of carbon dioxide tension during withdrawal from mechanical ventilation. Crit Care Med 15:764-768
16. Withington DE, Ramsay JG, Saoud AT, Bilodeau J (1991) Weaning from ventilation after cardio-pulmonary bypass: evaluation of a noninvasive technique. Can J Anaesth 38:15-19
17. Hess D, Schlottag A, Levin B, Mathai J, Rexrode WO (1991) An evaluation of the usefulness of end-tidal PCO_2 to aid weaning from mechanical ventilation following cardiac surgery. Respir Care 36:837-843
18. Morley TF, Giaimo J, Maroszan E et al (1993) Use of capnography for assessment of the adequacy of alveolar ventilation during weaning from mechanical ventilation. Am Rev Respir Dis 148:339-344
19. Saura P, Blanch Ll, Fernández R, Lucangelo U, Artigas A (1994) Usefulness of capnography to detect hypercapnic episodes during weaning. Int Care Med 20:S53
20. Meyer M, Mohr M, Schulz H, Piiper J (1990) Sloping alveolar plateaus of CO_2, O_2, and intravenously infused C_2H_2 and $CHClF_2$ in the dog. Respir Physiol 81:137-152
21. You B, Mayeux D, Rkiek B, Autran N, Dang Vu V, Grilliat JP (1992) La capnographie dans l'asthme: perspectives d'utilisation comme méthode de monitorage. Rev Mal Respir 9:547-552
22. You B, Peslin R, Duvivier C, Dang Vu V, Grilliat JP (1994) Expiratory capnography in asthma: evaluation of various shape indices. Eur Respir J 7:318-323
23. Watson R, Benumof J, Clausen J, Ozaki G (1989) Expiratory CO_2 plateau slope predicts airway resistance. Anesthesiology 71:A1072
24. Milic-Emili J (1989) Pulmonary flow resistance. Lung 167:141-148
25. Smith TC, Marini JJ (1988) Impact of PEEP on lung mechanics and work of breathing in severe airflow obstruction. J Appl Physiol 65:1488-1499
26. Blanch Ll, Fernandez R, Saura P, Baigorri F, Artigas A (1994) Relationship between expired capnogram and respiratory system resistance in critically ill patients during total ventilatory support. Chest 105:219-223
27. Chopin C, Fesard P, Mangalaboyi J et al (1990) Use of capnography in diagnosis of pulmonary embolism during acute respiratory failure of chronic obstructive pulmonary disease. Crit Care Med 18:353-357
28. Yamanaka MK, Sue DY (1987) Comparison of arterial-end-tidal PCO_2 difference and dead space/tidal volume ratio in respiratory failure. Chest 92:832-835
29. Blanch Ll, Fernandez R, Benito S, Mancebo J, Net A (1987) Effect of PEEP on the arterial minus end-tidal carbon dioxide gradient. Chest 92:451-454
30. Falk JL, Rackow EC, Weil MH (1988) End-tidal carbon dioxide concentration during cardiopulmonary resuscitation. N Engl J Med 318:607-611

Chapter 18

Face mask ventilation in acute exacerbations of chronic obstructive pulmonary disease

L. BROCHARD

Introduction

Acute exacerbation of chronic obstructive pulmonary disease (COPD) constitutes a frequent cause of admission in intensive care units. All patients require specific medical therapy, including oxygen, and many of them eventually require endotracheal intubation and mechanical ventilation with the aim of improving gas exchange, rest the respiratory muscles and avoid exhaustion and respiratory arrest. This technique is considered as invasive because it bypasses natural airway protective mechanisms in order to give access to the lower airways, often necessitates sedation and can be associated with traumatic or infectious complications [1, 2]. Non-invasive ventilation constitutes a way of delivering mechanical ventilation avoiding the use of endotracheal intubation. After being used in the setting of home mechanical ventilation [3, 4], it is now proposed for patients with acute respiratory failure [5-13].

Although the final objective is to try to reduce complications associated with mechanical ventilation, three different goals can be identified [14]. First, non-invasive ventilation can be delivered with the aim of replacing machanical ventilation in patients who would need endotracheal intubation. Second, it may be proposed at an earlier stage to avoid further deterioration of the patient and avoid the need for eventual endotracheal intubation. In fact, these two goals are often difficult to differentiate but may imply different action mechanisms. Similarly, this technique may be used to postpone intubation in patients in whom the decision of performing endotracheal intubation has not been firmly decised. Third, non invasive ventilation has been used as a way to deliver ventilatory support in patients with respiratory failure in whom intubation was considered as questionable, such as elderly patients.

Techniques of non invasive ventilation

The patient-ventilator interface has an important influence on the efficacy of the technique. Because direct access to the lower airways is not possible, nasal or facial masks have to be used. Although a mouth-piece costitutes a feasible alternative, it is rarely used in acute respiratory failure bacause of its frequent discomfort and the need for active cooperation of the patient. Nasal or full face masks have both been used successfully [5, 6] and both present advantages and disadvantages. An ideal mask should be easy to handle and to fit to the patient's face, it should have a low internal volume, prevent leaks as far as possible and be comfortable, avoiding pain created by localized zones of compression. Nasal masks offer many advantages compared to full face masks in this respect but one major drawback is the possibility of leakage through the mouth in the case of patients who mouth breathe or simply do not close their mouth. This can induce patient-ventilatory asynchrony and impedes the action of noninvasive ventilation [15]. Nasal masks, therefore, might be reserved for instance, for cooperative patients or after an initial phase of treatment with a full face mask.

Different ventilatory modes have been used, mainly distributed between pressure-targeted modes, like pressure support ventilation, and volume controlled modes. Both types of ventilatory modes may result in successful ventilation. In both types, the quality of the triggering mechanism may play an important role in the efficacy of the technique. Also, the characteristics of pressure and flow contour may influence the results (rate of rise of pressure, peak flow rate, flow-impeding characteristics). Although some special ventilators have been proposed for this purpose, most of them were proposed for long term home ventilation [16]. Only very few have been developed to meet requirements encountered in patients with respiratory failure [10]. One prospective study compared assist-control and pressure support ventilation delivered noninvasively [13]. No difference was found in the efficacy of the technique with regards to the need for endotracheal intubation, although only small groups of patients were studied. Patient's comfort, however, was poorer with assist-control and the number of side effects was significantly greater with this mode. This was probably explained by the higher peak mask pressure with assist-control which can induce discomfort, gastric insufflation, provide leaks around the mask and imposes the mask to be fitted more tightly and favors pressure skin lesions.

Lastly, the combination of pressure support and positive end-expiratory pressure seems to be one of the most attractive modalities of ventilation to reduce respiratory efforts in COPD patients [17]. Although the technique may not be crucial for the immediate efficacy of this therapy, it may play a role in the time-consuming aspects of this procedure and its acceptance by patients and nursing staff [18].

Physiological effects

Meduri and coworkers initially described the efficacy of the technique in a small group of hypercapnic patients rapidly improving gas exchange under face mask ventilation [6]. Most of the failures of the technique were not due to ventilatory inefficiency. Later on they suggested that a rapid improvement in PCO_2 and pH assessed after one hour of treatment was a good predictor of the ultimate success of the technique [19]. They also used this technique in a group of seven patients who presented ventilatory failure early after tracheal extubation. They were able to compare the efficacy of the same ventilatory support delivered either invasively or non-invasively at a few hours interval. They found no difference in expired ventilation or gas exchange with the two different ways of delivering the ventilatory support.

Several studies assessed the physiological effects of pressure support ventilation delivered non invasively in patients with stable COPD [20] or acute exacerbation [10]. Results similar to those observed in intubated patients have been reported. On short periods of time (about one hour), an improvement in oxygenation is combined with a decrease in $PaCO_2$ and a rise in pH, together with a reduction of respiratory muscle activity assessed by transdiaphragmatic pressure or diaphragm EMG. Most studies performed in this situation showed that non invasive ventilation usually constitutes a partial ventilatory support unloading the respiratory muscles, but not taking the whole respiratory work. Because the degree of assistance is usually limited, this may represent a cause of failure in patients with high levels of respiratory activity.

One interesting effect, reported in several studies [8, 21], is to allow a correction of hypoxemia without inducing worsening of hypercapnia, as often observed in COPD patients with acute exacerbation.

Clinical results

Assessment of the efficacy of non invasive ventilation has been performed using different methodologies. The first open uncontrolled studies described improvement in gas exchange and functional parameters, all results suggesting benefitial effects of the technique [6-8, 16, 19, 22]. Several authors used historical or non randomized control groups to evaluate the efficacy of this form of therapy. Foglio and co-workers found no benefit with non invasive ventilation delivered to patients with COPD by comparision to the evolution of similar patients who refused to be ventilated with the technique [9]. No randomization was performed in this study. In addition, only one patient required intubation in the whole group suggesting a mild severity of the exacerbation. Later the same group used non invasive ventilation delivered via a full face mask, instead of the nasal mask previously used, and found a significant reduction in the number of patients requiring intubation compared to an historical control group [13]. Fernandez and coworkers recently showed the effects of pressure support delivered via a full face mask in COPD patients describing a progressive worsening under oxygen therapy [8]. The initial oxygen-induced hypercapnia observed in these patients was rapidly corrected under pressure support and most patients avoided endotracheal intubation.

We previously compared the results obtained in 13 patients admitted for acute exacerbation of COPD and treated with pressure support ventilation delivered via a full face mask to a carefully matched historical control group in a case-control study [10]. Both groups had comparable severity on admission and similar mortality. The number of patients requiring intubation, however, was markedly reduced from almost 80 % to 10 %, together with a reduced duration of ventilatory assistance and a marked reduction in the length of hospital stay.

Recently, a multicenter randomized prospective study was performed by a British group [11]. Bott and co-workers studied 60 patients with acute respiratory failure on COPD and compared a standard medical therapy to the same treatment with the addition of nasal intermittent positive pressure. In the new therapy group several physiological parameters were significantly improved compared to the control group, as well as the breathlessness score. The authors also compared mortality between the two groups and found a significant reduction in the non-invasive ventilation group (29 % to 10 %, $p < 0.05$) when the 4 patients who did not tolerate non invasive ventilatory support were excluded from the analysis. It should be noted, however, that most of the patients in the control group died without being intubated, which reflects specific therapeutic attitudes compared to other approaches.

We recently completed a multicenter randomized study comparing standard therapy to face mask pressure support in 80 COPD patients [21]. Patients were in severe respiratory distress with tachypnea (mean respiratory rate 35 breaths/min), hypoxemia (mean PO_2 40 mmHg) and respiratory acidosis. Most patients presented signs of encephalopathy. A major reduction in the need for endotracheal intubation (74 % to 26 %, $p < 0.05$), a reduction in the length of hospital stay and a decrease of in-hospital mortality (29 % to 10 %, $p < 0.05$) was observed in the new therapy group. This benefit resulted from a marked reduction in the number of patients presenting complications during the ICU stay. It is important to note that patients with a clear cause for decompensation requiring a specific therapeutic approach, such as pneumothorax, lung abcess, need for surgery, etc., were not included in the study. These benefitial results were therefore obtained in a selected group of patients.

Conclusion

In Intensive Care Units non invasive ventilation seems to constitute an important advance for the management of acute exacerbation of chronic obstructive pulmonary disease. After an initial training in the technique, major benefitial results can be obtained in selected patients using pressure support ventilation via a full face mask. Further studies are needed to better delineate indications and to understand mechanisms of failure.

References

1. Pingleton SK (1988) Complications of acute respiratory failure. Am Rev Respir Dis 137:1463-1493
2. Fagon JY, Chastre J, Hance AJ, Montravers P, Novara A, Gibert C (1993) Nosocomial pneumonia in ventilated patients: a cohort study evaluating attributable mortality and hospital stay. Am J Med 94:281-288
3. Garay SM, Turino GM, Goldring RM (1981) Sustained reversal of chronic hypercap-

nia in patients with alveolar hypoventilation syndromes: long-term maintenance with non invasive mechanical ventilation. Am J Med 70:269-274
4. Bach JR, Alba A, Mosher R, Delaubier A (1989) Intermittent positive pressure ventilation via nasal access in the management of respiratory insufficiency. Chest 92:168-170
5. Leger P, Jennequin J, Gaussorgues P, Robert D (1988) Acute respiratory failure in COPD patients treated with non invasive intermittent mechanical ventilation (control mode) with nasal mask. Am Rev Respir Dis 137:A63
6. Hill NS (1993) Non invasive ventilation Does it work, for whom and how? Am Rev Respir Dis 147:1050-1055
7. Meduri GU, Conoscenti CC, Menashe P, Nair S (1989) Non invasive face mask ventilation in patients with acute respiratory failure. Chest 95:865-870
8. Benhamou D, Girault C, Faure C, Portier F, Muir JF (1992) Nasal mask ventilation in acute respiratory failure. Experience in elderly patients. Chest 102:912-917
9. Fernandez R, Blanch LP, Valles J, Baigorri F, Artigas A (1993) Pressure support ventilation via face mask in acute respiratory failure in hypercapnic COPD patients. Int Care Med 19:465-461
10. Foglio C, Vittaca M, Quadri A, Scalvini S, Marangoni S, Ambrosino N (1992) Acute exacerbations in severe COLD patients. Treatment using positive pressure ventilation by nasal mask. Chest 101:533-538
11. Brochard L, Isabey D, Piquet J, Amaro P, Mancebo J, Messadi AA, Brun-Buisson C, Rauss A, Lemaire F, Harf A (1990) Reversal of acute exacerbations of chronic obstructive lung disease by inspiratory assistance with a face mask. N Eng J Med 323:1523-1530
12. Bott J, Carroll MP, Conway et al (1993) Randomised controlled trial of nasal ventilation in acute ventilatory failure due to chronic obstructive airways disease. Lancet 341:1555-1557
13. Wysocki M, Tric L, Wolff MA, Gertner J, Millet H, Herman B (1993) Non invasive pressure support ventilation in patients with acute respiratory failure. Chest 103:907-913
14. Vitacca M, Rubini F, Foglio K, Scalvini S, Nava S, Ambrosino N (1993) Non invasive modalities of positive pressure ventilation improve the outcome of acute exacerbations in COPD patients. Int Care Med 19:450-455
15. Brochard L (1993) Non invasive ventilation: practical issues. Int Care Med 19:431-432
16. Carrey Z, Gottfried SB, Levy RD (1990) Ventilatory muscle support in respiratory failure with nasal positive pressure ventilation. Chest 97:150-158
17. Pennock BE, Kaplan PD, Carlin BW, Sabangan JS, Magovern JA (1991) Pressure support ventilation with a simplified ventilatory support system administered with a nasal mask in patients with respiratory failure. Chest 100:1371-1376
18. Appendini L, Patessio A, Zanaboni S, Carone M, Gukov B, Donner C, Rossi A (1994) Physiologic effects of positive end-expiratory pressure support during exacerbations of chronic obstructive pulmonary disease. Am J Respir Crit Care Med 149:1069-1076
19. Chevrolet JC, Jolliet P, Abajo B, Toussi A, Louis M (1991) Nasal positive pressure ventilation in patients with acute respiratory failure. Difficult and time-consuming procedure for nurses. Chest 100:775-782
20. Meduri GU, Abou-Shala N, Fox RC, Jones CB, Leeper KV, Wunderig RG (1991) Non invasive face mask mechanical ventilation in patients with acute hypercapnic respiratory failure. Chest 100:445-454
21. Nava S, Ambrosino N, Rubini F, et al (1993) Effect of nasal pressure support ventilation and external PEEP on diaphragmatic activity in patients with severe stable COPD. Chest 103:143-150
22. Brochard L, Wysocki M, Lofaso F, et al (1993) Face mask inspiratory positive airway pressure for acute aexacerbation on chronic respiratory insufficiency. A randomized multicenter study. Am Rev Respir Dis 147:A984

23. Elliott MW, Steven MH, Philipps GD, Branthwaite MA (1990) Non invasive mechanical ventilation for acute respiratory failure. B Med J 300:358-360

Chapter 19

Proportional assist ventilation (PAV)

R. Giuliani, V.M. Ranieri

Introduction

Proportional assist ventilation (PAV) [1-3] is an innovative ventilatory assistance technique devised by Dr. Magdy Younes of Manitoba University and intended for clinical use in patients who, though having an adequate respiratory "drive", are not capable of "sustaining" the respiratory work completely.

First of all, it should be stressed that this *ventilatory assistance mode* has not yet found a proper role in clinical use, and some technical and design solutions of the product are still awaiting definition. At present PAV is implemented on prototype respirators which associate it with the more traditional assisted or controlled ventilation techniques.

Proportional assist ventilation is the most advanced achievement of an evolutional process concerning all modern ventilation techniques and is characterized by an increasing adjustment of the respirator to the patient's ventilatory requirements.

The classical constant-flow and "cycled" controlled ventilation (by now confined to the cases with total loss of the neuro-muscular function) has given way to ventilation techniques capable of "assisting" the patient's ventilation by exclusively integrating the ventilatory activity component that the patient lacks, while respecting all the components that have remained intact.

This partial and "targeted" level of ventilatory assistance pursues two objectives:

1. maintain the utmost physiological conditions in both the ventilation and the interactions between ventilation and haemodynamics;
2. reduce the time of weaning from the ventilator.

In the light of these considerations, *optimal* ventilation and *minimal* ventilation coincide. According to a modern view of ventilatory assistance, weaning from the respiratory prosthesis begins when the patient is connected to the respirator.

The goal of "minimizing the ventilatory support" is completely absent in controlled ventilation (CV), in which both the respiratory rate and the various phases of the cycle (inspiration, pause and expiration) are the responsibility of the automatic ventilator. Under these circumstances should the patient's own ventilatory activity be inadequate, it is usually advisable to suppress it pharmacologically in order to reduce the risk of barotrauma.

The clinical choice of CV is, therefore, based on the evaluation of inadequacy of the patient's respiratory "drive" and on the decision to replace it with a more appropriate respiratory pattern for the patient's pulmonary conditions. This logic is best expressed by the inverted I:E ratio ventilation, in which low inspiration flows and short expiration times are the best strategy for a more homogeneous ventilation of the pulmonary parenchyma.

A first attempt to "adjust" the respirator to the patient's spontaneous activity is made whenever venturing into the rather difficult procedure improperly defined "patient's adjustment to the machine": the shortening of the inspiration time, the subsequent increase of the inspiration flow and the search for the optimal respiratory rate are mere attempts to "adjust the machine to the patient".

According to this logic of respirator-patient adjustment (of which PAV is the most advanced goal), the high-sensitivity trigger has turned the beginning of the inspiration cycle from a passive (time-dependent) into an "intelligent" condition (rapid response to the patient). Thanks to the trigger, not only can the patient increase the respiratory rate, but also the beginning of inspiration is synchronous with the patient's spontaneous activity. The "flow-by" trigger represents a further step forward, since it promptly responds to the patient's ventilatory requirements by reducing both the barotrauma and the energy expenditure [4].

A review of the various phases of this evolutional process is not the aim of this presentation, but emphasis should be laid on its logic being based on the ever improving discrimination of the various components of the ventilatory activities, and on the selective "support" of those that have been actually impaired.

Pressumetric ventilation (PV), characterized by a flow having an initial peak and a downward trend, ensures a flow a more similar to the physiological one. Nevertheless, PV, whether controlled or assisted, entrusts the respirator with the control of the in- and expiration time, maintaining the typical prerogative of "rigid", "time-cycled" ventilations.

Synchronized intermittent mandatory ventilation (SIMV) aims at reducing the number of acts "imposed by the machine", allowing the patient to breathe spontaneously between two respirator-controlled acts.

Ventilation by Pressure Support (PS), among the various systems adopted in clinical use, is characterized by the very limited level of respiratory assistance (continuous positive airway pressure - CPAP - cannot be regarded as a real ventilation as, per se, it does not ensure the patient any gas exchange). At present PS is, therefore, the most advanced mechanical ventilatory support mode in the weaning process. PS (like PV) guarantees a constant pressure value at the mouth throughout the inspiration. However, unlike the PV, PS gives back the patient the possibility of timing the phases of the respiratory cycle. The patient, by modifying the flow morphology with his/her own ventilatory activity, determines the change from the inspiratory to the expiratory phase (flow cycling). PS must therefore be used in those patients whose neuro-muscular function is "adequate".

During inspiration, PS increases the pressure gradient between mouth and alveolus. This gradient has two components: [1] the patient's inspiratory effort and [2] the support pressure set on the respirator. The gradient is, of course, at its maximum value at the beginning of the inspiration and then progressively decreases. Thanks to the "flow cycling" feature, the alveolar pressure will never reach the PS value, as the expiratory phase will surely be activated before such a condition occurs.

Let us analyse the pressure gradients during PS.
1. The mouth-alveolus gradient is mainly determined by the PS level and, to a very small extent, by the patient's effort.
2. The support pressure level set on the respirator remains constant and is independent from the patient's "respiratory effort" variations. This means that even significant percentage variations of the latter will only slightly affect the total gradient. For instance, let us suppose that a support pressure of 18 cm H_2O has been set on the respirator and that the patient makes an inspiratory effort creating a negative pressure of 2 cm H_2O. The total gradient will be equal to 20 cm H_2O. Should the patient double his/her "effort" (for example, owing to increased metabolic requirements) taking it to 4 cm H_2O, the total gradient will go from 20 (18+2) to 22 (18+4) cm H_2O. The real flow increase, therefore, is 10 %, as against an increase in the patient's activity of 100 %. In this situation the patient restores an adequate volume/minute by increasing the respiratory rate.
3. As the mouth-alveolus gradient at the beginning of the inspiration is heavily determined by the support pressure, the maximum flow is directly proportional to the latter. Subsequently, the gas going into the alveoli reduces the inspiratory flow to the "cycling" threshold value. Whatever the technical features determining the "cycling" process, at the end of the inspiration the tidal volume is directly proportional to the set pressure support level.

PS, therefore (and all constant pressure ventilations), not only allows the patient very limited variations of flow and tidal volume, but also entrusts these two variables (maximum flow and tidal volume) to the setting of a single parameter (pressure support). In patients with a selectively "resistive" or "compliance" pathology (an altered time constant) - not infrequent during weaning - the flow and/or tidal volume values can turn out not to be optimal if determined through the same parameter.

In the presence of increased resistances, without a parallel increase in elastance, an optimal inspiratory flow can only be guaranteed by an increase in the support pressure, which will be followed by pulmonary hyperinflation (since compliance is less compromised). Conversely, in situations of limited compliance and fundamentally "normal" resistances, a support pressure providing a moderate inspiratory flow peak will be inadequate to guarantee a sufficient tidal volume.

These aspects of PS can lead to clinical failures by blocking the weaning process.

The purpose of PAV is to overcome these limitations

PAV is a type of ventilation (belonging to the pressometric group) intended for those patients who, though having a substantially intact "respiratory drive", require ventilatory assistance owing to their inability to entirely sustain the work of breathing, more specifically elastic and/or resistive work. PAV can integrate the patient's inspiratory effort whenever this is quantitatively insufficient, although qualitatively adequate.

PAV can also optimize the ventilatory support in the presence of an impairment of the pulmonary time constant.

The innovative aspect of this technique consists in the continuous adjustment of the pressure support value, by distinguishing a "resistive" and an "elastic" component within the latter. At any instant, the pressure gradient (ΔP) governing the respiratory act is equal to the difference between the pressure generated by the respirator (P_{aw}) and the pleural pressure determined by "the activity" of the patient's respiratory muscles (P_{pl}), ($\Delta P = P_{aw}$-P_{pl}). The ΔP gradient can also be regarded as the sum of four pressure components: resistive, elastic, inertial and end expiratory pressure (Motion equation):

$$\Delta P = P_{res} + P_{el} + P_{in} + EEP \quad (1)$$

Leaving aside P_{in} (inertial pressure) (normally regarded as negligible and, at least, absorbable into the other terms) and zeroing the EEP value (end expiratory pressure), the equation can be appropriately simplified as follows:

$$\Delta P = P_{res} + P_{el} \quad (2)$$

By replacing the values of resistive and elastic pressure with their respective determinants, one can write:

$$\Delta P = R \bullet \dot{V} + E \bullet V \quad (3)$$

where R and E are the values of pulmonary resistance and elastance respectively, while $\dot{V}$ and V respectively express the "instantaneous" values of flow and tidal volume (pulmonary volume above the end expiratory volume = LV-EELV).

Breaking down of ΔP into P_{aw} and P_{pl} allows to identify the R_{vent} and R_{pat} percentages in the R value and the E_{vent} and E_{pat} percentages in the E value, there by identifying the R and the E fractions respectively "supported" by the ventilator (R_{vent} and E_{vent}) and by the patient (R_{pat} and E_{pat}). Hence:

$$(P_{aw} - P_{pl}) = (R_{vent} + R_{pat}) \bullet \dot{V} + (E_{vent} + E_{pat}) \bullet V \quad (4)$$

and by separating the two components:

$$- P_{pl} = R_{pat} \bullet \dot{V} + E_{pat} \bullet V \quad (5)$$
$$P_{aw} = R_{vent} \bullet \dot{V} + E_{vent} \bullet V \quad (6)$$

By analogy with [2]:

$$- P_{pl} = P_{pl\text{-}res} + P_{pl\text{-}el} \quad (7)$$
$$\text{where } - P_{pl\text{-}res} = R_{pat} \bullet \dot{V} \quad (8)$$
$$- P_{pl\text{-}el} = E_{pat} \bullet V \quad (9)$$

and again by analogy with [2]:

$$P_{aw} = P_{aw\text{-}res} + P_{aw\text{-}el} \quad (10)$$

where:

$$P_{aw\text{-}res} = R_{vent} \cdot \dot{V} \quad (11)$$
$$P_{aw\text{-}el} = E_{vent} \cdot V \quad (12)$$

where the letters "-res" and "-el" refer to the two different resistive and elastic components respectively.

Thanks to its ability to measure the instantaneous flow ($\dot{V}$) and to calculate the inspired volume (V), at each instant and through equation (6), PAV calculates the pressure support (P_{aw}) to be provided. The R_{vent} and E_{vent} values (of which the patient is to be "relieved" and the machine is to be loaded) must be set on the respirator. The remaining R_{pat} (= R-R_{vent}) and E_{pat} (= E-E_{vent}) percentages are the resistance and elastance values that have to be sustained by the patient (Eq. 5).

To summarize, according to the pre-set resistance and elastance values (R_{vent} and E_{vent}), the machine generates a pressure at the mouth (P_{aw}), equal to the sum of two pressure components (Eq. 6): a) one capable of guaranteeing the instantaneous flow through a resistance value equal to the set value ($\dot{V}$ R_{vent}); b) the other capable of offsetting, for each instantaneous tidal volume, an elastance value equal to the set value ($\dot{V}$ E_{vent}).

The remaining R_{pat} and E_{pat} percentages will remain the patient's responsibility. The larger the E_{vent} and R_{vent} values (*as set on the machine*), the smaller the respiratory effort made by the patient, of course. In the theoretical case in which the set values were exactly to coincide with the patient's values (R_{vent} = R and E_{vent} = E) all the work of breathing would be carried out by the machine. However, for the correct operation of the latter, the R_{vent} and E_{vent} values will always have to be lower than the respective R and E values.

A concrete example will clarify a few doubts. Let us suppose that the patient has a pulmonary elastance (E) of 20 cm H_2O/l and inspiratory resistances (R) equal to 10 cm H_2O/l/sec. In the absence of any ventilatory support the patient carries out all the work of breathing entailed by that particular anatomo-pathologic condition. Should we decide to use PAV to relieve the patient from half of the elastic effort and 3/4 of the resistive effort, an E_{vent} value of 10 (= 50 % of 20) and a R_{vent} of 7.5 (= 75 % of 10) would be set on the respirator. This would imply, during the inspiratory phase, the application of a pressure value at the mouth that is a function of the set R_{vent} and E_{vent} values, and continuously modified according to the instananeous flow and the already insufflated volume (Eq. 6).

When the patient starts a flow $\dot{V}$ (instantaneously equal to P_{pl}/R) the respirator begins to compensate for the patient's effort, by supplying a ($P_{aw\text{-}res}$) pressure equal to $\dot{V}$ R_{vent}. 3/4 of the resistive pressure P_{res} will now be sustained by the respirator ($P_{aw\text{-}res} = 7.5 \cdot \dot{V}$) and only 1/4 of its total value (equal to 10) by the patient ($P_{pl\text{-}res} = 2.5 \cdot \dot{V}$). At the same time, the machine determines the insufflated volume (V) and calculates the $P_{aw\text{-}el}$ value according to Eq [12] ($P_{aw\text{-}el} = V \cdot 10$). The other half of the elastic pressure ($P_{pl\text{-}el} = V \cdot 10$) will be sustained by the patient.

At each instant pressure P_{aw}, supplied by the respirator, is equal to the sum of the resistive (P_{aw-res}) and the elastic component (P_{aw-el}) (Eq 10, 11 and 12). The patient will have to take charge of a respiratory work that is the function of the resistive (P_{pl-res}) and elastic pressure (P_{pl-el}) percentages concerning the patient (Eq 7, 8 and 9).

While the machine applies pressure P_{aw} systematically and without exceptions, the patient is capable of modifying at any instant his/her own inspiratory effort P_{pl}. A part of P_{pl}, must, however, be "spent" as elastic pressure (in the example $P_{pl-el} = V \cdot 10$). The remaining P_{pl-res} value is the pressure which, with P_{aw-res} (supplied by the respirator), maintains the flow through resistance R. Any variation in P_{pl-res} (ΔP_{pl-res}) causes a flow variation ($\Delta \dot{V}$) (according to the formula $\Delta \dot{V} = \Delta P_{pl-res} / R$). The flow variation thus induced by the patient will be followed by a new calculation of the P_{aw-res} pressure and, as a consequence, a new flow value ($\dot{V}$). Thus, the patient, by varying his/her inspiratory effort, can bring about variations in the pressure support supplied by the respirator.

When the patient zeroes his/her resistive P_{pl-res} effort, the machine also ceases its resistive support, while the new calculations of Eq. 11 are being carried out (more numerous in the case of a sudden flow variation).

The elastic load sustained by the machine (P_{aw-el}) is continuously calculated on the basis of the instantaneous value of V and the E_{vent} constant (set on the respirator). The remaining percentage of elastic pressure P_{pl-el} must necessarily be sustained by the patient.

In short:

1. the pressure at the mouth (P_{aw}) applied by PAV is the sum of two components (P_{aw-res} and P_{aw-el});
2. the elastic component (P_{aw-el}) increases with the insufflated volume (V), according to a multiplying factor equal to the elastance value set on the respirator (E_{vent});
3. the resistive component (P_{aw-res}) is determined, instant by instant, by flow ($\dot{V}$) and by a multiplying factor equal to the resistance value set on the respirator (R_{vent});
4. any variation of the patient's inspiratory effort (P_{pl-res}) leads to a coherent and proportional variation in the pressure support of the respirator;
5. the pressure supplied by the respirator is, therefore, constantly adjusted to the ventilatory requirements of the patient, who will maintain an optimal ventilation, exclusively taking charge of the elastance and resistance percentages assigned to him/her.

In connection with the statements made on PS, the following observations can be made:

1. with PAV the patient can change the support supplied by the machine, which changes as a function of the insufflated volume;
2. the patient's inspiratory effort significantly modifies the alveolus-mouth pressure gradient (and therefore the flow). Each time that the patient modifies his/her "effort" (e.g. the patient doubles it), the machine changes in the same proportion. The entire ΔP gradient is thus "piloted" by the patient;

3. thanks to PAV, an end inspiratory elastic pressure adequate to the desired pulmonary volume can be achieved, while maintaining an optimal inspiratory flow.

Unfortunately, the clinical studies for the validation of this technique are still few. It is not possible, therefore, to confirm that excellent clinical use can be summed to its conceptual value. In our view, the clinical validation of this technique can only be attained through two complementary procedures:
- verification that such a sophisticated approach is useful and easy to manage in clinical practice;
- search for innovative technological solutions.

Among the critical aspects found during the experimental use of the machine, attention should be paid to the following:
1. mention has already been made of the difficulties in measuring the patient's pulmonary resistance and elastance values. The automation of measurements would certainly simplify the use of this technique. By means of this automatic calculation, the values that are set on the respirator could be expressed in percentage units or in values to be sustained by the patient;
2. an incorrect setting of the R_{vent} and E_{vent} values (particularly if in excess) causes the machine to malfunction dramatically and the immediate patient's disadjustment. In addition to phenomena of non-linearity or time variance of the pulmonary mechanics parameters, each subject with spontaneous ventilatory activity periodically modifies the depth of his/her breathing (and therefore the values of E), so impairing the adequacy of the set values;
3. the cycling mode between the inspiratory and expiratory phase is an extremely critical aspect. It is evident that, for the machine to start the expiratory phase, the patient must actively oppose the pressure supplied by the respirator. This procedure surely brings discomfort and an additional effort to the patient.

For iconographic purposes only, we shall present three figures which, as Claude Bernard would say, can succeed in "stimulating the researcher's imagination".

Figure 1 shows the curves regarding flow, volume, pressure at the mouth and esophageal pressure recorded in a patient ventilated with PS and PAV, both in basic conditions and after the introduction of a dead space with the aim of simulating a variation of the patient's ventilatory requirements [5].
Figure 2 which concerns the same subject during ventilation with PS shows emblematically that after the application of a dead space the patient does not modify his/her own inspiratory effort - which, moreover, is already rather high - and cannot therefore increase the tidal volume. The adjustment response is obtained by increasing the respiratory rate (see Fig. 1). Conversely, under basic conditions, PAV (Fig. 3) brings about a lower inspiratory effort which is increased with the tidal volume after applying the dead space.

We may conclude by saying that, if on the one hand PAV is a promising technique and has clearly shown to be an undeniable step forward compared with the clinically validated ventilatory support techniques, there are still some practical

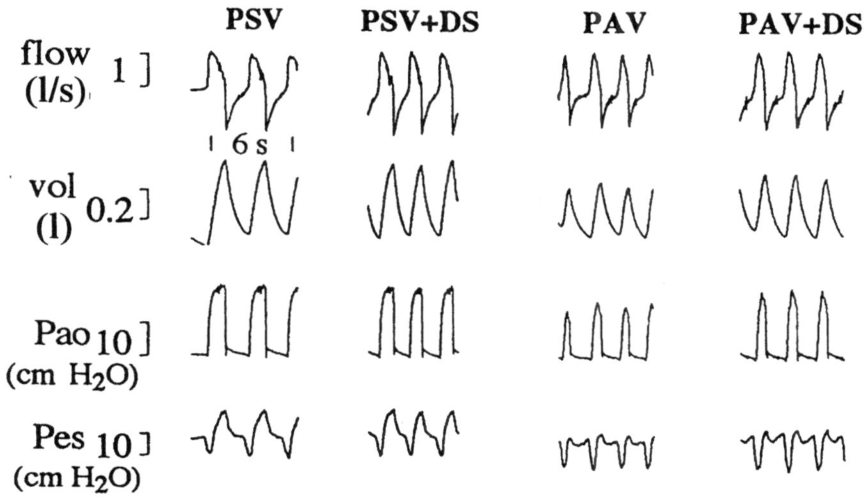

Fig. 1. Flow, volume, pressure at the mouth, and espophageal pressure in a basically ventilated patients and after the application of a dead space (DS)

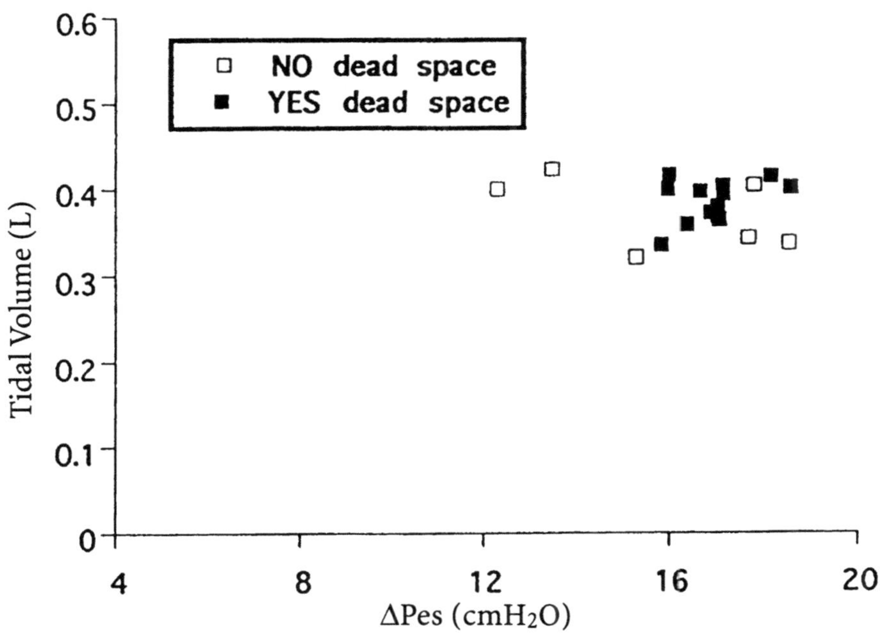

Fig. 2. Relationship between tidal volume and ΔP_{es} with and without application of a dead space in the same patient of Fig. 1 during PS ventilation

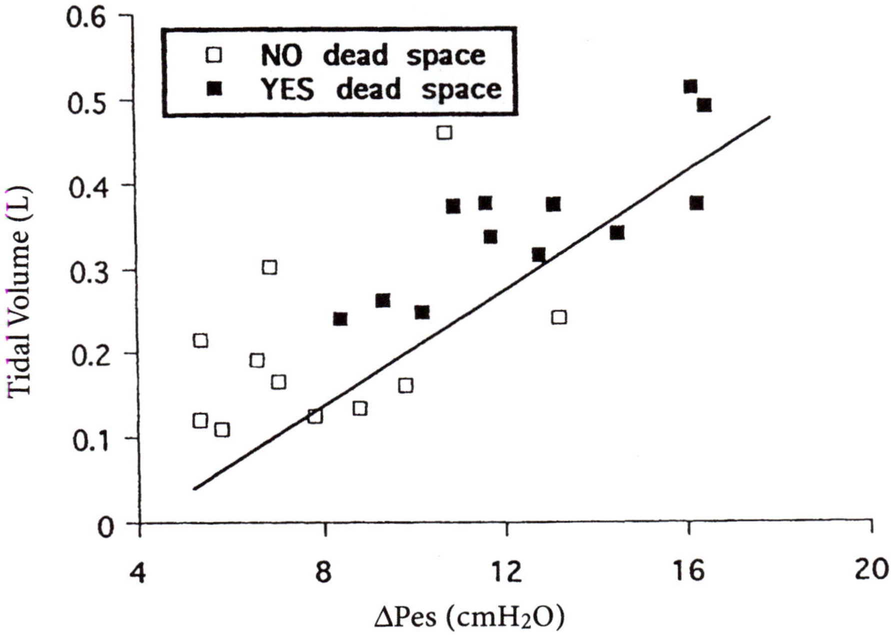

Fig. 3. Relationship between tidal volume and ΔP_{es} with and without application of a dead space in the same patient of Fig. 1 during PAV ventilation

difficulties preventing its widespread clinical use at present. In our opinion, these difficulties can be overcome by means of technologically advanced solutions, but also by means of compromise solutions involving theoretical and conceptual aspects.

References

1. Younes M (1992) Proportional assist ventilation, a new approach to ventilatory support theory. Am Rev Respir Dis 145:114-120
2. Younes M, Puddy A, Roberts D, Light RB, Quesada A, Taylor K, Oppenheimer L, Cramp H (1992) Proportional Assist Ventilation - Results of an initial clinical trial. Am Rev Respir Dis 145:121-129
3. Younes M (1991) Proportional assist ventilation and pressure support ventilation: similarities and differences. In: Marini JJ and Roussos C (eds) Ventilatory Failure Springer-Verlag, Berlin, Heidelberg, New York
4. Giuliani R, Mascia L, Recchia F, Caracciolo A, Fiore T, Ranieri VM (1996) Patient-Ventilator interaction during SIMV: effect of flow-triggering. Am J Respir Crit Care Med 151:1-9
5. Mascia L, Caracciolo A, Cinnella G, Grasso S, Petruzzelli V, Giuliani R, Ranieri M (1994) Pressure Support Ventilation (PSV) vs Proportional Assist Ventilation (PAV): effects of changes in respiratory drive. Int Care Med: 20 [Suppl. 2]S 51

Chapter 20

Pulmonary mechanics beyond peripheral airways

P.V. Romero, J. Lopez Aguilar, L. Blanch

Introduction

Lung mechanics is often introduced by means of the monoalveolar model. It presumes a simplified system composed by a newtonian or flow-independent resistance (R) and a linear or volume-independent compliance (C) placed in series. This is a convenient model to express lung mechanics in a simple way and is easy to handle in clinical situations, where complex patho-physiological interpretations are not needed. Usually the resistive term is referred to airways and defined as the pressure drop between alveoli and trachea or mouth in phase with airflow. Airways resistance can be assessed in different ways, high frequency oscillation and interrupter methods being usual in ventilated patients. As long as airways resistance behaves as a newtonian resistance, and alveolar pressure is adequately estimated after interruption, both methods should give similar results. Lung compliance is measured as the slope of a line drawn between the end inspiratory and end expiratory levels of tidal volume versus transpulmonary pressure loop (dynamic compliance). Dissipative forces acting in lung parenchyma (tissue resistance) are not considered in this simplified model of lung mechanics, lung compliance illustrating the mechanical behaviour of lung parenchyma. However, there is increasing evidence on the importance of tissue resistance in the overall lung mechanical behaviour [1, 2]. As pointed out in another chapter of this book, tissue resistance has a different nature than airways resistance. Both dissipative processes are mechanically in series and combine additivelly to generate total lung resistance.

Even though the non-linearity of pressure-volume and pressure-flow relationships is well known, lung mechanical behaviour is considered in practice to be linear. Linearity assumes a direct proportion between related parameters and the reliability of the principle of superposition. In general fewer parameters are needed to define a system under the assumption of linearity than if non-linearities are to be considered. Many non-linear models are theoretically able to improve information respective to a linear model. However, the lack of agreement on a single reliable model limits the application of non-linear analysis to mechanical lung behaviour. On the other hard parameters expressing non-linearity often lack clear physical or physiological correlation. These reasons favour the choice of linear analysis provided that a minimal linearity can be assumed at least in the operative range. Variations of linear parameters with volume or flow must be taken into account to compare data when different experimental approaches are used.

In many pathophysiological situations the monoalveolar lung model is no longers useful. We have then to account for differences between alveolar territories as well as for mechanical interactions between them. In these situations lung periphery, normally considered as the "silent" part of the lung, should be taken into account in the models used to describe the mechanical behaviour of the whole system. A plurialveolar more realistic model has to account for parenchymal characteristics derived from non-uniformity like alveolar heterogeneity or alveolar instability. Alveolar mechanical heterogeneity usually refers to differences in motion between alveolar areas and to out-of-phase behaviours. Alveolar instability is related to opening and closing phenomena as well as to alveolar recruitment.

At the alveolar level, mechanical forces are conservative. Therefore, they tend to maintain a given architecture and structure of airspaces and oppose any deformation or change in shape or volume. A series of interactions tend to keep or restore the equilibrium and act in favour of homogeneity and isotropy. These interactions can be summarized in three main mechanisms:

1. the balance between surface and tissue forces that prevents distortion or anisotropy;
2. the mechanical interaction between adjacent regions that tend to prevent or absorb out-of-phase behaviours;
3. the interaction between parenchyma and airways that helps to keep airways patency.

These mechanical interactions depend largely on alveolar structure and are conservative. Any distortion of alveolar shape, especially if not isotropic, generates restoring forces that tend to recover equilibrium [3].

Lung tissue mechanical behaviour and lung homogeneity

Alveolar expansion in homogenous lungs depends basically on the arrangement of the two main force bearing elements at alveolar level: the complex fibre system and the surface lining. The pleural pull is transmitted to the acini through the connective elements that form the peripheral fibre system. This volume dependent traction is evenly distributed throughout the lung. Only gravitational forces induce small differences between the upper and lower lung regions.

In an isolated lung a relaxed configuration is obtained in the absence of flow when alveolar pressure equilibrates with atmospheric pressure. This configuration is reached at a volume somewhat less than FRC. Figure 1 shows the amount of elastic energy stored in lung parenchyma and related to lung surface area ($A = k \cdot V$ [2, 3]) from the experimental results of Bachofen [4]. Elastic energy stored by lung parenchyma (Total) is non-linearly related to alveolar surface, in such a way that is minimum at a value corresponding to the lung relaxed configuration (Cnf_L). In isotropic deformation total elastic stress comes from the sum of the elastic fibres storage and surface forces at the air liquid interface [5]

Elastic energy stored in connective fibres is minimum (Cnf_t) at an alveolar surface (and therefore to a volume level) somewhat higher than the lung relaxed

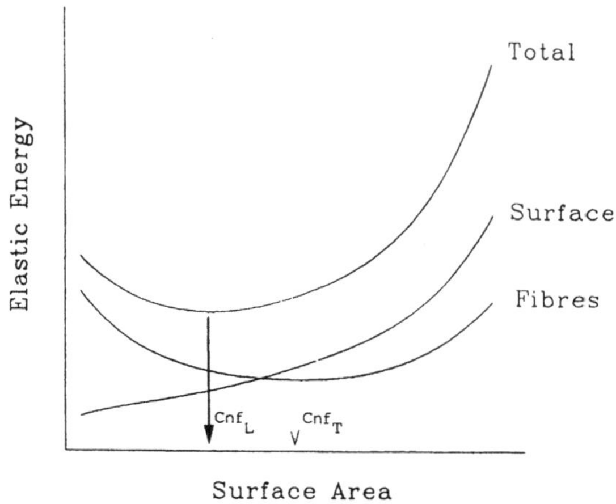

Fig. 1. Relationship between elastic energy stored by lung parenchima (total) and alveolar surface. In isotropic deformation total elastic stress comes from the sum of the elastic fibres storage and surface forces at the air liquid interface

configuration. Both distension and compression of alveoli tend to bring out recovery forces from the fibre structure. Surface forces increase non-linearly with alveolar surface, the slope increasing as lung volume approaches TLC. The net force acting at alveolar level tends to avoid any shift from the relaxed configuration. In the whole system the resting configuration is somewhat different from the relaxed configuration of the alveolar spaces. The equilibrium is kept by the opposing action of the chest wall.

Parenchymal distortion generates energy dissipation due to internal frictional processes. Forces opposing tissue motion are called tissue viscance or resistance, the term viscance refering to the peculiar characteristics of tissue resistive behaviour. For a given alveolar basal configuration, tissue resistance is highly dependent on the amplitude of the changes in alveolar volume and especially on the frequency and speed at which such changes are made; increasing with slow movements and high amplitudes. Tissue resistance is also dependent on lung volume, being higher as lung volume increases. This resistive behaviour of lung tissue also acts in favour of a more homogeneous alveolar filling. Decrease of tissue viscance with frequency has the effect of reducing the time constant and favouring alveolar filling. Increase of resistance with increased alveolar volume tends to load overdistended areas and favour alveolar filling in areas with low tidal excursion and low FRC.

To study lung tissue behaviour in homogeneous lungs a direct measurement of alveolar pressures (P_{alv}) is generally needed. The alveolar capsules technique allows the direct recording of alveolar pressure in experimental settings [6]. Measurement of Palv in different locations allows to inquire about homogeneity of lung behaviour. Alveolar capsules consist in small trumpet-like plastic pieces with a flat bottom that is glued to the pleural surface with cyanoacrilate glue (Fig. 2). The capsule chamber is connected to the subtended alveoli by gently

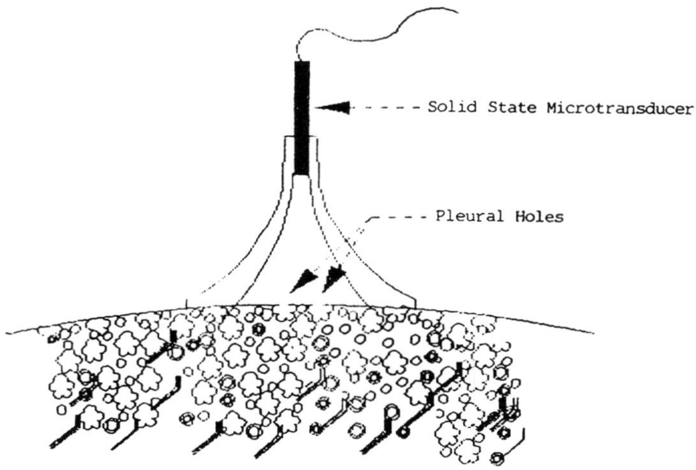

Fig. 2. Schematical representation of alveolar capsule

puncturing the pleura. On the free port of the capsule a small piezoelectric pressure transducer is either directly plugged in or connected by means of a flexible piece of small capacity tube. Recordings of alveolar pressure should fit tracheal pressure at the end of tidal volume excursions and hysteresis between different capsules should not exist or be negligible in an homogeneous lung.

Tissue fibres transmit tension generated at the pleura to the whole lung. But they also act as direct transmitters of forces generated by the distortion of an acinar area by the adjacent ones, this phenomenon being called alveolar interdependence [7]. Tissue forces are equally transmitted to the periphery of bronchi and vessels trough the adventitial attachments (tissue-airways interdependence) [8]. In this way any change of shape in a lung region gives rise to forces in the boundary that oppose the direction of the distortion. Tissue forces act specifically against atelectasis or airways narrowing, but also against not isotropic or out-of-phase motion of adjacent areas in order to keep homogeneity and airways patency.

Although lung tissue behaviour is non-linear in nature, linear models are usually applied to describe its mechanical properties [9]. The linear approach assumes homogeneity and is generally described by the following equation:

$$\Delta P_{tis} = (P_{alv}\text{-}P_{pl}) = E_{tis} \cdot V + R_{tis} \cdot (dV/dt) + PEEP_{alv} \quad (1)$$

In the case of alveolar capsules, Ppl is atmospheric pressure and hence $\Delta P = P_{alv}$. The nature of E_{tis} and R_{tis} is discussed elsewhere in this book. E_{tis} is assumed to be the dynamic elasticity of lung tissue and R_{tis} corresponds to tissue viscance; both defining together the viscoelastic behaviour of lung parenchyma. We can calculate mechanical parameters for the whole lung by applying the linear equation to fit transpulmonary pressure (P_{tp}) swings:

$$\Delta P_{tp} = (P_{tr}\text{-}P_{pl}) = E_{dyn} \cdot V + R_{tot} \cdot (dV/dt) + PEEP_{tr} \quad (2)$$

where E_{dyn} (dynamic elastance measured for the whole lung) and E_{tis} should be identical, except for gas compression in airways, and PEEP should be roughly the same either measured at alveolar or at tracheal level. Airways resistance (R_{aw}) is then calculated by subtracting R_{tis} from total pulmonary resistance (R_{tot}):

$$R_{aw} = R_{tot} - R_{tis} \quad (3)$$

Assessment of lung tissue mechanical properties requires that alveolar pressure adequately represent alveolar territories that fill and empty with a pattern of volume and flow roughly identical to that observed at tracheal level. No direct evidence of this is usually available because alveolar volume and flow cannot be directly measured. However, as long as dynamic elastance obtained from alveolar pressure (E_{tis}) and from tracheal pressure (E_{dyn}) differ by less than a 10 %, and PEEP obtained from equations (1) and (2) are similar (less than 0.5 hPa is acceptable for a $PEEP_{tr}$ of 5 hPa), measured alveolar pressure can be assumed to reflect alveolar filling pressure in phase with overall lung volume and flow changes. Figure 3 shows superimposed recordings of pressures from four alveolar capsules placed in different lobes of an homogeneous rabbit lung. The narrow fit of alveolar pressures can be appreciated.

Digital sampling of alveolar pressure at different subpleural regions allows to estimate alveolar heterogeneity by calculating the coefficient of variation of alveolar pressure at each sampling time CV %(t) [1].

Usually tidal variations of CV %(t) are maximum at end expiration or early in inspiration and minimum at end inspiratory level.

Alveolar heterogeneity depends largely on the patency of airways supplying the different alveolar territories. During lung challenge with agonists of smooth muscle, the interalveolar mean coefficient of variation varies in a dose dependent manner. If agonists of airways constriction are administered intravenously in rabbits (Fig. 4) we observe a sudden increase in total lung resistance and elastance reflecting biomechanical changes in airways and lung parenchyma. Lung heterogeneity, represented by the maximum and minimum value of CV % for each cycle, is delayed respective to changes in elastance and resistance. This delay reflects the action of forces that oppose lung heterogeneity which are overwhelmed only after a certain level of reaction is reached.

The first consequence of mechanical heterogeneity is the wide and uneven distribution of alveolar time constants and consequently the out-of-phase behaviour of areas with different time constants. The frequency dependence of lung elastance arise from a preferent distribution of inspired volume to the areas with a short time constant (faster areas) which became overventilated with respect to the areas with longer time constant. A second consequence of the out of phase behaviour is due to the different filling and emptying rates of different territories which causes the development of intrinsic or auto PEEP [10, 11, 12]. Figure 5 shows the development of intrinsic PEEP in an alveolar territory during the inhalation of increasing concentrations of methacholine in a responsive open

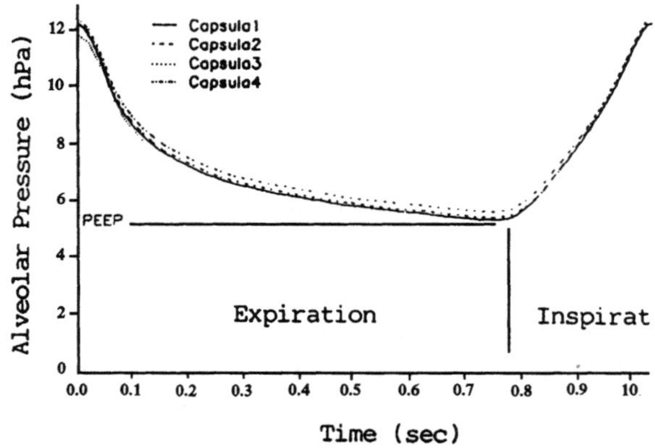

Fig. 3. Time course of the alveolar pressure from four alveolar capsules in an homogenous rabbit lung

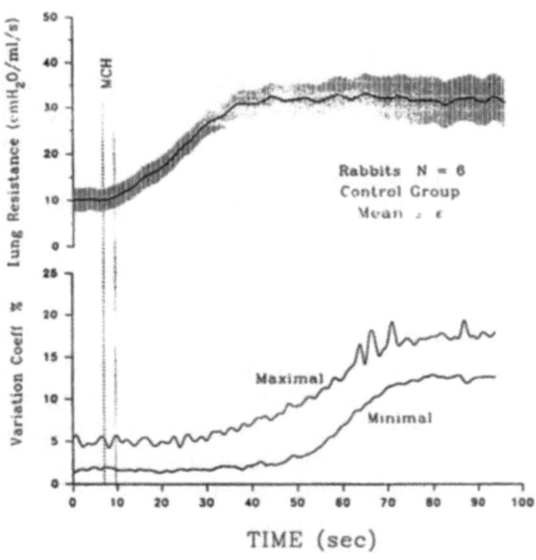

Fig. 4. Changes of lung resistance and maximum and minimum value of CV% of P_{alv} after methacholine

chested, ventilated and anaesthetized rabbit. Only the expiratory limbs of alveolar pressure at different increasing concentrations of methacholine (Mch) are shown. A timid response can be appreciated at 4 and 8 mg/ml, without a marked change in the pattern of the curve. Inhalation of 16 mg/ml induce a sudden and huge increase in the dynamic elastance (tidal volume remaining constant throughout trial), accompanied by a faster lung decompression during expiration

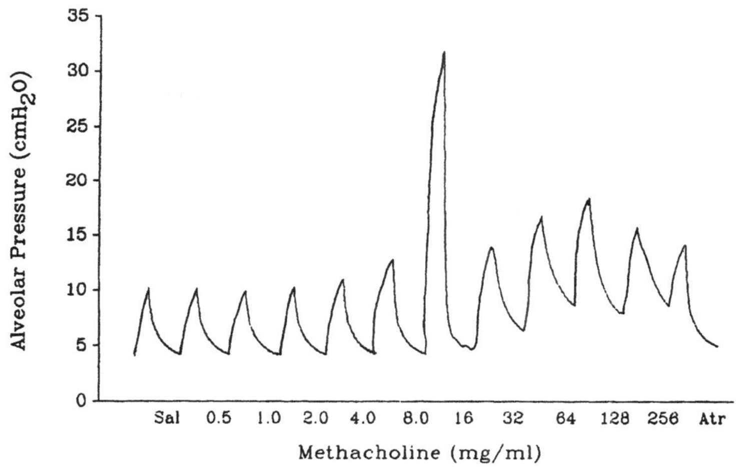

Fig. 5. Expiratory pattern of $P_{alv}(1)$ during Mch challenge (average of 10 breaths)

that reflects an important parenchymal reaction due to constriction of peripheral smooth muscle and to a paradoxical decrease of the local airways resistance because the negative interaction between lung tissue and airways [8]. Increasing Mch concentrations induce an important airways narrowing that reduces alveolar volume filling and therefore tidal alveolar pressure shifts. The development of intrinsic PEEP reflects the increase in the alveolar end expiratory volume due to the incomplete emptying of the slow air-trapped territory. The flat shape of the expiratory limb of alveolar pressure is related to the increase of the time constant of that territory, and therefore to the impairment of alveolar emptying. After atropine inhalation expiratory alveolar pressure recovers a more normal shape. PEEP comes back to previous values, therefore reflecting the reversibility of the response [2].

The estimation of pulmonary or parenchymal mechanical properties is often confused by the presence of out-of-phase alveolar behaviour due to alveolar pressure no longer representing the driving pressure of the system in phase with volume (elastic pressure) or flow (resistive pressure). In the presence of alveolar heterogeneity different alveolar territories are at different points on the breathing cycle, depending on the degree of phase lag. This phenomenon, called the pendelluft effect, is especially notorious immediately after interruption of airflow. Shortly after flow has been stopped alveolar pressure equilibrates all over the lung if the alveoli are homogeneous or if time constants are narrowly distributed. Therefore, in the presence of a wide distribution of time constants, alveolar equilibrium is reached progressively as slower alveoli empty into faster ones [13]. This process dissipates gradually until alveolar pressure becomes the same in all communicated areas. Collateral ventilation is of great importance in this alveolar equilibration especially in adjacent territories [14].

Figure 6 shows the behaviour of three alveolar territories during an expiratory interruption of airflow in an open chest dog in basal condition and after histamine inhalation. After an inspiratory pause that equilibrates alveolar pressures, the airway is opened and a free expiration takes place, tracheal pressure (P_{tr}) falls rapidly whereas alveolar pressure (a, b and c) decrease slowly due to airways resistance. The time course of expiratory decay of alveolar pressure is similar under the basal condition. Histamine inhalation induces big differences, which reflect dissimilarities in the mechanical behaviour of the respective territories. When flow is abruptly interrupted (dotted line), alveolar pressures tend to join tracheal pressure. Therefore, even in the basal condition the equilibration is delayed a short period after occlusion, faster territories (c) having lower pressures than slower ones (a) by the time of interruption. After histamine challenge heterogeneity increases the difference between the emptying rates of different territories. The pendelluft effect is accentuated in the sense that a longer time is needed to equilibrate alveolar pressures after occlusion.

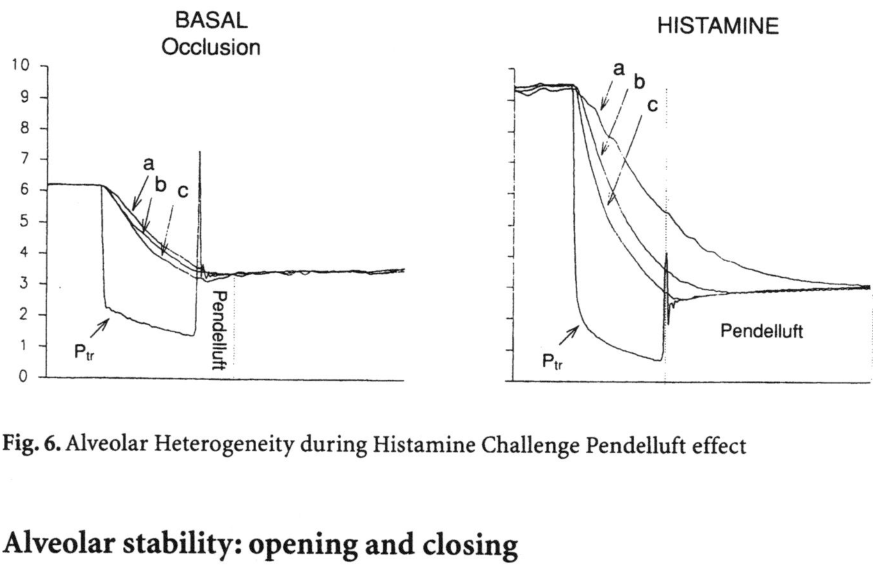

Fig. 6. Alveolar Heterogeneity during Histamine Challenge Pendelluft effect

Alveolar stability: opening and closing

In normal lungs alveoli remain permanently opened at FRC and only if volume is reduced forcibly to near RV are peripheral airways seen to close. An airspace is opened if communicated with the atmosphere through the conducting airways. Surface forces, airways patency and interdependence account for alveolar stability.

In some circumstances mechanisms that guarantee alveolar stability are overwhelmed and peripheral airspaces can close at volumes above FRC. This happens especially when there is increased fluid in the airspaces or impaired surface-lining properties [15]. Instability implies a region of negative lung compliance on the pressure-volume curve. During inflation increase of total volume of lung beyond a critical point tends to decrease pressure because of the unstable alveolar units that pop out and open as a critical point of pressure is reached.

To observe the dynamics of alveolar opening and closing in unstable lungs a group of rabbits were treated with i.v. ethclorovynol (ECV) a substance known to induce a permeability interstitial oedema [16, 17]. Several capsules were placed at different locations and lung volume was changed by slowly changing PEEP between 3 and 15 hPa. Tidal volume was kept constant. Figure 7 shows an alveolar territory opening at a critical opening pressure, then closing when pressure falls under a second critical level somewhat lower than opening pressure. As alveolar pressure swings after opening are not different from opened territories, it can be argued that elastic behaviour after opening is not different in the previously closed territories. This allows to determine the relative alveolar volume by taking into account the pressure-volume characteristics of alveolar territories when opened. Figure 8a shows the behaviour of two alveolar territories, both closed at the end expiratory pressure of about 5 hPa. One of them opens at a pressure of about 10 hPa and closes again at 5 hPa, the second territory does not open even at pressures as higher as 45 hPa. The first alveoli constitute an unstable territory because they open and close at physiological levels of pressure. The second territory remains permanently closed and is stable in this condition. Therefore, in the presence of alveolar instability three situations should be considered: a) alveoli can be permanently opened and so are stable in the opening condition; b) alveoli can be unstable and open and close in the range of physiological or applied pres-

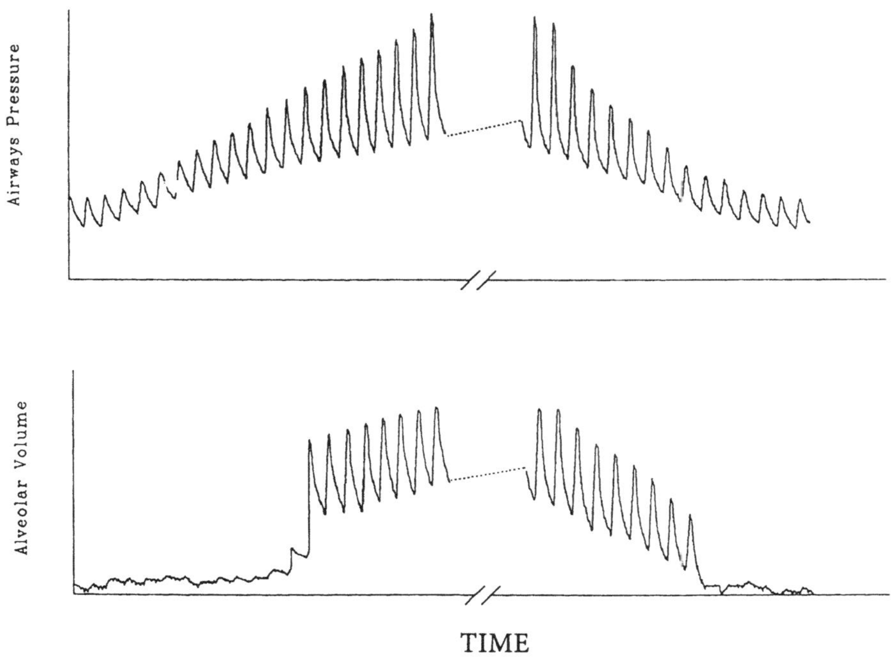

Fig. 7. Time course of the airway pressure and alveolar volume at critical opening and closing points

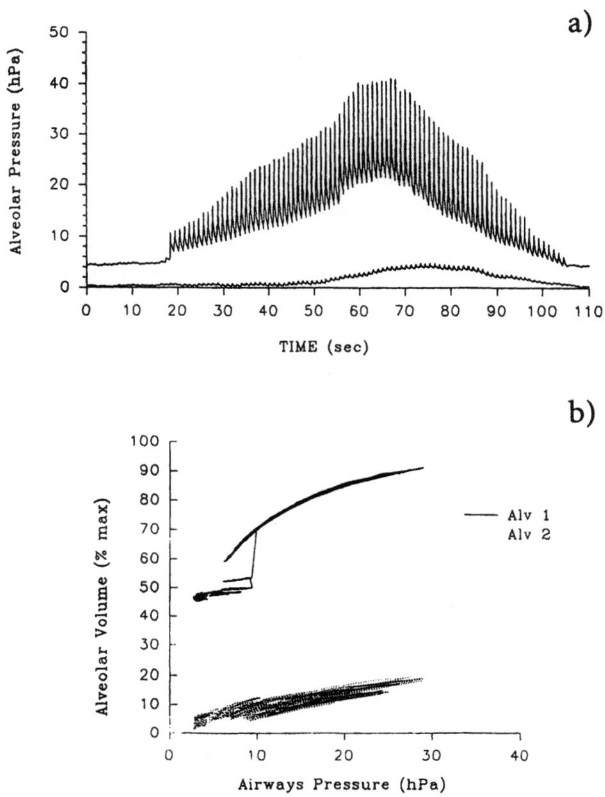

Fig. 8. Time course P_{alv} and relationship between P_{aw} and V_{alv} of two alveolar territories with different critical opening pressure points

sures and c) alveoli can be steady closed in the range of applied pressures. It follows that the state of an unstable territory will depend on the range of pressure applied in tidal excursions either as negative pleural-transmitted pressure in spontaneous ventilation or as airways positive pressure in ventilated patients. Figure 8b shows the pressure-volume behaviour of two territories closed at the tidal operative range in a ventilated rabbit. When airways pressure is increased over a threshold level Alv 1 opens whereas Alv 2 remains closed. Unstable alveoli (alv 1) show a tendency to trap air when closed. The amount of air trapped can vary as shown by the different levels of volume observed. Conversely, alv 2 seems to be atelectasic. Figure 9 shows the pressure-volume behaviour of another territory closed at the level of tidal volume (PEEP = 3 cm H_2O). Three status can be depicted in this unstable territory as a function of the pressure applied. Under a critical pressure (Zone C) alveoli are permanently closed, some air can be trapped as far as airway closing is reversible and/or no atelectasis has developed. The pressure-volume slope probably reflects the interaction with surrounding alveoli. A second Zone (Zone B) is characterized by the unpredicted configura-

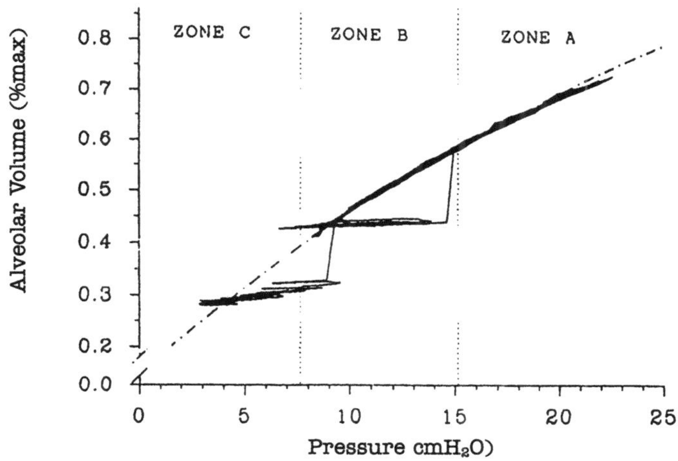

Fig. 9. Pressure-volume behaviour of a territory closed at the level of tidal volume

tion of unstable alveoli under the action of applied pressure in a range between the critical point of opening and a maximal point from which the alveolus remains permanently opened. This second zone admits several configurations as alveoli can either remain opened or close, then trapping a different amount of air inside. Finally, Zone A defines the opened stable status.

Opening of unstable alveoli can occur at different critical pressures, depending on the degree of local impairment. Therefore, a sequential recruitment is possible in lungs with unstable alveolar territories. Operating volume at a given pressure is no more directly dependent on elastic properties of the lung but on the number of units that are working at a that given level of pressure [18]. This phenomenon is called alveolar recruitment.

References

1. Ludwig MS, Romero PV, Bates JHT (1989) A comparison of dose-response behaviour of canine airways and parenchyma. J Appl Physiol 67:1220-1225
2. Romero PV, Robatto FM, Simard S, Ludwig MS (1992) Lung tissue behaviour during methacholine challenge in rabbits in vivo. J Appl Physiol 73:207-212
3. Greaves IA, Hildebrandt J, Hoppin FG Jr (1986) Micromechanics of the lung. In Fishman AP, Macklem PT, Mead J, Geiger SR (eds) Handbook of Physiology. The Respiratory System. Mechanics of Breathing. Sect. 3, Vol. III, Pt. 1, Chap 14. American Physiological Society, Bethesda, pp 217-229
4. Bachofen H, Hildebrandt J, Bachofen M (1970) Pressure-volume curves of air and liquid-filled excised lungs: surface tension in situ. J Appl Physiol 29:422-431
5. Goerk J, Clements JA (1986) Alveolar surface tension and lung surfactant. In Fishman AP, Macklem PT, Mead J, Geiger SR (eds) Handbook of Physiology. The Respiratory System. Mechanics of Breathing. Sect. 3, Vol. III, Pt. 1, Chap 16. American

Physiological Society, Bethesda, pp 247-261

6. Fredberg JJ, Keefe DH, Glass GM, Castle RG, Frantz ID III (1984) Alveolar pressure nonhomogeneity during small amplitude high-frequency oscillation. J Appl Physiol 57:788-800
7. Mead J, Takishima T, Leith D (1970) Stress distribution in lungs: a model of pulmonary elasticity. J Appl Physiol 28:596-608
8. Romero PV, Ludwig MS (1991) Maximal methacholin-induced constriction in rabbit lung: interaction between airways and tissues. J Appl Physiol 46:1251-1262
9. Mead J (1961) Mechanical properties of the lung. Physiol Rev 41:281-330
10. Blanch L, Fernandez R, Romero PV (1992) Hiperinsuflacion pulmonar dinàmica en el enfermo crìtico. Med Clin 99:627-635
11. Gottfried SB, Rossi A, Milic-Emili J (1986) Dynamic hyperinflation, intrinsic PEEP, and the mechanically ventilated patient. Int Crit Care Digest 5:30-33
12. Pepe PE, Marini JJ (1982) Ocult positive end-expirtory pressure in mechanically ventilated patients with airflow obstruction. Am Rev Respir Dis 126:166-170
13. Ludwig MS, Romero PV, Sly PD, Fredberg JJ, Bates JHT (1990) Interpretation of interrupter resistance after histamine-induced constriction in the dog. J Appl Physiol 68:1651-1656
14. Tsuzaki K, Hales CA, Strieder DJ, Venegas JG (1993) Regional lung mechanics and gas transport in lungs with inhomogeneous compliance. J Appl Physiol 75:206-216
15. Otis DR Jr, Johnson M, Pedley TJ, Kamm RD (1993) Role of pulmonary surfactant in airway closure: a computational study. J Appl Physiol 75:1323-1333
16. Blanch L, Roussos C, Brotherton S, Michel RP, MR Angle (1992) Effect of tidal volume and PEEP in ethclorovynol-induced asymmetric lung injury. J Appl Physiol 73:108-116
17. Wylsormerski R, Lagunoff D, Dahms T (1974) Ethclorovynol-induced pulmonary edema in rats. An ultrastructural study. Am Rev Respir Dis 110:49-55
18. Rainieri VM, Eissa NT, Corbeil C, Chassé M, Braidy J, Matar N, Milic-Emili J (1991) Effects of positive end-expiratory pressure on alveolar recruitment and gas exchange in patients with the adult respiratory distress syndrome. Am Rev Respir Dis 144:544-551

Chapter 21

Oscillatory mechanics

D. NAVAJAS

Introduction

Normal tidal breathing is generated by cyclic muscular pressure applied to the chest wall. Mechanical ventilation is produced by cyclic pressure applied to the airway opening. In both situations tidal volume generated by the driving pressure is determined by the mechanical load of the respiratory system. In general, for a given driving pressure, higher mechanical load results in lower ventilatory out put. The mechanical load as computed from the pressure-flow relationship of the respiratory system undergoing sinusoidal oscillation is called respiratory impedance (Z_{rs}), because of the complex structure of the respiratory system Z_{rs} varies markedly with oscillatory frequency. Mechanical properties of the airways and the lung and chest wall tissues can be estimated by fitting suitable physiological models to Z_{rs} measured at different frequencies. Therefore, the study of oscillatory mechanics in a wide range of frequencies is of clinical interest in the assessment of respiratory mechanics in spontaneously breathing and mechanically ventilated patients.

Equipment

Oscillatory mechanics is commonly studied in spontaneously breathing patients by applying low-amplitude pressure oscillations at the mouth. Forced oscillation frequencies usually span from $\simeq$ 2 Hz to $\simeq$ 30 Hz. Measurements at frequencies close to that of spontaneous breathing are difficult to obtain because of the superposition of breathing flow. Figure 1 describes the standard equipment used to measure Z_{rs} by forced oscillations in spontaneously breathing patients. The excitation pressure (peak-to-peak amplitude $\simeq$ 2 hPa) is generated by a loudspeaker attached to a chamber. Flow is measured with a pneumotacograph connected to a differential pressure transducer. Pressure is measured with a similar pressure transducer. A bias tube ($\simeq$ 1 m long, $\simeq$ 2 cm ID) allows the patient to breath. The gas inside the equipment is renewed by means of a constant flow of air ($\simeq$ 0.3 l/s). Flow and pressure signals are recorded with a microcomputer which is also used to generate the excitation signal to the loudspeaker. The equipment must be designed in accordance with published recommendations [1].

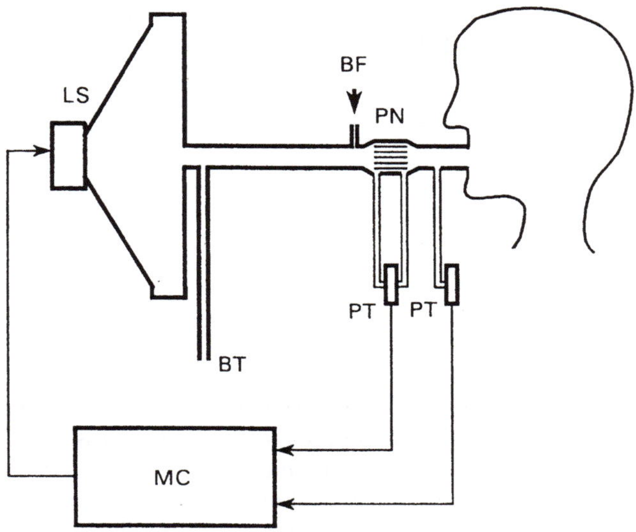

Fig. 1. Standard equipment to measure respiratory impedance by forced oscillation. LS: loudspeaker; PN: pneumotachograph; PT: pressure transducers; MC: microcomputer; BT: bias tube; BF: bias flow

Data processing and modelling

The oscillatory behaviour of the respiratory system is interpreted by means of mechanical models. At spontaneous breathing frequencies and normal tidal volumes, respiratory mechanics of healthy subjects can be roughly represented by a series combination of a resistance (R) and an elastance (E). The driving pressure (P) required to overcome the resistive and elastic loads of this R-E model is:

$$P = R \cdot \dot{V} + E \cdot V$$

where $\dot{V}$ and V are flow and volume respectively. When such a linear system is subjected to sinusoidal driving pressure, sinusoidal flow and volume oscillations of the same frequency result (Fig. 2). For a given peak-to-peak pressure amplitude (P) the peak-to-peak flow ($\dot{V}$) and volume (V) amplitudes are determined by the mechanical load of the model.

In sinusoidal oscillation minimum and maximum of sinusoidal flow occur at mid tidal volume (Fig. 2). The pressure difference between these isovolume points (Pr) accounts for the resistive pressure change ($Pr = R \cdot \dot{V}$). Hence,

$$Pr/\dot{V} = R$$

The ratio $Pr/\dot{V}$ is called effective resistance (R_{ef}). R_{ef} reflects the resistive load which, in this model, does not depend on frequency ($R_{ef} = R$).

At points of minimum and maximum volume flow is zero and the pressure dif-

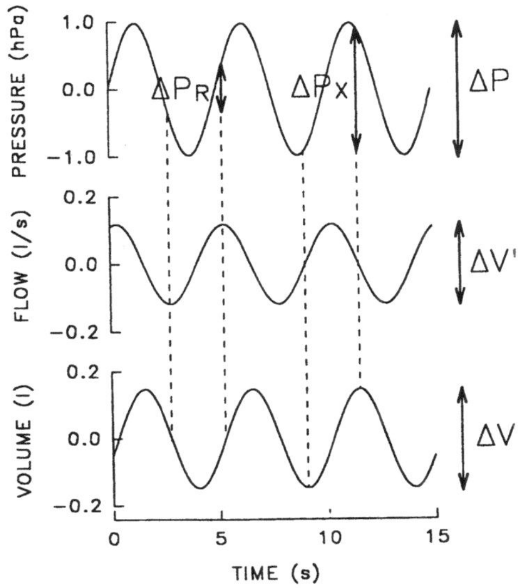

Fig. 2. Sinusoidal response at 0.2 Hz of a series combination of a resistance (R = 3 hPa • s • l^{-1}) and an elastance (E = 10 hPa/l). ΔP, $\Delta\dot{V}$ and ΔV are peak-to-peak amplitudes of pressure, flow and volume, respectively. Pr: pressure difference between minimum and maximum flow; Px: pressure difference between minimum and maximum volume

ference between them (Px) accounts for the elastic pressure change (Px = E • V). Since in sinusoidal oscillation $V = \dot{V}/2\pi f$ (f = frequency) the elastic load is usually expressed in terms of pressure and flow changes as follows:

$$-\Delta Px/\dot{V} = -\Delta E/2\pi f$$

The ratio $-\Delta Px/\dot{V}$ is called reactance (X) and in this model X corresponds exclusively to the elastic load ($X = -E/2\pi f$) which depends inversely on frequency. From this definition X of an elastic load is negative indicating that flow leads pressure.

The oscillatory response of any linear system is fully described at each frequency by R_{ef} and X, these two variables together defining its mechanical impedance.

R_{ef} and X of the respiratory system exhibit frequency dependencies which cannot be adequately interpreted in terms of a resistance-elastance combination. In particular, at frequencies greater than ≃ 2 Hz inertial properties of airways and tissues cannot be neglected. The R-E model can be completed with an inertance (I) to account for these additional features. Figure 3 plots the two parts (R_{ef} and X) of the impedance of a model made up of a series combination of a resistance (R = 3 hPa • s • l^{-1}), an elastance (E = 10 hPa/l) and an inertance (I = 0.01 hPa • s^2 • l^{-1}). R_{ef} of this R-E-I model does not vary with frequency and coincides with that of the R-E combination (R_{ef} = R). X is the addition of the inertial and elastic loads ($X = 12\pi f - E/2\pi f$). At low frequencies the inertial load ($12\pi f$) is negligible and, therefore, X mainly reflects the elastic load ($X \simeq -E/2\pi f$) which is negative (flow leads pressure). At high frequencies X is positive (flow lags pressure) and mostly accounts for the inertial load. The frequency where elastic and inertial loads are compensated and X = 0 (flow is in phase with pressure) is called frequency of resonance (fr).

Respiratory impedance

In healthy subjects Ref ≃ 2.5 hPa • s • l^{-1} and varies little with frequency in the conventional forced oscillation range (≃ 2 - 30 Hz). On the other hand, X shows a marked positive frequency dependence with fr ≃ 8 Hz. Normal values of respiratory impedance have been published recently [2, 3]. Respiratory impedance of healthy subjects exhibits a pattern similar to that of a R-E-I model (Fig. 3) and for this reason, it is usual to compute R, E and I by fitting the model to R_{ef} and X measured between ≃ 2 - 30 Hz. Fitted values of R and I are reasonable and interpreted as the resistance and inertance of the total respiratory system. By contrast, E fitted from frequencies > 2 Hz is substantially greater (about a factor of 3) than values reported at spontaneous breathing frequencies. This difference could reflect pendelluft and tissue viscoelasticity.

Patients with airway obstruction show higher R_{ef} with a marked negative frequency dependence and a shift in X to lower values with increased fr [4]. Studies

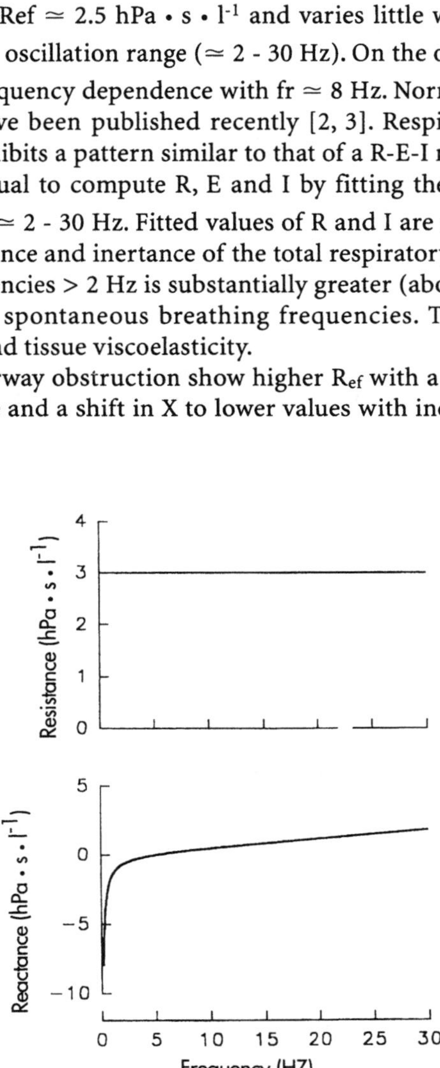

Fig. 3. Effective resistance and reactance of a model composed by a series combination of a resistance (R = 3 hPa • s • l^{-1}), an elastance (E = 10 hPa/l) and an inertance (I = 0.01 hPa • s^2 • l^{-1})

in patients with restrictive lung diseases reported a similar pattern but with a smaller rise in R_{ef} [5]. The negative frequency dependence of R_{ef} has been attributed to mechanical inhomogeneties between lung compartments [6], however, this could be in part due to extrathoracic airway shunt. To minimize this artefact Peslin et al. [7] suggested the application of pressure oscillations by means of a head generator.

Lung impedance

Oscillatory mechanics can be partitioned into lung and chest wall compartments by measuring pleural pressure with an oesophageal balloon [8]. Farrè et al. [9] combined forced oscillation and breathing signals to measure lung impedance of healthy subjects in a frequency range extended down to spontaneous breathing frequencies. They observed a slight negative dependence of R_{ef} of the lung at low frequencies ($\simeq$ 0.2 - 2 Hz), which could be explained by lung tissue viscoelasticity. By using the same approach Navajas et al. [10] studied lung impedance in patients with obstructive disease and found a large R_{ef} ($\simeq$ 11 hPa • s • l^{-1}) which varied little between spontaneous breathing and forced oscillation frequencies.

Respiratory impedance measurements in mechanically ventilated patients

The most direct approach to measure respiratory impedance in mechanically ventilated patients would be to connect a standard pressure generator in parallel with the ventilator. However, this cannot be done because conventional loudspeakers do not withstand the high pressures produced by the ventilator. One solution is to disconnect the patient from the ventilator for a few seconds and apply pressure oscillations with a loudspeaker attached to the inlet of the endotracheal tube. By using this method Navajas et al. [11] measured total respiratory impedance from 0.25 to 32 Hz in anaesthetized paralysed patients. They found a strong negative frequency dependence of R_{ef} between 0.25 and 2 Hz. At higher frequencies R_{ef} showed a modest negative frequency dependence. They attributed the high values of R_{ef} found at spontaneous breathing frequencies to chest wall viscoelasticity. To avoid disconnecting the patient from the ventilator, Navajas et al. [12] connected a standard pressure generator to the expiratory outlet of the ventilator. During the inspiratory phase the expiratory valve of the ventilator is occluded and, as a result, the loudspeaker is not subjected to the high pressures applied to the patient. During the expiratory phase the valve is opened and the pressure oscillation generated by the loudspeaker is transmitted to the patient through the expiratory tubing. This method allows us to measure respiratory mechanics during expiration by means of standard equipment in paralysed as well as in non-paralysed patients. To measure oscillatory mechanics during all the ventilatory cycle, Peslin et al. [13] designed a pressure generator based on a loudspeaker enclosed in a small box and shunted by a tube. They measured respiratory impedance from 5 to 20 Hz in patients with acute respiratory failure without disturbing mechanical ventilation. These authors found large cyclic changes in R_{ef} and X which were consistent with airflow nonlinearities and dynamic airway compression, respectively. Therefore, measuring respiratory impedance at different points in the respiratory cycle may be helpful in assessing flow dependence of resistance and in detecting expiratory flow limitation in mechanically ventilated patients.

References

1. Van de Woestijne KP, Desager KN, Duiverman EJ, Marchal F (1994) Recommendations for measurement of respiratory input impedance by means of the forced oscillation method. Eur Respir Rev 4:19 235-237
2. Peslin R, Teculescu D, Locuty J, Gallina C, Duvivier C (1994) Normal values of total respiratory input impedance with the head generator technique. Eur Respir Rev 4:19 138-142
3. Pasker HG, Mertens I, Clèment J, Van de Woestijne KP (1994) Normal values of total respiratory input resistance and reactance for adult men and women. Eur Respir Rev 4:19 134-137
4. Van Noord JA, Clèment J, Van de Woestijne KP, Demedts M (1991) Total respiratory resistance and reactance in patients with asthma, chronic bronchitis, and emphysema. Am Rev Respir Dis 143:922-927
5. Van Noord JA, Clèment J, Cauberghs M, Mertens I, Van de Woestijne KP, Demedts M (1989) Total respiratory resistance and reactance in patients with diffuse interstitial lung disease. Eur Respir J 2:846-852
6. Michaelson ED, Grassman ED, Peters WR (1975) Pulmonary mechanics by spectral analysis of forced random noise. J Clin Invest 56:1210-1230
7. Peslin R, Duvivier C, Didelon J, Gallina C (1985) Respiratory impedance measured with head generator to minimize upper airway shunt. J Appl Physiol 59:1790-1795
8. Peslin R, Navajas D, Rotger M, Farrè R (1993) Validity of the esophageal balloon technique at high frequencies. J Appl Physiol 74:1039-1044
9. Farrè R, Peslin R, Rotger R, Navajas D (1994) Human lung impedance from spontaneous breathing frequencies to 32 Hz. J Appl Physiol 76:1176-1183
10. Navajas D, Farrè R, Barber JA, Roca J, Rotger M (1994) Lung impedance in COPD patients. Am J Respir Crit Care Med 149:4 A222
11. Navajas D, Farrè R, Canet J, Rotger M, Sanchis J (1990) Respiratory input impedance in anesthetized paralyzed patients. J Appl Physiol 69:1372-1379
12. Navajas D, Farrè R, Rotger D, Torres A (1994) Monitoring respiratory impedance by force oscillation in mechanically ventilated patients. Eur Respir Rev 4:19 216-218
13. Peslin R, Felicio da Silva J, Duvivier C, Chabot F (1993) Respiratory mechanics studied by forced oscillations during artificial ventilation. Eur Respir J 6:772-784

Chapter 22

Experimental and clinical research to improve ventilation

R.J. HOUMES, D. GOMMERS, K.L. SO, B. LACHMANN

Introduction

A common finding in patients with acute respiratory failure or acute lung injury (ALI) is a reduced lung distensibility (Fig. 1). It has been shown that this decrease in lung compliance is due to a disturbed pulmonary surfactant system, resulting in an increased surface tension.

In turn, increased surface tension leads to an increase in retractive forces acting at the alveolar air-liquid interface which in turn leads to end-expiratory alveolar collapse, atelectasis and an increase in right to left shunt, resulting in a decrease in PaO_2. The only rational therapy to treat this condition consists of:

1. counterbalancing the increased collapse tendency by applying positive airway pressure to prevent end-expiratory collapse (mechanical gas ventilation);
2. decreasing alveolar surface tension by application of exogenous surfactant;
3. eliminating the air-liquid interface by filling the lung with a fluid that is capable of maintainig gas exchange at the alveolar capillary membrane.

This paper will briefly review the rationale for these three therapeutic approaches.

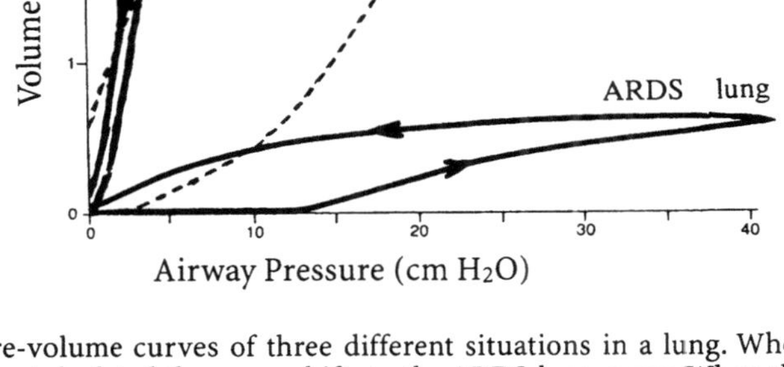

Fig. 1. Pressure-volume curves of three different situations in a lung. When the healthy lung is surfactant depleted the curve shifts to the ARDS-lung curve. When this ARDS-lung is filled with fluid (elimination of the alveolar air-liquid interface) the curve shifts to the fluid-filled curve

Improvement of ventilation by optimal ventilator settings

Since its introduction into clinical practice more than 40 years ago, artificial ventilation has proven to be a life-saving method or therapy in intensive care. Yet it has remained a topic of much discussion and controversy as it involves a disturbance to normal respiratory and cardiovascular function [2, 3, 4, 5]; that is why the adult respiratory distress syndrome (ARDS) may be, in part, a product of our therapy - rather than the progression of the underlying disease.

To date no adequate explanation of the pathophysiologic basis of these changes caused by artificial ventilation has been documented. The main contributing factors which emerge from almost all the above-mentioned studies seem to be the ventilatory modes which fail to prevent partial (or complete) end-expiratory lung collapse combined with high pressure amplitudes during the ventilatory cycle.

More than twenty years ago Mead et al. stated that: "at a transpulmonary pressure of 30 cm H_2O, the pressure tending to expand on atelectatic region surrounded by a fully expanded lung would be approximately 140 cm H_2O" [6].

Such forces may be the major cause of structural damage (especially to bronchiolar epithelium, alveolar epithelium and capillary endothelium) and may be the basis not only for formation of hyaline membranes but may also cause the release of mediators from the disrupted parenchyma, so triggering the pathophysiological mechanisms of ARDS [7].

During ventilation of patients with ARDS, who almost always have atelectatic lung regions, pressure differences of 30 cm H_2O or higher are quite common. We have to understand, however, that it is not the 30 cm H_2O pressure difference that damages the lungs but rather the resulting shear forces of more than 140 cm H_2O which are responsible for the barotrauma. It must be concluded that in order to prevent lung damage due to high shear forces between open and closed lung units, only ventilation modes that result in an open lung and keep that lung open with the smallest possible pressure amplitudes should be used.

The Laplace law ($P=2g/r$, where P is the pressure to stabilize a bubble/alveoli; g is surface tension at the air-liquid interface; r, the radius of the bubble/alveolus) offers an explanation as to why in ALI-lungs that are not prevented from end-expiratory collapse, high pressure amplitudes appear during the respiratory cycle. However, if this end-expiratory collapse is prevented and the functional residual capacity (FRC) is normal, the injured lungs can be ventilated with small pressure amplitudes (Fig. 2).

In other words, to get a certain volume change in larger alveoli the necessary pressure changes are much smaller compared to alveoli which are collapsed or have a lower volume. It can further be derived from the law of Laplace that the pressure necessary to keep the alveoli open is smaller at a high FRC level. Therefore, the PEEP necessary to stabilize the end-expiratory volume can be minimized if the lungs are totally opened to an FRC level of a healthy lung.

Another reason why the lung should be kept open is the fact that under certain circumstances artificial ventilation affects the pulmonary surfactant system.

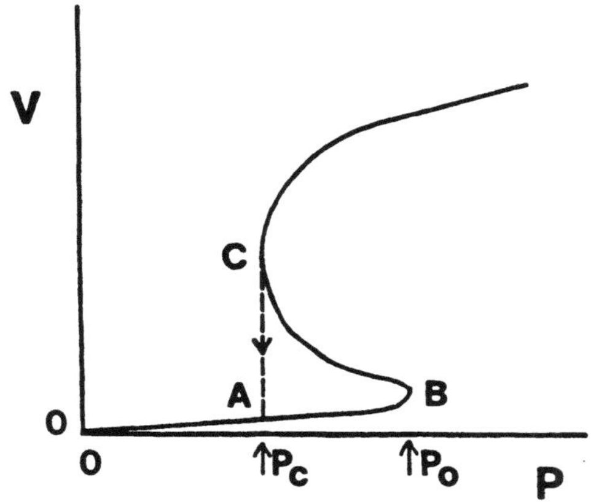

Fig. 2. Pressure-volume relation (P-V) showing the pressure needed to inflate a total airless lung to the total lung capacity. B indicates the opening pressure (P_0) which has to be overcome to inflate the lung. Once the lung is inflated to the FRC (C) only a pressure P_C is needed to stabilize this lung. A shows that without opening the lung, pressure P_C does not result in volume increase

In normal healty lungs, during end-expiration the surfactant molecules are compressed on the small alveolar area (leading to a low surface tension or a high surface pressure) thus preventing the alveoli from collapse. If the surface of the alveolus becomes smaller than the total surface of the surfactant molecules, the molecules are squeezed out of the surface and forced towards the airway and thus lost for the alveoli. During the following inflation of alveoli, the surface is replenished with surfactant molecules that were in the hypophase. During the next expiration, the same mechanism continues to work and surfactant molecules are forced into the airways; this a continuing cycle (Fig. 3) [8].

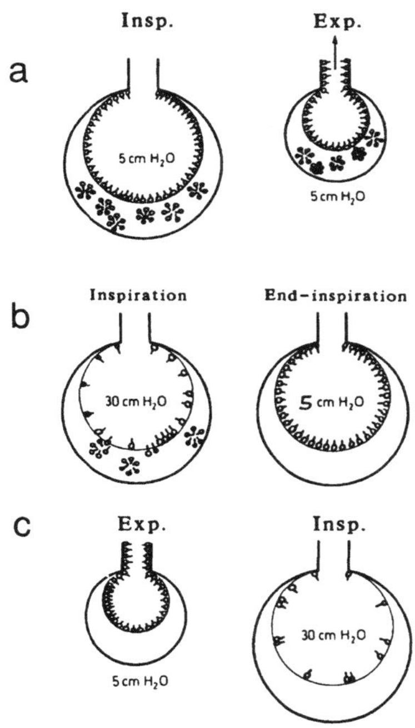

Fig. 3. a: shows the balance between synthesis, release and consumption of surfactant in the healthy lung. The intrapulmonary pressures values to stabilize the lung are indicated. b: shows an imbalance between synthesis, release and consumption of surfactant due to artificial ventilation. At the beginning of inspiration, there exists an apparent deficiency of surfactant molecules but due to respreading of stored surfactant molecules the surfactant layer is restored at end inspiration. c: shows the effect of depletion of the stored surfactant molecules due to continuous squeezing out of surfactant, resulting in a serious surfactant deficiency

With large tidal volume and/or high rates, surfactant molecules are lost into the airways rather rapidly, as demonstrated by Faridy [9].

This mechanism explains how loss of surfactant by artificial ventilation can be caused by the rhythmic compression (expiration) and decompression (inspiration) of the alveolar liming, especially when the compression is far below the static state of the surfactant layer, which is normal equal to or just above the FRC level [10].

Thus, to prevent loss of surfactant by artificial ventilation one should maintain aeration of as large parts of the lung as possible without allowing either hyperdistention or lung collapse.

Improving ventilation by exogenous surfactant

Pulmonary surfactant is a complex of phospholipids (80-90 %), neutral lipids (5-10 %) and at least four specific surfactant-proteins (5-10 %) (SP-A, SP-B, SP-C and SP-D) syntesized and secreted from the alveolar type II cells, lying as a monolayer at the air-liquid interface in the lung [11, 12].

One of the functions of the pulmonary surfactant system is to lower the surface tension at the alveolar surface and small airways, which reduces the muscular effort necessary to ventilate the lungs and, due to this lowering of surface tension prevents end-expiratory collapse when, during expiration, the alveolar radius decreases [6, 12]. Surfactant also plays a role in maintaining the fluid balance in the lung and in the lung's defence against infection. In addition, surfactant, and in particular SP-A, enhance the antibacterial and antiviral defence of alveolar macrophages [13].

When considering the main physiologic functions of the alveolo-bronchial surfactant system (*i.e.* surfactant keeps the lungs open, surfactant keeps the lungs dry, surfactant keeps the lungs clean) it can easily be understood that alteration in its functional integrity will lead to:

- decreased lung distensibility and thus to increased work of breathing and increased oxygen demand by the respiratory muscles;
- atelectasis;
- transudation of plasma into the interstitium and into the alveoli with decreased diffusion for O_2 and CO_2;
- inactivation of the surfactant by plasma and specific surfactant inhibitors;
- hypoxaemia and metabolic acidosis secondary to increased production of organic acids under anaerobic conditions;
- enlargement of functional right-to-left shunt due to increased perfusion of non-ventilated alveoli (the von Euler-Lijestrand reflex does not "work" in surfactant deficient alveoli);
- decreased production of surfactant as a result of hypoxaemia, acidosis and hypoperfusion. This will lead to a vicious circle and the lung will fail as a gas exchange organ.

The central role of surfactant deficiency can further be illustrated by recent studies in animal models of ARDS which demonstrated that exogenous surfactant instillation dramatically improved blood gases and lung mechanics. The models of surfactant deficiency in which these improvements could be demonstrated include acute respiratory failure due *in vivo* whole-lung lavage, neurogenic ARDS, respiratory failure after intoxication with N-nitroso-N-methylurethane or paraquat. Evidently, it is rational to administer exogenous surfactant in ARDS patients, but the question the arises why is this not yet a reality. Surfactant has been commercially available for neonates for about six years. Surfactant therapy in patients other than neonates with RDS is almost impossible due to the fact there is not enough surfactant available and current prices are too high (1g of surfactant costs about US $ 3,000-5,000). Therefore, only a few case reports have been performed up to now. (For review see [16]).

The impact and importance of exogenous surfactant therapy was recently demonstrated by Gregory and colleagues [17].

Were the first to demonstrate decreased lung compliance and increased minimal surface tension in lung extracts from two ARDS patients. Since then, several studies have demonstrated qualitative and quantitative changes of surfactant in BAL fluid from ARDS patients (for review see [15]). Recently Gregory et al. demonstrated that several of these alteration already occur in patients at risk of developing ARDS, suggesting that these abnormalities of surfactant occur early in the disease process.

Analyses of lung surfactant recovered in BAL from patients with ALI, or from animal models of acute respiratory failure, demonstrate disturbances of the lung surfactant system. Reduction on surfactant activity is associated with increased minimal surface tension of lung extracts or lung homogenates, and compositional changes of surfactant and/or decreased surfactant content of the lungs. Ashbaugh and colleagues [14]. In a pilot study on ALI, showing a reduction of mortality from 43.8 to 17.6 % by instillation of 400 mg surfactant per kg body weight.

Thus, surfactant therapy seems a promising approach for the treatment of acute respiratory failure in ARDS and ARDS-like syndromes. However, from experimental and clinical experience, it has been seen that the impact on the magnitude of the response after exogenous surfactant therapy, depends not only on the course of the injury but also on the timing of surfactant therapy, the used dose of exogenous surfactant, the type of surfactant preparation, the ventilator settings of the mechanical ventilation; and especially the level of PEEP, and the method of administration surfactant which is important for its distribution. The rationale for giving surfactant is to improve ventilation by recruiting collapsed alveoli and to stabilize them with the applied ventilator settings. Thus, before exogenous surfactant therapy is applied, one has to evaluate by lung function tests whether or not sufficient parts of recruitable lung areas are still available. Thus, one should not give surfactant to patients with heavily consolidated and/or fibrotic lungs in which surfactant could not effectively improve lung function. As soon as surfactant preparations become more widely available at lower costs, trials should begin to define the role of surfactant treatment in adults.

Improving ventilation by eliminating the air-liquid interface

In 1929 von Neergaard demonstrated that lungs that were collapsed would open up more readily if the effect of surface tension was completely nullified by using liquid rather than air as the expanding medium, i.e. by eliminating the alveolar gas-liquid interface [18] (Fig. 1).

In this respect, the findings of Clark et al. in 1966 were of utmost importance, which demonstrated the ability of healthy small mammals to successfully breathe while sumberged in oxygenated perfluorocarbon (PFC); moreover these animals could even be reconverted to air breathing [19].

These findings are explained by the special properties of PFCs: a high ability to dissolve respiratory gases and a low surface tension; furthermore, in the physiologic range PFCs do not show any in vivo metabolisation (Table 1).

Table 1. Physical properties of some PFC liquids

	Perflubron	FC-77	RM-101
Density (g/ml)	1.92	1.75	1.77
Vapor pressure (mmHg at 37°C)	10.5	75	64
Surface tension (dynes/cm)	18	14	15
O_2 solubility (ml/100 ml)	53	56	52
CO_2 solubility (ml/100 ml)	210	198	160

Since this publication, extensive research has been performed to study the efficacy of PFCs in liquid breathing techniques; furthermore, it would be rational to apply these techniques in diseases characterized by high alveolar surface forces.

Initial work was directed towards total fluid ventilation, using PFCs oxygenated outside the body. This type of liquid ventilation is a process in which the gaseous FRC of the lung is filled with PFCs, and gas exchange is accomplished by pumping tidal volumes of PFCs in and out of the lung, which are guided through a membrane lung outside the body, where oxygen is added and CO_2 removed. Greenspan et al. successfully ventilated preterm using this principle [20].

Besides its technical complexity, total liquid ventilation causes the movement of liquid tidal volumes through the airway and generates high viscous resistive forces, rendering the work of spontaneous liquid breathing prohibitive.

Fuhrman et al. demonstrated the feasibility of liquid ventilation without the need of a modified liquid breathing system [21]. This technique combined intratracheal PFC administration with conventional ventilation, which brought the use of PFC for liquid ventilation closer to clinical practice. Fuhrman's group named this type of oxygenation: "in vivo bubble oxygenation".

It is established that increased alveolar surface tension plays a central role in the pathophysiology of the respiratory distress syndrome of prematurity; furthermore, it is thought to contribute to lung dysfunction in ARDS [12, 16]. Therefore, our group investigated the efficacy of partial fluid ventilation in an animal model of acute respiratory failure.

Thus, we were the first to demonstrated in adult animals with acute respiratory failure, using a combination of conventional mechanical ventilation and intratracheal PFC administration in increasing doeses (yet below FRC), that oxygenation can be improved in a dose-dependent manner at reduced airway pressure [22, 23] (Fig. 3).

Subsequently, we further demonstrated in the same animal model, using the same technique yet with PFC doses approximating functional residual capacity volume, that pulmonary gas exchange was improved and maintained stable throughout the observation period at lower airway pressures; also respiratory lung compliance improved; discernible treatment-related alveolar damage was not seen on histological analysis [24].

From these studies we concluded that the dose-dependent improvement of gas exchange supported that large doses of PFC, approaching normal FRC of the animal, are required to correct hypoxia as fully as possible. On the other hand, respiratory system compliance and airway pressures can be improved even with a low dose of PFC, and further doses do not make significant changes in the lung mechanical properties of lung-lavaged animals.

As for the different mechanisms involved, we proposed that even low doses of PFCs diminish the surface tension forces that oppose lung inflation, but that the space- occupying characteristics of the PFCs play a major role in its restoration of FRC and gas exchange (*e.g.* recruitment of previously collapsed alveoli, thus preventing end- expiratory collapse) (Fig. 4).

The described studies demonstrate the feasibility of partial fluid ventilation in improving pulmonary gas exchange and respiratory mechanics in animals with ALI. Moreover this technique, considering the remarkable reductions in airway pressures during partial fluid ventilation, appears to be an alternative modality to minimize or prevent the progress of lung injury (*e.g.* ventilator-induced injury). Now clinical studies are warranted in order to investigate the clinical efficacy of this new technique.

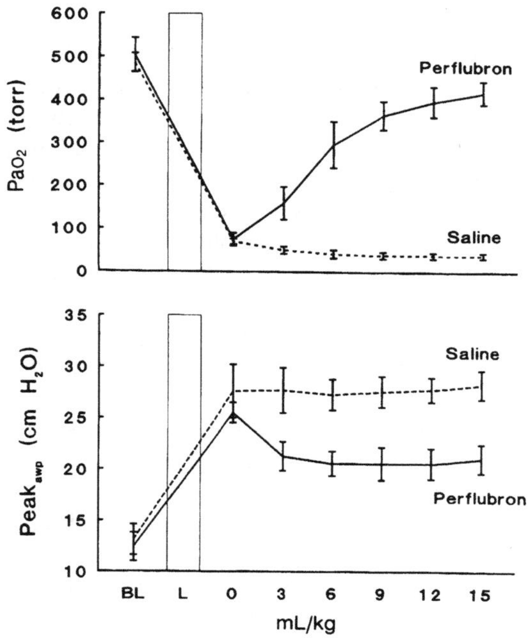

Fig. 4. PaO_2 (top), and P_{eak} airway pressure $Peak_{awp}$ at a PEEP of 6 cm H_2O (bottom), before lavage (BL), after lavage (0), and after treatment with perfluorocarbon (PFC) or saline. The bar represents the lavage procedure (L). Mean PaO_2 increases significantly with each increasing dose of PFC, while in the saline group oxygenation, is severely impaired at the same ventilatory settings. Peakawp shows a significant drop from pretreatment values after the first PFC dose and remains stable during the study period, whereas in the saline treated group $Peak_{awp}$ remains at pretreatment values. (From [22])

Conclusion

The forms of therapy discussed in this paper have been shown in experimental and clinical reports to be promising therapies for improvement of ventilation and to prevent and/or minimize the progress of lung injury in patients suffering from acute respiratory failure.

References

1. Gregory TJ, Longmore WJ, Moxley MA, Whitsett JA, Reed CR, Fowler AA, Hudson LD, Maunder RJ, Crim C, Hyers TM (1991) Surfactant chemical composition and biophysical activity in acute respiratory distress syndrome. J Clin Invest 88:1976-1981
2. Lachmann B, Danzmann E, Haendly B, Jonson B (1982) Ventilator settings and gas exchange in respiratory distress syndrome. In: Prakash O (ed) Applied Physiology in Clinical Respiratory Care. Martinus Nijhoff Publishers, The Hague, pp 141-176
3. Froese AB (1989) Role of lung volume in lung injury: HFO in the atelectasis-prone lung. Acta Anaesthesiol Scand 33 [Suppl 90]:126-130
4. Sykes MK (1991) Does mechanical ventilation damage the lung? Acta Anaesthesiol

Scand 35 [Suppl 95]:35-39
5. Hickling KG (1990) Ventilatory management of ARDS: can it affect the outcome? Int Care Med 16:219-226
6. Mead J, Takishima T Leith (1970) Stress distribution in lungs: a model of pulmonary elasticity. J Appl Physiol 28:596-608
7. Spragg RG, Smith RM (1991) Biology of acute lung injury. In: Crystal RG, West JB, et al (eds) The Lung: Scientific Foundation. Raven Press Ltd, New York, pp 2003-2017
8. Bos JAH, Lachmann B (1992) Effects of artificial ventilation on surfactant function. In: Rügheimer E (ed) New Aspects on Respiratory Failure. Springer-Verlag, Berlin Heidelberg New York, pp 194-208
9. Faridy EE (1976) Effect of distension on release of surfactant in excised dogs' lungs. Respir Physiol 27:99-114
10. Benzer H (1969) Respiratorbeatmung und Oberflächenspannung in der Lunge. In: Frey R, Kern F, Mayrhofer O (eds) Anaesthesiologie und Wiederbelebung, Springer-Verlag, Berlin Heidelberg New York, p 38
11. van Golde LMG, Batenburg JJ, Robertson B (1988) The pulmonary surfactant system: biochemical aspects and functional significance. Physiol Rev 68:374-455
12. Lewis JF, Jobe AH (1993) Surfactant and the adult respiratory distress syndrome. Am Rev Respir Dis 147:218-233
13. van Iwaarden F (1992) Surfactant and the pulmonary defense system. In: Robertson B, Van Golde LMG, Batenburg JJ (eds) Pulmonary surfactant. Elsevier, Amsterdam, pp 215-253
14. Ashbaugh DG, Bigelow DB, Petty TL, Levine BE (1967) Acute respiratory distress in adults. Lancet 2:319-323
15. Spragg RG, Giliiard N, Richman P, Smith RM, Hite D, Pappert D, Heldt GP, Merritt TA (1992) The adult respiratory distress syndrome: clinical aspects relevant to surfactant supplementation. In: Robertson B, Van Golde LMG, Batenburg JJ (eds) Pulmonary Surfactant. Elsevier, Amsterdam, pp 685-703
16. Gommers D, Lachmann B (1993) Surfactant therapy: does it have a role in adults? Clin Int Care 4:284-295
17. Gregory TJ, Gadek JE, Hyers TM et al (1994) Survanta supplementation in patients with acute respiratory distress syndrome (ARDS). Am J Respir Crit Care Med 149[Suppl]:A567
18. Von Neergaard, K (1929) Neue Auffassungen über einen Grundbegriff der Atemmechanik. Die Retraktionskraft der Lunge, abhängig von der Oberflachenspannung in den Alveolen. Ges Exp Med 66:373-394
19. Clark LC, Golan F (1966) Survival of mammals breathing organic liquids equilibrated with oxygen at atmosphere pressure. Science 152:1755-1756
20 Greenspan JS, Wolfson MR, Rubenstein SD, Shaffer TH (1990) Liquid ventilation of human preterm neonates. J Pediatr 17:106-111
21. Fuhrman BP, Paczan PR, DeFrancis M (1991) Perfluocarbon-associated gas exchange. Crit Care Med 19:712-722
22. Tütüncü AS, Faithfull NS, Lachmann B (1993) Intratracheal perfluorocarbon administration combined with artificial ventilation in experimental respiratory distress syndrome: dose-dependent improvement of gas exchange. Crit Care Med 21:962-969
23. Tütüncü AS, Akpir K, Mulder P, Erdmann W, Lachmann B (1993) Intratracheal perfluorocarbon administration as an aid in the ventilatory mangement of respiratory distress syndrome. Anesthesiology 79:1083-1093
24. Tütüncü AS, Faithfull NS, Lachmann B (1993) Comparison of ventilatory support with intratracheal perfluorocarbon administration and conventional mechanical ventilation in animals with acute respiratory failure. Am Rev Respir Dis 148:785-792

Main Symbols

$AaPO_2$	alveolar-arterial differencew of PO_2
ACV	assisted control ventilation
AMV	assisted mechanical ventilation
APCV	assisted pressure control ventilation
C	compliance
C_{cw}	chest wall compliance
$C_{dyn,L}$	dynamic lung compliance
CL	lung compliance
COPD	chronic obstructive pulmonary disease
CPAP	continue positive airway pressure
C_{rs}	respiratory system compliance
$C_{st,L}$	static lung compliance
ΔE	additional elastance
ΔR	additional resistance
ΔVL	volume change of the lung
ΔV_W	volume change of the chest wall
ΔW_L	additional work of the lung
E	elastance
E_{dyn}	dynamic elastance
$E_{dyn,L}$	dynamic elastance of the lung
$E_{dyn,rs}$	dynamic elastance of the respiratory system
$E_{dyn,w}$	dynamic elastance of the chest wall
EELV	end expiratory lung volume
E_{st}	static elastance
$E_{st,rs}$	static elastance of the respiratory system
E_{tis}	tissue elastance
E_{visc}	viscoelastic elastance
F	force
f	frequency
F_{max}	maximal force
FRC	functional residual capacity
FVC	forced vital capacity
G	conductance
G_{aw}	airway conductance

I	inertance
L	lung
NTS	nucleus of tractus solitarius
P	pressure
$P_{0.1}$	airway occlusion pressure $_{0.1}$ after onset of inspiration
$P_{1,aw}$	zero flow airway pressure
$P_{2,aw}$	plateau airway pressure
P_A	alveolar pressure
P_{ab}	abdominal pressure
$PaCO_2$	partial pressure of CO_2 in arterial blood
P_{ao}	pressure at the airway opening
P_AO_2	alveolar partial pressure of O_2
PaO_2	partial pressure of O_2 in arterial blood
PAV	proportional assisted ventilation
P_{bs}	body surface pressure
P_{cv}	central venous pressure
$P_{cv,tm}$	transmural central venous pressure
P_{di}	mean transdiaphragmatic pressure
$P_{eak,aw}$	peak airway pressure
PEEP	positive end expiratory pressure
$PEEP_i$	intrinsic positive end expiratory pressure
$PEEP_{i,dyn}$	dynamic intrinsic positive end expiratory pressure
P_{es}	esophageal pressure
$PetCO_2$	end-tidal PCO_2
PFC	perflurocarbon
P_{mus}	muscles pressure
P_{pa}	pulmonary arterial pressure
$P_{pa,tm}$	transmural pulmonary arterial pressure
PP_ACO_2	alveolar partial pressure CO_2
P_{pl}	pleural pressure
P_{res}	resistive pressure
$P_{st,L}$	static pressure of the lung
$P_{st,re}$	static pressure of the respiratory system
$P_{st,w}$	static pressure of the chest wall
PSV	pressure support ventilation
PTP	pressure-time product
P_{tr}	tracheal pressure
$PvCO_2$	partial pressure of CO_2 in venous blood
P_{visc}	viscoelastic pressure
PvO_2	partial pressure of O_2 in venous blood
Qp	hematic pulmonary volume
R	resistance
R_{aw}	airway resistance
R_{ef}	effective resistance
R_{ex}	expiratory resistance

$R_{int,L}$	interrupter resistance og the lung
$R_{int,rs}$	interrupter resistance of the respiratory system
$R_{int,w}$	interrupter resistance of the chest wall
R_L	total pulmonary resistance
R_{min}	minimal resistance
$R_{min,L}$	minimal resistance of the lung
$R_{min,rs}$	minimal resistance of the respiratory system
R_{tis}	tissue resistance
RV	residual volume
R_{visc}	viscoelastic resistance
R_w	total chest wall resistance
SaO_2	saturation of hemoglobin with O_2 in arterial blood
SIMV	synchronized intermittent mandatory ventilation
t	time
T_E	expiratory time
T_I	inspiratory time
T_I/T_{TOT}	duty cicle
TLC	total lung capacity
τ_{rs}	standard time constant of the respiratory system
TT_{di}	tension-time index
T_{TOT}	total respiratory cycle time
τ_{visc}	viscoelastic time constant
V	volume
VC	vital capacity
V_d	dead space
V_r	relaxation volume
V_T	tidal volume
V_T/T_I	mean inspiratory flow
$\dot{V}_A/Q$	ventilation-perfusion ratio
$\dot{V}_E$	expired minute ventilation
$\dot{V}$	flow
W	work
ω	angular frequency
W_{aw}	airway resistive work
$W_{dyn,rs}$	dynamic work of the respiratory system
$W_{I,rs}$	inspiratory work of the respiratory system
$W_{i,st,rs}$	static inspiratory work of the respiratory system
WOB	work of breathing
Z	impedance
Z_{rs}	resoiratory impendance

Subject index

MIX
Papier aus verantwortungsvollen Quellen
Paper from responsible sources
FSC® C105338

If you have any concerns about our products,
you can contact us on
ProductSafety@springernature.com

In case Publisher is established outside the EU,
the EU authorized representative is:
Springer Nature Customer Service Center GmbH
Europaplatz 3, 69115 Heidelberg, Germany

Printed by Libri Plureos GmbH
in Hamburg, Germany